Taylor's Family Medicine Review

Springer
New York
Berlin
Heidelberg
Barcelona
Budapest
Hong Kong
London
Milan
Paris
Singapore
Tokyo

Taylor's Family Medicine Review

Robert B. Taylor

With 30 Illustrations

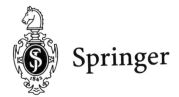

Springer

Editor:

Robert B. Taylor, M.D.
Professor and Chairman
Department of Family Medicine
Oregon Health Sciences University
School of Medicine
Portland, OR 97201, USA

Associate Editors:

Alan K. David, M.D.
The Fred Lazarus, Jr.
Professor and Director
Department of Family Medicine
University of Cincinnati College of Medicine
Cincinnati, OH 45267, USA

Thomas A. Johnson, Jr., M.D.
Chairman
Department of Family Medicine
St. John's Mercy Medical Center
St. Louis, MO 63141, USA

D. Melessa Phillips, M.D.
Professor and Chairman
Department of Family Medicine
University of Mississippi School of Medicine
Jackson, MS 39216, USA

Joseph E. Scherger, M.D., M.P.H.
Associate Dean for Clinical Affairs
and
Chair
Department of Family Medicine
University of California—Irvine
College of Medicine
Orange, CA 92868, USA

Contributor:

Gerald K. Goodenough, M.D., M.S.P.H.
Family Physician and Practicing Geriatrician
St. Mark's Senior Health Center
Columbia H.C.A.
Salt Lake City, UT 84124, USA

Library of Congress Cataloging in Publication Data
Taylor's family medicine review / [edited by] Robert B. Taylor.
      p.   cm.
   Referenced to: Family medicine / Robert B. Taylor, editor, 5th ed.
c1998
   Includes bibliographical references and index.
   ISBN 0-387-98569-7 (softcover : alk. paper)
   1. Family medicine—Examinations, questions, etc. I. Taylor, Robert B.
   [DNLM: 1. Family Practice—examination questions. 2. Clinical Medicine—
examination questions. WB 18.2 T247 1998]
RC46.F36   1998 Suppl.
616'.0076—dc21

                                                          98-21884

Printed on acid-free paper.

Production coordinated by Princeton Editorial Associates and managed by Theresa Kornak; manufacturing supervised by Jacqui Ashri.
Typeset by Princeton Editorial Associates, Scottsdale, AZ, and Roosevelt, NJ.
Printed and bound by Maple-Vail Book Manufacturing Group, York, PA.
Printed in the United States of America.

9 8 7 6 5 4 3 2 1

ISBN 0-387-98569-7 Springer-Verlag New York Berlin Heidelberg SPIN 10682317

Preface

Test taking does not end upon completion of formal medical training. With certification, recertification, and licensure examinations, test taking is as much a part of modern clinical practice as medical records and quality assurance. For example, during my career I have taken all three parts of what is now called the United States Medical Licensure Examination (USMLE), one state licensing board examination, plus the specialty certification exam and four periodic recertification examinations of the American Board of Family Practice (ABFP). Periodic examinations demonstrate the examinee's current fund of knowledge, and are important to maintaining the highest standards of medical practice. For the physician personally, it is reassuring to validate that, when measured against peers (and even the bright young recent graduates), one can achieve a respectable score on a standardized examination.

Taylor's Family Medicine Review is intended to help the reader review the full scope of family medicine, whether to prepare for a broad-based clinical examination or simply to enhance one's clinical knowledge. The book contains **more than 1200 questions**, each followed by a discussion explaining the correct response. The questions are based on the all-new Fifth Edition of *Family Medicine: Principles and Practice*. The discussion following each question is taken directly from the Fifth Edition, with notations of the source chapter and page. The reader will find that, in many instances, the discussion goes beyond validating the correct response and expands upon the clinical approach to the problem presented. Questions have been grouped by area (e.g., preventive care, care of the elderly, and the female reproductive system) to allow focused review of selected topics.

The book begins with a chapter on "Test Taking Techniques," by Gerald Goodenough, M.D., M.S.P.H. I am the author of all questions, which allows uniformity of style and the exercise of my bias toward clinically pertinent family medicine topics. I have attempted to write questions that address *key points* for each clinical problem.

I have used the two most common question types: multiple choice and multiple true–false, and avoided the less-often-used question types that may not reflect what the examinee actually knows. Whenever appropriate, questions are framed in a "case-based" format. The result, I hope, is a book that can help the reader become both a better test-taker and a more knowledgeable physician.

I gratefully acknowledge the contributions of Dr. Goodenough, all authors in the Fifth Edition of *Family Medicine: Principles and Practice*, and the Fifth Edition Associate Editors: Alan K. David, M.D., Thomas A. Johnson, M.D., D. Melessa Phillips, M.D., and Joseph E. Scherger, M.D., M.P.H. Thanks are also due Harmony Matthews, Coelleda O'Neil, Laretta Borg, and Laurie Charron for their assistance in manuscript preparation. I appreciate the work of family physicians Keith A. White, M.D., John V. Mackel, M.B., and Laura E. Holmes, M.D., who reviewed all questions in this manuscript in preparation for their own ABFP examinations.

This is a new book. As readers take examinations after using this book in preparation, I would welcome comments and suggestions that could make ours the very best Family Medicine Review.

Robert B. Taylor, M.D.
Portland, Oregon, USA

Contents

Leading numbers in italics indicate the relevant chapter number in *Family Medicine: Principles and Practice* (Fifth Edition) for each chapter in this book.

Contributors to Fifth Edition of *Family Medicine: Principles and Practice*

Abbott, Allan V., M.D., Professor, Department of Family Medicine, University of Southern California School of Medicine, Los Angeles, CA

Abboud, Cheryl, M.P.A., Coordinator, Rural Health Programs, Department of Family Medicine, University of Nebraska College of Medicine, Omaha, NE

Acheson, Louise S., M.D., M.S., Associate Professor, Department of Family Medicine, Case Western Reserve University School of Medicine, Cleveland, OH

Adelman, Alan M., M.D., M.S., Professor, Department of Family and Community Medicine, Penn State University College of Medicine, Hershey, PA

Alexander, Beth, M.D., M.S., Professor, Department of Family Practice, Michigan State University College of Human Medicine, East Lansing, Ml

Allen, John, Ph.D., M.P.A., Chief, Treatment Research Branch, National Institute on Alcohol Abuse and Alcoholism, Rockville, MD

Ambuel, Bruce, Ph.D., M.S., Assistant Professor, Department of Family and Community Medicine, Medical College of Wisconsin, Milwaukee, WI; Behavioral Science Coordinator and Research Director, Waukesha Family Practice Residency, Waukesha Memorial Hospital, Waukesha, WI

Andolsek, Kathryn M., M.D., M.P.H., Clinical Professor, Department of Community and Family Medicine, Duke University School of Medicine, Durham, NC

Apgar, Barbara S., M.D., M.S., Clinical Associate Professor, Department of Family Practice, University of Michigan Medical School, Ann Arbor, MI

Arevalo, Jose A., M.D., Associate Clinical Professor, Department of Family Practice, University of California, Davis School of Medicine; Associate Medical Director, Planned Parenthood of Sacramento, Sacramento, CA

Bachman, John W., M.D., Consultant, Department of Family Medicine, Mayo Clinic and Mayo Foundation; Parker D. Sanders and Isabella G. Sanders Professor of Primary Care, Mayo Medical School, Rochester, MN

Bailey, Boyd L., Jr., M.D., Associate Professor, Department of Family Medicine, University of Alabama School of Medicine at Birmingham, AL; Clinic Director, Selma Family Medicine Residency Program, Selma, AL

Baird, Macaran A., M.D., M.S., Clinical Professor, Department of Family Medicine and Community Health, University of Minnesota School of Medicine; Associate Medical Director for Primary CareHealth Partners, Minneapolis, MN

Baumgardner, Dennis J., M.D., Associate Professor, Department of Family Medicine, University of Wisconsin Medical School, Madison, WI; Family Practice Residency Director, St Luke's Medical Center, Milwaukee, WI

Beebe, Diane K., M.D., Associate Professor, Department of Family Medicine, University of Mississippi School of Medicine; Director of Residency Training, Vice Chairman for Academic Programs, University of Mississippi Medical Center, Jackson, MS

Berg, Alfred O., M.D., M.P.H., Professor, Associate Chair, and Affiliated Residency Network Director, Department of Family Medicine, University of Washington School of Medicine, Seattle, WA

Bielak, Kenneth M., M.D., Assistant Professor, Department of Family Medicine, University of Tennessee Medical Center of Knoxville, Graduate School of Medicine, Knoxville, TN

Birrer, Richard B., M.D., M.P.H., Associate Professor, Department of Family Medicine, State University of New York, Health Sciences Center at Brooklyn, Brooklyn, NY; Chairman, Family Medicine Department, Catholic Medical Center of Brooklyn and Queens, Jamaica, NY

Blondell, Richard D., M.D., Professor, Department of Family and Community Medicine, University of Louisville School of Medicine, Louisville, KY

Boken, Patricia Ann McGuire, M.D., Private Practice, Portland, OR

Bracker, Mark D., M.D., Clinical Professor, Director of Sports Medicine Fellowship Program, Department of Family and Preventive Medicine, University of California, San Diego School of Medicine, La Jolla, CA

Breuner, Cora Collette, M.D., Clinical Assistant Professor, Department of Family Medicine, University of Washington School of Medicine; Faculty, Swedish Family Medicine Residency, Swedish Medical Center, Seattle, WA

Brody, Howard, M.D., Ph.D., Professor, Department of Family Practice, Director, Center for Ethics and Humanities in the Life Sciences, Michigan State University College of Human Medicine, East Lansing, MI

Brotzman, Gregory L., M.D., Associate Professor, Department of Family and Community Medicine, Medical College of Wisconsin, Milwaukee, WI

Brownlee, H. James, Jr., M.D., Professor and Chair, Department of Family Medicine, University of South Florida College of Medicine; Chair, Department of Family Medicine, Tampa General Hospital, Tampa, FL

Brummel-Smith, Kenneth, M.D., Associate Professor, Department of Family Medicine and Department of Medicine, Oregon Health Sciences University School of Medicine; Medical Director, Long Term Care Division, Providence Health Systems, Portland, OR

Brunton, Stephen A., M.D., Clinical Professor, Department of Family Medicine, University of California–Irvine, Irvine, CA; Director, Family Medicine Residency Program, Long Beach Memorial Medical Center, Long Beach, CA

Buckley, Robert L., M.D., Clinical Professor, Department of Family Medicine, Loyola University Stritch School of Medicine, Maywood, IL; Director, Family Practice Residency Program, Resurrection Medical Center, Chicago, IL

Calmbach, Walter L., M.D., Assistant Professor, Department of Family Practice, The University of Texas Health Science Center; Director, Sports Medicine Training Program, University Hospital, San Antonio, TX

Calvert, James F., Jr., M.D., Assistant Professor, Department of Family Medicine, Oregon Health Sciences University School of Medicine, Portland, OR; Director, Cascades East Family Practice Residency Program, Merle West Medical Center, Klamath Falls, OR

Campbell, Bryan, M.D., Assistant Professor, Department of Family and Preventive Medicine, University of Utah School of Medicine, Salt Lake City, UT; McKay-Dee Hospital, Ogden, UT

Campbell, Thomas L., M.D., Associate Professor, Department of Family Medicine and Department of Psychiatry, University of Rochester School of Medicine and Dentistry, Rochester, NY

Carden, Ann D., Ph.D., Staff Psychologist, Clinical Supervisor, Child and Family Intervention Team, Medina, OH

Celestino, Frank S., M.D., Associate Professor, Director of Geriatrics, Department of Family and Community Medicine, Bowman Gray School of Medicine, Winston-Salem, NC

Chessare, John B., M.D., M.P.H., Associate Professor, Department of Pediatrics, Albany Medical College, Albany, NY

Clarity, Greg, M.D., Assistant Professor, Department of Family Medicine, East Tennessee State University, James H. Quillen College of Medicine, Johnson, TN

Clement, Kathi D., M.D., Associate Professor, Department of Family Medicine, University of Wyoming School of Medicine, Cheyenne, WY

Coleman, George C., M.D., Associate Professor, Department of Family Practice, Medical College of Virginia of Virginia Commonwealth University; Coordinator, Clinical Programs, Department of Family Practice, Medical College of Virginia Hospitals, Richmond, VA

Connor, Pamela D., Ph.D., Associate Professor, Director of Research, Department of Family Medicine, The University of Tennessee, Memphis College of Medicine, Memphis, TN

Copeland, Joyce A., M.D., Clinical Assistant Professor, Director of Family Medicine Clerkship, Department of Community and Family Medicine, Duke University School of Medicine, Durham, NC

Corey, George A., M.D., Assistant Professor, Department of Family Medicine, University of Vermont School of Medicine, Burlington, VT

Cross, Gerald M., M.D., Commander, 86th Combat Support Hospital, Fort Campbell, KY

Cullen, Paul T., M.D., Clinical Assistant Professor, Department of Family and Community Medicine, Pennsylvania State University College of Medicine, Hershey, PA; Residency Program Director, The Washington Hospital, Washington, PA

Cullom, Susan C., D.O., Assistant Professor, Department of Family Medicine, Uniformed Services University of the Health Sciences, Bethesda, MD

Culpepper, Larry, M.D., M.P.H., Professor and Chair, Department of Family Medicine, Boston University School of Medicine, Boston, MA

Curry, R. Whit, Jr., M.D., Professor and Chairman, Department of Community Health and Family Medicine, University of Florida College of Medicine, Gainesville, FL

Curry, William J., M.D., Assistant Professor, Department of Family and Community Medicine, Pennsylvania State University College of Medicine, Hershey, PA; Medical Director, Penn State Family Health, Middletown; University Hospital, Penn State University, Hershey, PA

Cutlip, Anne Cather, M.D., Associate Professor, Department of Family Medicine, West Virginia University School of Medicine; Department of Family Medicine, Ruby Memorial Hospital, Morgantown, WV

Cutlip, William D. II, M.D., Associate Professor, Departments of Neurology and Behavioral Medicine and Psychiatry, West Virginia University School of Medicine;

Director, Thought Disorders Program, Chestnut Ridge Hospital, Morgantown, WV

Daly, Mel P., M.D., Associate Professor and Director, Division of Geriatrics, Department of Family Medicine, University of Maryland School of Medicine; J.L. Kernan Hospital, University of Maryland Hospital, Baltimore, MD

Deckert, James J., M.D., Associate Director, Family Practice Residency Program, St. John's Mercy Medical Center, St. Louis, MO

DeWitt, Donald E., M.D., Clinical Professor and Procedural Skills Coordinator, Department of Family Medicine, East Carolina University School of Medicine, Greenville, NC

Driscoll, Charles E., M.D., Clinical Professor, Department of Family Medicine, University of Iowa College of Medicine; Mercy Hospital of Iowa City, IA

Driscoll, Jacquelyn S., R.N., Iowa City, IA

Duckett, Charles H., M.D., Professor, Department of Family Medicine; Chairman, Department of Physical Medicine, East Carolina University School of Medicine, Greenville, NC

Edwards, Rita K., Pharm. D., Pharmacist, Long Beach Memorial Medical Center, Long Beach, CA

Elizondo, Margaret V., M.D., Director, Perinatal Education, Sharp Grossmont Family Practice Residency, La Mesa, CA

Evans, Paul, D.O., Associate Clinical Professor, Department of Family Medicine, University of Washington School of Medicine, Seattle, WA; Chief, Department of Family Practice, Madigan Army Medical Center, Tacoma, WA

Felmar, Eugene, M.D., Clinical Professor, Department of Family Medicine, University of California, Los Angeles School of Medicine, Los Angeles, CA; Director, Family Practice Residency Program, Santa Monica-UCLA Medical Center, Santa Monica, CA

Fernandez, Enrique S., M.D., M.S.Ed., Director, Division of Medicine, Health Resources and Services Administration, Silver Spring, MD

Fields, Scott A., M.D., Associate Professor, Department of Family Medicine, Oregon Health Sciences University School of Medicine, Portland, OR

Fisher, Judith A., M.D., Assistant Professor, Department of Family and Community Medicine, University of Pennsylvania School of Medicine; Director, Family Practice Residency Program, University of Pennsylvania Health Systems, Philadelphia, PA

Fowler, Grant, M.D., Associate Professor, Department of Family Practice and Community Medicine, The University of Texas Health Science Center Medical School at Houston; Director, Hermann/LBJ Family Practice Residency Program, Hermann Hospital, Houston, TX

Fuller, Steven H., Pharm.D., B.C.P.S., Associate Professor, Department of Pharmacy Practice, Campbell University School of Pharmacy, Buies Creek, North Carolina; Kaiser Permanente, Cary, NC

Gilchrist, Valerie J., M.D., Professor, Department of Family Medicine, Northeastern Ohio Universities College of Medicine, Rootstown, OH; Associate Director, Family Practice Residency Program, Aultman Hospital, Canton, OH

Gjerdingen, Dwenda K., M.D., Associate Professor, Department of Family Practice and Community Health, University of Minnesota School of Medicine, Minneapolis, MN; Acting Residency Unit Director, St. Joseph's Hospital, St. Paul, MN

Goetz, Rupert R., M.D., Assistant Professor, Department of Psychiatry, Oregon Health Sciences University School of Medicine, Portland, OR

Goldberg, Bruce W., M.D., Associate Professor, Department of Family Medicine and Department of Public Health and Preventive Medicine, Oregon Health Sciences University School of Medicine, Portland, OR

Goldschmidt, Ronald H., M.D., Professor and Vice Chair, Department of Family and Community Medicine, University of California, San Francisco School of Medicine; Director, Family Practice Inpatient Service, San Francisco General Hospital, San Francisco, CA

Gonzalez, Eduardo C., M.D., Assistant Professor, Department of Family Medicine, University of South Florida College of Medicine; Faculty Physician, Tampa General Hospital, Tampa, FL

Grant, William D., Ed.D., Research Professor, Department of Family Medicine, State University of New York Health Science Center at Syracuse, Syracuse, NY

Gravel, Joseph W., Jr., M.D., Assistant Clinical Professor, Department of Family Medicine, Boston University School of Medicine, Boston, MA; Director, The Malden Hospital Family Practice Residency Program, The Malden Hospital, Malden, MA

Gude, James K., M.D., Clinical Professor, Department of Family and Community Medicine, University of California, San Francisco, School of Medicine, San Francisco, CA; Coordinator of Internal Medicine, Family Practice Residency Program, Community Hospital of Sonoma County, Santa Rosa, CA

Haas, Leonard J., Ph.D., Professor and Director of Behavioral Sciences Section, Department of Family and Preventive Medicine, University of Utah School of Medicine, Salt Lake City, UT

Hale, Frank A., Ph.D., Professor and Director of Faculty Development Program, Department of Family and Community Medicine, University of Arizona College of Medicine, Tucson, AZ

Hall, Karen L., M.D., Associate Professor and Family Practice Residency Program Director, Department of Community Health and Family Medicine, University of Florida College of Medicine, Gainesville, FL

Ham, Richard I., M.D., Professor, Department of Family Medicine and Department of Medicine, SUNY Distinguished Chair in Geriatric Medicine, State University of New York Health Science Center at Syracuse, College of Medicine, Syracuse, NY

Harper, Michael B., M.D., Professor, Department of Family Medicine, Louisiana State University Medical Center, Shreveport, LA

Herbst, Michael M., M.D., Assistant Clinical Professor, Department of Family Medicine, University of California, Los Angeles, CA; Residency Faculty, Santa Monica-UCLA Medical Center, Santa Monica, CA

Herman, James M., M.D., M.S.P.H., Professor and Chair, Department of Family and Community Medicine, Associate Dean for Primary Care, Pennsylvania State University School of Medicine, Hershey, PA

Hermann, Denise, M.D., Assistant Clinical Professor, Division of Cardiology, University of California, San Diego; Assistant Director, Heart Failure and Cardiac Transplantation Program, University of California, San Diego Medical Center, San Diego, CA

Hirsch, Kenneth A., M.D., Ph.D., Faculty and Staff Psychiatrist, Naval Medical Center, San Diego, CA

Hobbs, Joseph, M.D., Professor and Vice Chair of Academic Affairs, Department of Family Medicine, Associate Dean for Primary Care, Medical College of Georgia School of Medicine, Augusta, GA

Hoffman, Richard H., M.D., Associate Clinical Professor, Department of Family Practice, Medical College of Virginia of Virginia Commonwealth University; Associate Director, Chesterfield Family Practice Center, Chippenham Hospital, Richmond, VA

Jack, Brian W., M.D., Associate Professor and Associate Chair, Department of Family Medicine, Boston University School of Medicine, Boston, MA

James, Robert E., M.D., Clinical Instructor, Department of Urology, University of California School of Medicine, San Francisco, CA

Jobe, Ann C., M.D., M.S.N., Associate Professor, Department of Family Medicine, Senior Associate Dean, East Carolina University School of Medicine, Greenville, NC

Johnson, Thomas A., Jr., M.D., Chairman, Department of Family Medicine, St. John's Mercy Medical Center, St. Louis, MO

Jones, Jeffrey G., M.D., M.P.H., Medical Director, St. Francis Occupational Health Centers, St. Francis Hospital and Health Care Centers, Beech Grove, IN

Katerndahl, David A., M.D., M.A., Professor and Director of Research and Education, Department of Family Practice, The University of Texas Health Science Center at San Antonio, San Antonio, TX

Kessel, Kenneth F., M.D., Professor, Department of Family Practice, Rush-Presbyterian St. Lukes Medical Center, Rush University School of Medicine, Chicago, IL; Associate Director, Family Practice Residency, Columbia/LaGrange Memorial Hospital, LaGrange, IL

Kimmel, Sanford R., M.D., Associate Professor of Clinical Family Medicine, Medical College of Ohio; Associate Director, Family Practice Residency, St. Vincent Medical Center, Toledo, OH

King, John G., M.D., Associate Clinical Professor, Department of Family Practice, Medical College of Virginia of Virginia Commonwealth University; Associate Director, Residency Program, Hanover Family Physicians, Medical College of Virginia Hospitals, Richmond, VA

Kirkpatrick, George L., M.D., Associate Professor, Department of Family Practice, University of South Alabama School of Medicine, Mobile, AL

Kleeberg, Paul, M.D., Private Practice, Saint Peter Clinic; Medical Advisor, Internet Services, Allina Health System, St. Peter, MN

Kligman, Evan W., M.D., Professor and Head, Department of Family Medicine, University of Iowa College of Medicine, Iowa City, IA

Klinkman, Michael S., M.D., M.S., Assistant Professor, Department of Family Practice, University of Michigan Medical School, Ann Arbor, MI

Knight, Aubrey L., M.D., Associate Professor of Clinical Family Medicine, University of Virginia School of Medicine, Charlottesville, VA; Associate Director of Family Practice Education, Roanoke Memorial Hospitals, Roanoke, VA

Koester, Donald R., M.D., Associate Professor, Department of Family Practice and Community Medicine, The University of Texas Southwestern Medical Center, Dallas, TX; Hillcrest Baptist Medical Center and Providence Health Center, Waco, TX

Kubala, Ginger S., M.D., Co-Chairman, Family Practice Department, Bethesda North Hospital; Community Preceptor for University of Cincinnati College of Medicine, Cincinnati, OH

Larsen, Lars C., M.D., Associate Professor, Department of Family Medicine, Assistant Dean for Generalist Programs, East Carolina University School of Medicine, Greenville, NC

Larsen, William G., M.D., Department of Family Medicine, The Nalle Clinic, Charlotte, NC

Lee, Daniel T., M.D., Assistant Clinical Professor, Department of Family Medicine, University of California at Los Angeles School of Medicine, Los Angeles, CA; Family Practice Residency Program, Santa Monica-UCLA Medical Center, Santa Monica, CA

Leslie, William T., M.D., Assistant Professor, Section of Medical Oncology, Rush Presbyterian St. Lukes Medical Center, Rush University School of Medicine, Chicago, IL

Lessenger, James E., M.D., Private Practice, Morinda Medical Group, Inc., Porterville, CA

Lewan, Richard B., M.D., Assistant Professor, Department of Family and Community Medicine, Medical College of Wisconsin, Milwaukee, WI; Director, Waukesha Family Practice Residency Program, Waukesha Memorial Hospital, Waukesha, WI

Lustig, Michael R., M.D., Associate Clinical Professor, Department of Family Practice, Medical College of Virginia of Virginia Commonwealth University, Richmond, VA; Associate Director, Riverside Family Practice Center, Riverside Hospital, Newport News, VA

MacDonald, David C., D.O., Clinical Assistant Professor, Department of Family Practice, University of Washington School of Medicine, Seattle, WA and the Uniformed University of the Health Sciences, Bethesda, MD; Director of Residency Training, Madigan Army Medical Center, Tacoma, WA

Magill, Michael K. M.D., Professor and Chairman, Department of Family and Preventive Medicine, University of Utah School of Medicine, Salt Lake City, UT

Marsland, David W., M.D., Professor and Chairman, Department of Family Practice, Medical College of Virginia of Virginia Commonwealth University, Richmond, VA

Matheny, Samuel C., M.D., M.P.H., Professor and Chair, Department of Family Practice, University of Kentucky College of Medicine, Lexington, KY

Mauer, Richard C., M.D., A.B.E.S., F.A.C.S., Director, Mauer Eye Center, Convenant Medical Center, Waterloo, IA

Mayeaux, Edward J., Jr., M.D., Associate Professor, Department of Family Medicine, Louisiana State University Medical Center, Shreveport, LA

McBride, Patrick E., M.D., M.P.H., Associate Professor, Department of Family Medicine, University of Wisconsin School of Medicine, Madison, WI

McCabe, Melvina, M.D., Associate Professor, Department of Family Medicine, University of New Mexico School of Medicine, Albuquerque, NM

McCahill, Margaret E., M.D., Associate Clinical Professor, Department of Family and Preventive Medicine, University of California, San Diego School of Medicine; Director, Combined Family Medicine-Psychiatry Residency Program, Associate Director, Family Medicine Residency Training Program, UCSD Medical Center, San Diego, CA

McDaniel, Susan H., Ph.D., Associate Professor, Departments of Family Medicine and Psychiatry, University of Rochester School of Medicine and Dentistry, Rochester, NY

McKenna, Marc W., M.D., University of Pennsylvania School of Medicine, Director of Family Practice Residency Program, Chestnut Hill Hospital, Philadelphia, PA

McSherry, James A., M.D., Ch.B., Professor, Department of Family Medicine, University of Western Ontario School of Medicine, London, Canada; Chief of Family Medicine, London Health Sciences Centre, London, Canada

Melvin, Susan Y., D.O., Associate Clinical Professor, Department of Family Medicine, University of California–Irvine School of Medicine, Long Beach, CA

Middleton, Donald B., M.D., Clinical Associate Professor, Department of Family Medicine and Clinical Epidemiology, University of Pittsburgh School of Medicine; Director, Family Practice Residency Program, St. Margaret Memorial Hospital, Pittsburgh, PA

Miser, William F., M.D., Clinical Associate Professor, Department of Family Medicine, University of Washington School of Medicine, Seattle, WA; Director, Faculty Development Fellowship, Madigan Army Medical Center, Tacoma, WA

Monroe, Alicia D., M.D., Assistant Professor, Department of Family Medicine, Brown University School of Medicine; Memorial Hospital of Rhode Island/Brown University, Pawtucket, RI

Murphy, John B., M.D., Associate Professor, Department of Family Medicine, Brown University School of Medicine; Director of Residency Training, Memorial Hospital of Rhode Island/Brown University, Pawtucket, RI

Nahlik, James E., M.D., Associate Clinical Professor, Department of Community and Family Medicine, Saint Louis University School of Medicine; Faculty Family Physician, Deaconess Health System, St. Louis, MO

Nasir, Laeth S., M.D., Assistant Professor, Department of Family Medicine, University of Nebraska College of Medicine, Omaha, NE

Nesbitt, Thomas S., M.D., M.P.H., Associate Professor, Department of Family Practice, University of California, Davis School of Medicine, Sacramento, CA

Newkirk, Gary R., M.D., Director, Family Practice Residency Program, Sacred Heart Medical Center, Spokane, WA

Nistler, Carole, M.D., El Camino Hospital, Mountain View, CA

Noll, Edmond C., M.D., Assistant Professor of Clinical Family Medicine, University of Southern California School of Medicine, Los Angeles, CA

Norcross, William A., M.D., Professor of Clinical Family Medicine, University of California, San Diego School of Medicine, La Jolla, CA; Director of Residency Training, University of California, San Diego Medical Center, San Diego, CA

Nuovo, Jim, M.D., Assistant Professor and Director of Residency Training, Department of Family Practice, University of California, Davis School of Medicine, Sacramento, CA

O'Dell, Michael L., M.D., Associate Professor, Department of Family Medicine, University of Texas Medical Branch, Galveston; Residency Program Director, John Sealy Hospital, Galveston, TX

Ostergaard, Daniel J., M.D., Vice President for Education and Scientific Affairs, American Academy of Family Physicians, Kansas City, MO

Parchman, Michael L., M.D., Associate Professor, Department of Family Medicine, Texas Tech University Health Sciences Center, El Paso, TX

Paul, Edward G., M.D., Assistant Professor, Department of Family and Community Medicine, Pennsylvania State University College of Medicine, Hershey, PA; Director of Residency Training, The Good Samaritan Hospital and Medical Center, Lebanon, PA

Paulman, Paul M., M.D., Associate Professor and Director of Undergraduate Education, Department of Family Medicine, University of Nebraska College of Medicine, Omaha, NE

Peterson, Dana W., M.D., Private Practice, Southwest Medical Associates, P.A., Albuquerque, NM

Petrie, Kent, M.D., Assistant Clinical Professor, Department of Family Medicine, University of Colorado Health Sciences Center, Denver, CO; Private Practice, Vail, CO

Pfenninger, John L., M.D., President, The National Procedures Institute, Midland, MI; Clinical Professor, Department of Family Medicine, Michigan State College of Human Medicine, East Lansing, MI; Private Practice, Midland, MI

Phelps, Gregory L., M.D., M.P.H., Medical Director, Fort Sanders Physician Group, Fort Sanders Hospital System, Knoxville, TN

Prest, Layne A., Ph.D., Assistant Professor and Director of Behavioral Medicine, Department of Family Medicine, University of Nebraska College of Medicine, Omaha, NE

Ratcliffe, Stephen D., M.D., M.S.P.H., Associate Professor and Division Chief, Department of Family and Preventive Medicine, University of Utah School of Medicine, Salt Lake City, UT

Realini, Janet P., M.D., M.P.H., Professor, Department of Family Practice, University of Texas Health Science Center at San Antonio; Director, Family Practice Residency Program, University Hospital, San Antonio, TX

Rhyne, Maureen C., Ph.D., Assistant Clinical Professor, Department of Family Medicine, University of California School of Medicine, Irvine, CA; Director, Behavioral Medicine, Family Practice Residency Program, Long Beach Memorial Medical Center, Long Beach, CA

Richardson, James P., M.D., M.P.H., Associate Professor, Departments of Family Medicine and Epidemiology and Preventive Medicine, University of Maryland School of Medicine, Baltimore, MD

Robertson, Russell G., M.D., Assistant Professor, Department of Family and Community Medicine, Medical College of Wisconsin; Director of Residency Training, Columbia Family Practice Program, Columbia Hospital, Milwaukee, WI

Robinson, Timothy T., D.O., Assistant Attending, Department of Medicine, North Shore University Hospital, New York College of Osteopathic Medicine, Old Westbury, NY; Affiliate Faculty, Idaho State University, Pocatello ID; Affiliate Clinical Instructor, St. John's University College of Pharmacy; Attending Physician, Department of Family Practice, Catholic Medical Center of Brooklyn and Queens, Jamaica, NY

Rodnick, Jonathan E., M.D., Professor and Chair, Department of Family and Community Medicine, University of California at San Francisco, San Francisco, CA

Rodriguez, Glenn S., M.D., Adjunct Associate Professor, Department of Family Medicine, Oregon Health Sciences University School of Medicine; Regional Director, Population Health Improvement Programs, Providence Health Systems, Portland, OR

Rosenfeld, Jo Ann, M.D., Associate Professor, Department of Family Medicine, East Tennessee State University School of Medicine, Bristol, TN

Ross, Joseph E., M.D., Assistant Clinical Professor, Department of Family Medicine, University of Illinois College of Medicine–Rockford, Rockford, IL

Saba, George, Ph.D., Associate Clinical Professor, Department of Family and Community Medicine, University of California, San Francisco School of Medicine; Associate Program Director, Behavioral Sciences, Family Practice Residency Program, San Francisco General Hospital, San Francisco, CA

Sander, Robert W., M.D., Assistant Professor, Department of Family and Community Medicine, Medical College of Wisconsin, Milwaukee, WI; Associate Director, Waukesha Family Practice Residency Program, Waukesha Memorial Hospital, Waukesha, WI

Saultz, John W., M.D., Professor, Department of Family Medicine, Oregon Health Sciences University School of Medicine, Portland, OR

Schaffer, Ted C., M.D., Clinical Assistant Professor, Department of Family Medicine and Clinical Epidemiology, University of Pittsburgh School of Medicine; Director,

Family Health Centers, Family Practice Residency Program, St. Margaret Memorial Hospital, Pittsburgh, PA

Scherger, Joseph E., M.D., M.P.H., Professor and Chairman, Department of Family Medicine, Associate Dean for Clinical Affairs, University of California, Irvine College of Medicine, Irvine, CA

Schmittling, Gordon, M.S., M.S., Director, Division of Research and Information Services, American Academy of Family Physicians, Kansas City, MO

Schulz, Jerome E., M.D., Associate Clinical Professor, Department of Family Medicine, East Carolina University School of Medicine, Greenville, NC

Scott, Robert H., M.D., Clinical Assistant Professor, Department of Family Medicine, University of Washington School of Medicine; Faculty, Family Medicine Residency, Swedish Medical Center, Seattle, WA

Seaburn, David B., M.S., Assistant Professor, Department of Family Medicine and Department of Psychiatry, University of Rochester School of Medicine and Dentistry, Rochester, NY

Searight, H. Russell, Ph.D., Adjunct Associate Professor, Department of Psychology and Department of Community and Family Medicine, Saint Louis University School of Medicine; Director of Behavioral Sciences, Deaconess Family Medicine Residency Program, St. Louis, MO

Sereno, Patricia A., M.D., M.P.H., Residency Faculty, The Malden Hospital Family Practice Residency Program, The Malden Hospital, Malden, MA

Sheehan, John P., M.D., Associate Clinical Professor, Department of Medicine, Case Western Reserve University School of Medicine, Cleveland, OH; Medical Director, North Coast Institute of Diabetes and Endocrinology, Inc., Westlake, OH

Sitorius, Michael A., M.D., Professor and Chairman, Department of Family Medicine, University of Nebraska Medical Center, Omaha, NE

Smith, Charles Kent, M.D., Professor and Chairman, Department of Family Medicine, Case Western Reserve University School of Medicine, Cleveland, OH

Smith, Mindy A., M.D., M.S., Associate Professor, Department of Family Practice, Michigan State University College of Human Medicine, East Lansing, MI

Snell, George F., M.D., Associate Professor, Department of Family and Preventive Medicine, University of Utah School of Medicine, Salt Lake City, UT; Director of Residency Training–Retired, McKay-Dee Hospital, Ogden UT

Solorio, Rosa, M.D., Acting Assistant Professor, Department of Family Medicine, University of Washington School of Medicine, Seattle, WA

South-Paul, Jeannette E., M.D., Associate Professor and Chair, Department of Family Medicine, Uniformed Services University of the Health Sciences, Bethesda, MD

Spees, David N., M.D., Clinical Instructor, Department of Family and Preventive Medicine, University of California School of Medicine, San Diego; Director, Travel Clinic, Sharp Rees-Stealy, Sharp Memorial Hospital, San Diego, CA

Spieker, Michael R., M.D., Assistant Professor, Department of Family Medicine, Uniformed Services University of the Health Sciences, Bethesda, MD

Squier, Harriet A., M.D., M.A., Assistant Professor, Department of Family Practice, Michigan State University College of Human Medicine, East Lansing, MI

Stange, Kurt, M.D., Ph.D., Associate Professor, Department of Family Medicine, Case Western Reserve University School of Medicine, Cleveland, OH

Stevens, Nancy G., M.D., M.P.H., Associate Professor, Department of Family Medicine, University of Washington School of Medicine, Seattle, WA

Sturgis, Thomas M., M.D., Assistant Professor, Department of Internal Medicine, East Carolina University School of Medicine, Greenville, NC

Suess, Judith A., M.D., M.P.H., Assistant Professor, Department of Family Practice, Michigan State University College of Human Medicine, East Lansing, MI

Supanich, Barbara, M.D., R.S.M., Assistant Professor, Department of Family Practice, Michigan State University College of Human Medicine, East Lansing, MI

Sur, Denise K.C., M.D., Assistant Clinical Professor, Department of Family Medicine, University of California, Los Angeles School of Medicine, Los Angeles, CA; Associate Director of Residency Training, Santa Monica-UCLA Medical Center Family Practice Residency, Santa Monica, CA

Sutherland, John E., M.D., Clinical Professor, Department of Family Practice, University of Iowa College of Medicine, Iowa City, IA; Director, Northeast Iowa Medical Education Foundation and Family Practice Residency Program, Allen Memorial Hospital, Covenant Medical Center, Waterloo, IA

Sweha, Amir, M.D., Assistant Clinical Professor and Family Practice Clinic Director, Department of Family Practice, Family Practice Clinic Director, University of California, Davis School of Medicine, Sacramento, CA

Tanji, Jeffrey L., M.D., Associate Professor, Department of Family Practice and Department of Exercise Science, University of California, Davis School of Medicine, Sacramento, CA

Tatum, Nancy O., M.D., Assistant Professor, Department of Family Medicine, University of Mississippi School of Medicine; Director of Clinical Ethics, University of Mississippi Medical Center, Jackson, MS

Taylor, Robert B., M.D., Professor and Chairman, Department of Family Medicine, Oregon Health Sciences University School of Medicine, Portland, OR

Tobin, Marla J., M.D., Private Practice, Warrensburg, MO

Toffler, William L., M.D., Professor, Department of Family Medicine, Oregon Health Sciences University School of Medicine, Portland, OR

Tronetti, Pamela S., D.O., Clinical Associate Professor of Geriatric Medicine, Lake Erie College of Osteopathic Medicine; Medical Director, Erie Center on Health and Aging, Hamot Medical Center, Erie, PA

Tuggy, Michael L., M.D., Clinical Assistant Professor, Department of Family Medicine, University of Washington School of Medicine; Faculty, Swedish Family Medicine Residency, Swedish Medical Center, Seattle, WA

Tunzi, Marc, M.D., Assistant Clinical Professor, Department of Family and Community Medicine, University of California School of Medicine, San Francisco, CA; Assistant Director, Family Practice Residency Program, Natividad Medical Center, Salinas, CA

Ulchaker, Margaret M., M.S.N., R.N., C.D.E., N.P-C., Clinical Instructor, Medical/Surgical Nursing, Case Western Reserve University School of Medicine, Cleveland, OH; Director of Patient Education/Research Coordinator, North Coast Institute of Diabetes and Endocrinology, Inc., Westlake, OH

Underbakke, Gail, R.D., M.S., Nutrition Coordinator, Department of Family Medicine, University of Wisconsin School of Medicine, Madison, WI

Van Durme, Daniel J., M.D., Associate Professor, Department of Family Medicine, University of South Florida College of Medicine, Tampa, FL

Vincent, E. Chris, M.D., Assistant Professor, Department of Family Medicine, University of Washington School of Medicine, Seattle, WA; Faculty Physician, Swedish Medical Center, Seattle, WA

Wallace, Mark E., M.D., Clinical Instructor, University of Colorado School of Medicine, Denver, CO; Director of Family Practice Residency Training, North Colorado Medical Center, Greeley, CO

Walling, Anne D., M.B., Ch.B., F.F.P.H.M., Professor, Department of Family Medicine, University of Kansas School of Medicine, Wichita, KS

Walsh, Eric, M.D., Assistant Professor, Department of Family Medicine, Oregon Health Sciences University School of Medicine; Director of Family Practice Residency Training, Oregon Health Sciences University Hospital, Portland, OR

Warshaw, Gregg, M.D., Professor, Department of Family Medicine, University of Cincinnati College of Medicine, Cincinnati, OH

Weinberg, Howard N., M.D., Private Practice, Virginia Beach, VA; SentaraHospitals, Norfolk, VA

Wilkinson, John M., M.D., Assistant Professor, Department of Family Medicine, Mayo Medical School; Consultant, Department of Family Medicine, Mayo Clinic and Mayo Foundation, Rochester, MN

Willard, Mary A., M.D., University of Medicine and Dentistry of New Jersey, Robert Wood Johnson School of Medicine, New Brunswick, NJ; Director, West Jersey Family Practice Residency, West Jersey Health System, Voorhees, NJ

Wooten, Wilma J., M.D., M.P.H., Assistant Clinical Professor, Department of Family and Preventive Medicine, University of California School of Medicine, San Diego, CA; SSPM Tract Coordinator, University of California, San Diego/General Preventive Medicine Residency, San Diego State University, LaJolla, CA

Wright, David W., M.L.S., Research Librarian, Huffington Library, American Academy of Family Physicians, Kansas City, MO

Zimmerman, Richard Kent, M.D., M.P.H., Assistant Professor, Departments of Family Medicine and Clinical Epidemiology and Health Services Administration, University of Pittsburgh School of Medicine, Pittsburgh, PA

Zuber, Thomas J., M.D., Assistant Clinical Professor, Department of Family Medicine, Michigan State University College of Human Medicine, East Lansing, MI; Program Director in Family Medicine, Saginaw Cooperative Hospitals, Saginaw, MI

1

Test Taking Techniques

Gerald K. Goodenough, M.D., M.S.P.H.

Test taking is necessary for all health care professionals. Like it or not, we must prove competency for licensure, and at continuing intervals in many specialties, by performing adequately on board exams. If you are already a health care professional, you have shown that you are able to master the field by performing adequately on examinations during training. This chapter addresses the unique testing style found on medical board exams.

Board exams test your ability to perform on board exams. Albeit, there is a general consistency between board scores and academic performance during training. However, the outcome of a board exam (the score) certainly reflects, most of all, the ability of the test taker to perform on a board exam. Some people seem to have a natural ability to do well on board exams. They appear to have a "sense" about which answer should be chosen. Most of us do not have this sense, but all of us can improve our scores by learning some techniques about taking board exams. If individuals fail on an exam, it is often because they fail to understand and apply one or more of the techniques discussed in this chapter.

It must be said, of course, that nothing will replace diligent study. One must know the information content of the exam or the whole purpose of the board exam will be distorted. The message of this introductory chapter is that the techniques discussed are not to replace timely study reviews, but rather to complement one's studies so that the best possible outcome is achieved on the exam.

The Exam

The traditional board exam will consist of one or more booklets of questions with answer sheets to match. Generally, there are 60 questions per book. Questions may be short or long, but they all count equally. Often, a clinical stem (a patient care scenario) will be followed by a specific question and answer choices.

Two types of answer choices are found on the typical exam. One type has four or five choices, with only one choice being correct. The other type has a series of choices, each of which may be true or false. The answer sheet will make obvious the type of question, but test takers may lose valuable time pondering over a "best choice," only to discover that the question is a multiple true–false-type question.

Scoring and establishing the pass/fail cutoff varies by the committee who plans the exam. Remember that scores are reported as "percentile" scores. A score does not denote the percentage of questions answered correctly. The percentile score reflects the test taker's standing in relation to all persons taking the exam. A score of 80th percentile means that 20% of individuals performed better and 80% scored worse than the test taker in question. A person could possibly answer 99% of the questions correctly but still be in a low percentile if most of the other test takers answered 99.1% or more of the questions correctly.

Pass/fail cutoffs vary widely by the test, the year, and the individual committee. Sometimes a "core" of questions is prepared that represents basic knowledge expected of a person who is a diplomate of the specialty. It is then expected that most, or nearly all, of these questions will be answered correctly. The remainder of the questions may be designed to uncover an unusual depth of knowledge, with the expectation that most test takers will not answer most of these questions correctly. A cutoff limit will be established for the must-do "core" of basic questions. Those failing to perform adequately on those questions will fail the exam, unless they do unusually well on the more esoteric questions.

Preparing for the Exam

Any test taker should have a well-rehearsed plan in preparing for taking the exam. This plan should include the following:

- Know the exact time and date of the exam. For Family Practice, the exam is always given on the second Friday in July. Be aware that the *certification* exam is different from the *recertification* exam, and prepare accordingly. By process A, in Family Practice, for example, the second half of the exam day consists of three preselected modules. Also, the general distribution of question types may help guide your preparation. For Family Practice, the distribution is as follows:

  40% Internal Medicine
  12% Pediatrics
  12% Surgery
  12% Psychiatry
  10% Obstetrics-Gynecology
  5% Geriatrics
  5% Community Medicine

- Remember that, because exam questions are written 1.5 to 2 years before the exam, new research findings from the latest articles are not pertinent to your board preparation study. Review articles and textbooks are the best sources. An excellent technique, also, is to use practice exams. This will inform you of your weak areas and will act as a study guide. There are practice exam references that can be purchased (such as this book), or one can review old copies of the in-training exams that are required of Family Practice residents.

- Write down selected lists or pieces of information for repeated reviewing just prior to the exam. Such topics as immunization schedules, hepatitis B antibody curves, side effect tables of certain classes of drugs (e.g., antidepressants), and Advanced Cardiac Life Support protocols are examples of areas with a high likelihood of appearing on the exam. A quick review of these lists may just give you the edge you need.

- Arrive early and be physiologically ready. A good night's sleep and a substantive breakfast are advised. The test taker should be familiar with the location of the bathrooms, the functions of the test monitors, and the rules for when to start and stop.

Taking the Exam

There are certain common-sense rules that bear reviewing:

- Do a relaxing activity the day before the exam as a preparation for a good night's sleep. Very seldom does last-minute "cramming" pay off, and the anxiety it can produce may be detrimental.

- Be certain to check, and double check, the time you are to arrive at the testing station. An alarm clock is a valuable asset.

- Comfort is an important consideration. Wear comfortable clothing and carry along that extra jacket just in case the examination room is cool. If you are prone to develop that "low blood sugar" feeling at times of stress, take along a high-energy snack.

- Listen carefully. The instructions will be reviewed prior to the exam. You should know the total duration of the exam so as not to leave after the first booklet of a two-booklet exam. Realize that when the proctor says, "Stop working," that is an absolute imperative. Do not have your exam seized because you broke a rule. The rules are clear and will be clearly repeated by the exam monitor.

- Apportion your time. Most often the 60 questions must be answered in 2 hours. This gives an average of 2 minutes per question. For most people, these exams are a race against the clock. It is a sad outcome for a test taker to be on question 46 when time is called. No credit is given for unanswered questions. It is a good idea to mark the time, in pencil, by landmark questions to be achieved (say, 15 should be marked at 8:30, and question 30 should be marked by 9:00). Remember to choose an answer for each question, even if it is only a guess. Unmarked choices are always wrong.

- Do not ponder. Do not spend excessive time over questions whose answers are not readily obvious. This is a waste of time. Place an "X" in the column of the question book so you may return if time permits, and then move on. Realize that many individuals will miss the difficult questions, so those will not have nearly the impact on your percentile score as will unanswered questions.

Board Exam Tips

The following are some tips for "second-guessing" the answer choices when you are uncertain of the correct answer or for saving time in dealing with long questions. There are 15 tips, with examples and discussions. During your preparation, practice using these tips and see how they work out.

Tip 1: When a question has a long stem, read the answer choices first. This will direct or focus your reading and speed up the process.

Example:
1. A 58-year-old man who had a recent CABG involving two vessels is complaining of a new-onset chest pain since 48 hours ago. He describes the pain as a

pressure on his chest with left arm radiation, related to exercise. He shows a family history of CAD with obesity, elevated triglycerides, and smoking. Laboratory data reveals WBC 11,900, Hb 12.2, Hct 38.6, RDW 12, Na 141, K 3.9, Cl 100, BUN 22, Ca 10.2, Alk Phos 150, and LDH 180. The electrocardiogram (ECG) shows a regular sinus rhythm with an occasional PVC and inverted T-waves in leads I, AVL, and the lateral limb leads. There is no ST elevation. He has a cough that causes chest discomfort that is not similar to the exertional pain. Lately, he has had a decreased appetite and mild shortness of breath. You should

(A) refer to the cardiologist for angiography
(B) treat symptomatically with nitroglycerin
(C) give codeine and see the patient in 2 weeks
(D) perform a treadmill stress test

Discussion—The stem contains much information not relevant to the choice of an answer. By knowing that the choices involve an action appropriate for the chest pain, much of the information in the stem can be skimmed and dismissed. This will save valuable time.

Tip 2: Typically, a question is based on a "principle." Try to identify what information or principle the test writers expect you to know.

Example:
2. An 82-year-old woman, hospitalized for pneumonitis, is weak, has a mild cough, and wants to return to her home. She says she will do just fine there. Her daughter has called from another state and feels that her mother belongs in a facility where care is available and meals are prepared. You should

(A) ask the daughter to clarify which facility she wishes for her mother
(B) ask the social worker to do an assessment of affordability of various facilities
(C) ask the social worker to help find the least restrictive facility that still prepares meals
(D) perform a functional assessment on the patient

Discussion—The first principle in disposition planning is to determine the function of the patient. The test writer wants to determine whether you know that no planning can go forward until you know how well the patient is able to perform. The will of the daughter should not supercede the wishes of a patient who is mentally capable of understanding and making choices.

Tip 3: Stick to standard, or "by the book," principles. Your own value system may be at variance with stand-

ard teaching, or you may have experiential knowledge that is not "textbook" information. Remember that most test writers will rely on the recommendations found in standard references.

Example:
3. A 14-year-old girl asks you to provide her with birth control pills. She is afraid to consult her parents, who are unaware that she is sexually active. She is not at all comfortable with letting her parents know of her choices. You would

(A) counsel her at length on the need to tell her parents of her choice and ask her to return with one or both parents
(B) take an appropriate history, perform an appropriate examination, educate the patient about safe sex, and give her a prescription for the pill, if no physical contraindications are found
(C) call her parents and inform them of her request, asking them to help in your decision process
(D) tell the patient that she is too young for sex and that she should stop her sexual activity

Discussion—The laws in most states allow a physician to dispense birth control to minors without parental consent. You may not feel comfortable in taking such action yourself. However, for purposes of answering this question on a board exam, you would go with the standard choice and allow her to have the pill.

Tip 4: Sometimes question stems contain information that may help in other questions. Go back and use such information if it is helpful.

Example:
4. A patient with a history of Wegener's granulomatosis confirmed in the past with a sedimentation rate of 107 and elevated c-antineutrophil cytoplasmic antibodies (c-ANCAs) now has a blood-tinged mucousy nasal discharge and a headache. He has been in remission since a course of cyclophosphamide and prednisone 2 years ago. You would

(A) treat for sinusitis and repeat the sedimentation rate
(B) refer to an ENT specialist
(C) refer to a rheumatologist for treatment of his Wegener's granulomatosis
(D) order a computed tomographic (CT) scan of his sinuses

Discussion—The stem tells you that Wegener's granulomatosis is accompanied by an elevated sedimentation rate and c-ANCAs. This may prove useful in another question about Wegener's granulomatosis or about c-ANCAs and what they indicate. You may use this information to your advantage.

Tip 5: Eliminate obviously incorrect answers to improve your chances at guessing.

Example:
5. A 45-year-old white man presents with a complaint of progressive arthralgia and deformities of the second and third M-P joints bilaterally. He has bronzing of his skin about the ankles and says he has chronic fatigue and occasional memory problems. For about 6 months, he has had occasional cardiac palpitations. Two older brothers died of cirrhosis of the liver and cardiomyopathy. Appropriate lab tests would include

- (A) transferrin saturation and serum ferritin, serum glucose, and liver enzymes
- (B) complete blood count (CBC), U/A, PFTs, and chest radiograph
- (C) bone biopsy, serum calcium and phosphorus, and parathyroid hormone
- (D) head CT scan, ALZ 50 cerebrospinal fluid (CSF) level, and CSF acetylcholine level

Discussion—Option D is obviously aimed at a primary dementia workup, and C would be directed at hypercalcemia. Both would be illogical in working up a case of a multiorgan genetic disease. This narrows the choices down to options A or B.

Tip 6: Be on the alert for "catch" words or phrases "that guide your selection."

Example:
6. An unresponsive man is brought to the emergency department where you work. He passed out 30 minutes ago and has remained unresponsive. There is no history of trauma. Vital signs are normal. The appropriate first step is to

- (A) obtain details of his activities of the past 24 hours
- (B) obtain a stat Chem-7, CBC, ABGs, and U/A
- (C) draw a tube of blood, then administer IV glucose $D_{50}W$ by push
- (D) obtain a head CT, neck films, and KUB of the abdomen

Discussion—Although each of the choices may be appropriate to work up the unresponsive patient, only one would be the appropriate *first step*. We may be tempted to pick a choice that seems the most extensive

or thorough. However, the stem asks the *first step*, which is to administer glucose. That step is immediate, is potentially life-saving, and would not significantly slow down any of the ensuing workup.

Other catch words or phrases are noteworthy. One should avoid answer choices that say "only," "never," "always," "all," or "no." Examples are

- (A) There are never adequate community services for these problems.
- (B) All are the result of irresponsible behavior.

Tip 7: If a choice is totally unfamiliar, it is probably not the correct choice. This may be a clever distractor, made up to lead you down a dangerous path.

Example:
7. A patient with moderately heavy epistaxis continues to bleed despite nasal compression, cold packs, and head positioning. Blood pressure (BP) is 130/72, pulse 92, and the patient's airway is unobstructed. There is no sign of trauma. The most appropriate next step is to

- (A) replace fluid as whole blood, 2 units
- (B) place an anterior pack to tamponade the bleeding nostril
- (C) use a directed laser beam anterior septolyzer at the bedside
- (D) cauterize all vessels in the nose

Discussion—A "directed laser beam anterior septolyzer" is a made-up term. If you have not heard of such a treatment, avoid the temptation to show that you are up to date with the latest advances by choosing an imaginary choice.

Tip 8: Choice sequences, such as a whole row of "B" choices, or all "true" choices, may be a clue that there are one or more incorrect choices. *If* you are totally guessing on a choice, steer away from perpetuating a run of identical letters.

Example and Discussion:
8. A row of "A's" is probably incorrect, as stated above. If you are confident in your choices, *DO NOT* change just to break up a pattern. If you are guessing and picking an arbitrary choice, however, pick one that breaks up the sequence.

Tip 9: Analyze answers comparatively. If one answer merely restates the other, both are wrong. If one is opposite another, one is apt to be correct. If two answers look similar but each has subtle differences, one is probably correct.

Example:
9. Benzodiazepines that depend primarily on the p-450 cytochrome oxidase system for metabolism are best avoided for daily use in the elderly because

(A) the half-life increases predictably with age, thus running a risk of accumulation
(B) the drug can never achieve therapeutic levels
(C) the serum level will remain too low to be effective
(D) they are relatively expensive, and they may be unaffordable for Medicare patients

Discussion—In this case, B and C say the same thing. Both are wrong. Because the p-450 cytochrome oxidase system declines predictably with aging, the half-life of drugs depending on oxidation for metabolism increases and may lead to accumulation.

Tip 10: Some stems are very confusing. Make quick notes to break down and clarify the question.

Example:
10. Pharmakotherapeutics in children requires special training. Which of the following most represents the principle brought to bear in pediatric practice and taught in most medical schools, that proportionality does not always dictate computation of quantitation for administration to younger individuals?

(A) Children require higher doses (in mg/kg) of opiates compared with adults.
(B) Children can be compared with adults on a kilogram-to-kilogram basis.
(C) Children excrete drugs faster because they have higher urine output.
(D) Most children tolerate drugs poorly.

Discussion—Some stems can ramble, have unclear syntax, or are not phrased in common parlance. In this stem, the question can be clarified if rephrased as: *Proportionality does not dictate [dosing], based on weight in children.* "A" exemplifies this.

Tip 11: For choices involving numbers or percentages, pick midrange values (if you are guessing).

Example:
11. The calculated creatinine clearance for a 70-kg male who is 80 years old with a serum creatinine of 2 is

(A) 2
(B) 10
(C) 30
(D) 90
(E) 150

Discussion—When you are making a guess because you are totally unfamiliar with the subject, pick a *midrange* choice or a *logical* choice. A creatinine clearance of 2 is low enough to be illogical. A choice of 10 is also very low. A value of 90 is high for an older person and 150 is higher than that for even young adults. You would choose 30 as representing the best guess.

Tip 12: Pick the "warm, fuzzy" choice if one is presented.

Example:
12. A 64-year-old woman visits your office. She is distraught because her husband is no longer able to perform sexually. She feels inadequate because she can no longer bring him to erection, and she expresses suspicion that he may be seeing another woman. She senses that he has begun to avoid her. You should

(A) refer the husband to a urologist for an impotency workup
(B) give the husband a trial of testosterone after ascertaining that he is not suffering from heart disease or vascular problems
(C) request that she and her husband schedule a session with you to discuss a work-up for erectile dysfunction and also to discuss methods of intimacy that may not include the traditional sex act
(D) refer the couple to a marital counselor

Discussion—Often if there is a choice that clearly portrays the provider as a caring, self-sacrificing, and concerned person, that will be the choice. For psychosocial problems, especially, referring to a specialist before the primary care physician has given the problem a reasonable effort is almost never the correct choice.

Tip 13: If a question involves a medication, the correct choice is usually to stop, rather than start, a medication.

Example:
13. A 72-year-old woman presents with a 3-month history of involuntary facial movements, difficulty walking, and diminished activity. Examination reveals mild rigidity of the extremities, vermicular tongue movements, and bradykinesia. Her history includes arthritis, constipation, and frequent nausea and dyspepsia, for which she takes metoclopramide. Her labs, including a CBC, chemistry 21, and sedimentation rate, are normal. You would

(A) prescribe L-Dopa 100 mg b.i.d. and see her in
1 month
(B) prescribe cogentin 1 mg qd and see her in
1 month
(C) prescribe diphenhydramine and see her in
2 weeks
(D) discontinue the metoclopramide and see the
patient in 1 month

Discussion—Often, the test writer will wish to make a point about a medication, especially if a serious side effect is not widely known. Look for any existing medication that may be creating the problem. Discontinue that medication if there is a chance that it is causing the problem.

Tip 14: Do not look for tricks. If a choice seems obvious, choose it. Do not overly analyze the question because it appears too obvious.

Example:
14. A 78-year-old woman complains of shortness of breath on mild exertion, ankle swelling, and fatigue. She has a history of hypertension and angina pectoris. Her BP is 158/84, her jugular veins are moderately distended, and she has an S_3 and an S_4 gallop, bibasilar rales, and 2+ peripheral edema. Her ECG shows a Q wave in leads II, III, and AVF. Her echocardiogram shows an ejection fraction of 30%, a thickened left ventricle, and normal diastolic function. Her cardiac enzymes are within normal limits, and BUN and electrolytes are normal. You should

(A) place the patient on an ACE inhibitor and a
diuretic and see in 2 weeks
(B) place the patient on a calcium channel blocker
and see in 1 week
(C) start the patient on digoxin and a diuretic and
see in 1 month
(D) begin nonpharmacologic management of her
hypertension

Discussion—Congestive heart failure based on systolic dysfunction is common. The initial treatment with an ACE inhibitor and diuretic is established practice. This may be one of those "core" questions to test basic knowledge in Family Practice. Choose the obvious answer.

Tip 15: Accept information in the stem as given. Do not question the information.

Example:
15. A 32-year-old woman presents with a red, swollen, tender calf, fever, and cough. The V/Q scan reports

high probability for PE. She has had two such episodes in the past involving the opposite leg. She denies using birth control pills or smoking. Along with treating the DVT and PE, you should

(A) check a CBC for polycythemia
(B) obtain a venogram of the pelvis
(C) workup for hypercoagulable state
(D) interview family members to verify that the
patient does not smoke or use oral contraceptives

Discussion—When you are told that the patient denies using birth control pills or smoking, you can accept that she does not use them. Do not doubt what you are told. Choose your answers based on the clues in the stem.

Practice Answers

Now, let's practice using the tips given above. Following are several sets of answers. Practice applying one or more of the tips to choose an answer, *even though there are no questions!*

Example 1

(A) Tell the patient that surgery is the only answer.
(B) Explain the options, giving the advantages and
disadvantages of each.
(C) Tell the patient that you are withdrawing from
the case because of his decision.
(D) Advise the patient that he should see a
psychiatrist.

Example 2

(A) 15
(B) 60
(C) 120
(D) 180
(E) 300

Example 3

(A) FSH, TSH, T4, serum glucose
(B) MEP, DSG, CARP
(C) Omeprazol level in the urine
(D) Hct and serum potassium *only*

Example 4

(A) Begin diazepam, 10 mg b.i.d. and see in 1 month.
(B) Begin amitriptyline 50 mg hs and see in
1 month.

(C) Discontinue the haloperidol and see in 2 weeks.

(D) Begin lorazepam and see in 2 weeks.

Summary

It must be restated that timely diligent study is the only reliable way to ensure passing a board exam. However, certain techniques of analyzing sets of answers and making a choice can be learned. In a case in which the topic is unfamiliar and the correct answer is not obvious, a good guess is the best alternative. The review and tips presented in this chapter may make that good guess as good as it can be.

Answer Key

For your interest, the answers the author chose for the practice questions were:

Example Answers

1. A
2. D
3. B
4. C
5. A
6. C
7. B
8. No question
9. A
10. A
11. C
12. C
13. D
14. A
15. C

Practice Answers

1. B (Tip 12)
2. C (Tip 11)
3. A (Tips 6 & 7)
4. C (Tip 13)

Acknowledgment

I am indebted to Lanyard K. Dial, M.D., of Ventura, California, for his assistance and earlier concepts in developing this topic.

2

Preventive Care

The questions in this chapter constitute a review of the following chapters in *Family Medicine: Principles and Practice, Fifth Edition:*
    Clinical Prevention (Chapter 7)
    Health Promotion (Chapter 8)
    Health Care of the International Traveler (Chapter 9)

DIRECTIONS (Items 2.1 through 2.28): Each of the questions or incomplete statements in this section is followed by five suggested answers or completions. Select the ONE that is BEST in each case.

2.1 A 54-year-old African American attorney comes for his first visit to your family practice office. He asks about the current status of various clinical preventive services. Your response might appropriately include which ONE of the following statements?

 (A) Clinical preventive services have not been found to be cost-effective and are no longer generally recommended.
 (B) The current recommendation is an annual comprehensive physical examination for all adults.
 (C) Specific clinical services are recommended by age group without consideration of high-risk patients, family history, or life-style behaviors.
 (D) Chronologic rather than physiologic age is used when customizing clinical preventive services.
 (E) Clinical preventive services involve the practice of conducting selective health maintenance procedures at periodic intervals based on rational guidelines.

Answer: (E). Clinical preventive services are an integral part of the patient care process. The traditional concept of the annual physical examination has been replaced by the practice of conducting selective health maintenance procedures at periodic intervals based on rational guidelines. Practice guidelines have been developed to reduce inappropriate services, control geographic variations in practice patterns, and encourage more efficient and effective use of resources. Efficient delivery of clinical preventive services means that not all patients need every clinical intervention. Identification of high-risk patients whether based on personal or family medical history (or both), a particular life-style behavior, or "physiologic" rather than "chronologic" age is important when customizing clinical prevention. (*Chapter 7, Page 38.*)

2.2 Following the usual immunizations of infancy and early childhood, a second measles/mumps/rubella (MMR) immunization is currently

 (A) not recommended
 (B) recommended for select populations at high risk such as immunocompromised patients or those receiving corticosteroid therapy
 (C) recommended only for patients planning overseas travel
 (D) recommended at 4 to 6 years of age
 (E) given with 1 ml of immune serum globulin (ISG)

Answer: (D). Universal immunization over the past 40 years has eliminated the threat of major infectious diseases to many children, a significant cause of mortality and morbidity in this age group. With the decrease in immunization rates among some groups of young children in the United States, there are regions with sporadic outbreaks of pertussis, measles, and other preventable communicable infectious diseases. Thus, a second MMR immunization is now recommended at 4 to 6 years. (*Chapter 7, Page 41.*)

2.3 Clinical preventive services identified by the U.S. Preventive Services Task Force (USPSTF) encompass all the following EXCEPT

(A) counseling
(B) screening
(C) immunizations
(D) coordination by a single government agency
(E) chemoprophylaxis

Answer: (D). The concept of offering clinical prevention to all patients based on their age, sex, and risk level is important for the family physician. Clinical preventive services identified by the USPSTF encompass four categories: counseling, screening, immunizations, and chemoprophylaxis agents. The task force's report, when combined with the preventive recommendations for asymptomatic adults generated by other groups and the work of individual clinicians, provides a database to justify the selection of appropriate preventive clinical services for individuals and families. (*Chapter 7, Page 37.*)

2.4 The major health problem for children in the age range from birth to 10 years is

(A) unintentional injuries
(B) lead poisoning
(C) child abuse
(D) human immunodeficiency virus and acquired immunodeficiency syndrome
(E) learning disorders

Answer: (A). Unintentional injuries are the major health problem for children in this age group. Periodic preventive interventions during this life period should focus on injury prevention. (*Chapter 7, Page 41.*)

2.5 The chief illness-related reason that young children miss school is

(A) respiratory disease
(B) injuries
(C) child abuse
(D) truancy
(E) psychological/social problems

Answer: (A). Respiratory problems such as influenza and asthma are the chief illness-related reasons young children miss school. The role of parental smoking and passive smoking exposure, a major trigger of these

illnesses, should be addressed periodically during this age period. Healthy child development depends on establishing healthy behaviors during this age period to avoid smoking and alcohol abuse and develop good nutrition and physical activity. (*Chapter 7, Page 41.*)

2.6 Screening for hypercholesterolemia in all children older than age 2 is

(A) recommended by the USPSTF
(B) recommended for children of northern European ancestry
(C) controversial
(D) contraindicated
(E) recommended beginning at age 12

Answer: (C). Screening for hypercholesterolemia in all children older than age 2 is controversial. The USPSTF has concluded that there is insufficient evidence to recommend for or against routine screening of children and adolescents for cholesterol and other lipid disorders. Without data on the costs, risk, and benefits of intervention strategies for children with high cholesterol concentrations, general screening of all children for total cholesterol values must be considered carefully. Many children with high cholesterol levels have normal levels during young adulthood in the absence of prescribed individual interventions. (*Chapter 7, Page 41.*)

2.7 In the United States, the average age of first use of alcohol and marijuana is

(A) 9 years
(B) 11 years
(C) 13 years
(D) 15 years
(E) 18 years

Answer: (C). Adolescence through early adulthood represents a time of changing health hazards. Major health impediments to screen for and counsel about include injuries, violence, tobacco use and substance abuse, school failure, delinquency, suicide, unwanted pregnancy, and sexually transmitted diseases. Three-fourths of children have smoked their first cigarette by grade 9, and the average age of first use of alcohol and marijuana is age 13. (*Chapter 7, Page 41.*)

2.8 The leading causes of death from ages 40 to 64 years include all the following EXCEPT

(A) heart disease
(B) infections
(C) cancer

(D)   stroke
(E)   chronic lung disease

Answer: (B). Heart disease, cancer, stroke, and chronic lung disease are the leading causes of mortality from age 40 to 64 years. Each entity is associated with precursor health behaviors that are totally preventable or modifiable through effective physician intervention. (*Chapter 7, Page 42.*)

2.9 In the United States, the percentage of deaths linked to smoking is

(A)   10%
(B)   30%
(C)   50%
(D)   75%
(E)   less than 5%

Answer: (B). More than 30% of cancer deaths are linked to smoking, and about 35% of deaths are associated with diet. Many primary and secondary prevention interventions are recommended by the National Cancer Institute and Healthy People 2000. Counseling regarding tobacco use with an integrated office-based program best supports physician activities: organized identification, progress records, brief physician messages, follow-up assistance, and a focus on those most interested in quitting. Passive smoking exposure is responsible for 3,000 lung cancer cases each year in the United States among never-smokers. (*Chapter 7, Page 44.*)

2.10 The patient is a 55-year-old white female bookkeeper, concerned about health maintenance and especially about cancer. She is curious about cancer risks. You can tell her that the most commonly diagnosed cancer is

(A)   breast
(B)   lung
(C)   prostate
(D)   pancreas
(E)   colon

Answer: (A). Breast cancer is the most commonly diagnosed cancer and the second leading cause of mortality due to cancer. Although there has been an increased incidence in recent years, perhaps because of improved screening, the death rate remains stable. Unalterable risk factors include family history and age at menarche and menopause. Other factors, such as parity and age at first pregnancy, are not easily modifiable. Thus primary prevention interventions such as maintaining a low-fat diet and secondary prevention screening by mammography are essential. (*Chapter 7, Page 44.*)

2.11 In the United States, the most rapid population increase during the 1990s is occurring among which of the following age groups?

(A)   childhood and adolescence
(B)   young adults
(C)   middle age
(D)   ages 60 to 85
(E)   ages 85 and older

Answer: (E). The most rapid population increase during the 1990s is occurring among those older than age 85. (*Chapter 7, Page 48.*)

2.12 The average cost of preventive service benefits for a U.S. family would be about

(A) $7.50 per month
(B) $20.00 per month
(C) $50.00 per month
(D) $100.00 per month
(E) $200.00 per month

Answer: (A). It has been estimated that comprehensive implementation of a basic prevention package for all Americans would boost the nation's net health care bill by an estimated $1 billion to $3 billion annually. Nevertheless, the average cost of preventive services benefits would only be about $7.50 per month for family coverage. (*Chapter 7, Page 53.*)

2.13 Five risk factors account for 90% of the potential benefit from risk factors that can be modified. These five factors, in descending order, are

(A)   hypertension, hypercholesterolemia, overweight, analgesic abuse, and sun exposure
(B)   hypertension, lack of regular exercise, exposure to sunlight, job-related stress, and industrial accidents
(C)   obesity, lack of regular exercise, alcohol use, vitamin deficiency, and hypercholesterolemia
(D)   smoking, obesity, lack of regular exercise, hypercholesterolemia, and hypertension
(E)   hypertension, alcohol consumption, traffic accidents, job-related stress, and nutritional deficiencies

Answer: (D). There are 524,000 excess deaths annually due to nine chronic diseases for which risk factors such as smoking could be modified! Five risk factors account for 90% of the potential benefit (in descending order): smoking, obesity, lack of regular exercise, hypercholesterolemia, and hypertension. If the benefits from risk reduction from smoking, cholesterol, obesity, sedentary lifestyle, and heavy alcohol consumption are calculated, life expectancy at birth in the United States would increase by 3.85 years. Thus, healthy lifestyles can result in significant gains in longevity. (*Chapter 8, Page 56.*)

2.14 How many deaths are caused by smoking each year in the United States?

   (A)   100,000
   (B)   400,000
   (C)   800,000
   (D) 1,200,000
   (E) 1,800,000

Answer: (B). Smoking causes more than 400,000 deaths annually in the United States, which is about one-fifth of all deaths. About 180,000 of these deaths are due to cardiovascular disease, 150,000 to neoplasms, and 84,000 to respiratory disease. In 1990, cigarette smoking resulted in 5 million estimated years of potential life lost prior to life expectancy. The USPSTF reported that the data show "consistent, convincing evidence" that links tobacco to a variety of serious diseases. (*Chapter 8, Page 56.*)

2.15 The FIRST intervention recommended for smokers is

   (A) nicotine gum
   (B) nicotine patches
   (C) group counseling
   (D) advice to quit smoking
   (E) bupropion (antidepressant) in an initial dose of 150 mg daily

Answer: (D). The first intervention recommended for smokers is advice to quit smoking, as many smokers are able to quit on their own. Counseling has been shown to increase cessation rates. About half (47.5%) of smokers who have attempted to quit on their own since the early 1980s have been successful. Counseling increases cessation rates by 3 to 7% when done by clinicians and by 8 to 25% when done in group sessions. Counseling and self-help materials also have been shown to increase the rate of quitting by 5 to 23% in pregnant women. Brief advice during routine physician visits is cost-effective at $705 to $998 for men and $1,204 to $2,058 for women per year of life saved. Despite these data, about half of smokers report that they have never been asked by their physicians if they smoke. The advice should include a statement on the need to stop and the health and social benefits of stopping. If the patient is considering quitting, the clinician should recommend that the patient set a quit date, advise the patient to develop a plan to deal with times of vulnerability, and offer to schedule follow-up visits to assist with cessation. (*Chapter 8, Page 57.*)

2.16 Physical exercise causes all the following EXCEPT

   (A) improved myocardial oxygen balance
   (B) improved fibrinolysis
   (C) increased platelet aggregation
   (D) lowered sensitivity to catecholamine
   (E) decreased insulin resistance

Answer: (C). Exercise improves cardiovascular fitness, lipoprotein profiles, insulin sensitivity, pulmonary physiology, and bone mass. The most important change is improved myocardial oxygen balance, which occurs by improved blood supply to the heart, reduced heart rate, reduced blood pressure, and improved stroke volume. Improved fibrinolysis, decreased platelet aggregation, lower sensitivity to catecholamine, and decreased insulin resistance also contribute to the decrease in mortality and morbidity from coronary heart disease. (*Chapter 8, Page 59.*)

2.17 Which of the following statements regarding exercise and arthritis is true?

   (A) Exercise is contraindicated with patients with a family history of osteoarthritis.
   (B) Most runners develop clinical arthritis of the knees and ankles following 10 years of running.
   (C) Running has not been shown to accelerate the development of radiographic or clinical osteoarthritis of the knees.
   (D) There is an increased incidence of lupus arthritis in long-distance runners.
   (E) Running has a protective effect against osteoarthritis of the knees.

Answer: (C). Running has not been shown to accelerate the development of radiographic or clinical osteoarthritis of the knees. Thus beginning an exercise program with more strenuous activities such as jogging may lead to an increased rate of injuries, especially in the elderly, but does not predispose to arthritis. (*Chapter 8, Page 59.*)

2.18 Total dietary fat intake should be restricted to what percentage of total calories?

   (A) 20%
   (B) 30%
   (C) 40%
   (D) 50%
   (E) 60%

Answer: (B). An average of 37% of the calories consumed by Americans comes from fat; by contrast, authorities recommend limiting fat intake to 30% of total calories to reduce the health risks. Following this recommendation could result in 42,000 fewer deaths annually and extend average life expectancy by 3 months in women and 4 months in men. (*Chapter 8, Page* 61.)

2.19 When bottled water is not available during international travel, the safest method of sterilizing water is

   (A) chlorine solution
   (B) iodine tablets
   (C) water filters
   (D) boiling
   (E) using water from the hot water tap that is steaming and then allowed to cool for 30 minutes

Answer: (D). The maxim is *"Cook it, boil it, peel it, or forget it."* Boiling clean water for 3 minutes at any altitude is sufficient and the safest form of any water. Bottled water is generally safe if the sealed cap is removed only in the tourist's presence. Chlorine and iodine tablets are available in camping stores and sufficiently kill organisms for the immunocompetent; iodine is more efficacious. Water filters are not recommended because of insufficient testing or inadequate filtering of viruses. Avoid all tap water and ice cubes, even if mixed in alcoholic beverages. (*Chapter 9, Page* 65.)

2.20 During travel to an area with a high risk of being bitten by an insect vector, applications of 30% DEET on all exposed surfaces may prevent bites of

   (A) mosquito
   (B) tick
   (C) sandfly
   (D) flea
   (E) all of the above

Answer: (E). The traveler cannot contract certain diseases, fortunately, unless bitten by the vector. Bites of the mosquito, tick, tsetse fly, sandfly, or flea are avoided by frequently applying a repellent containing around 30% DEET (e.g., Repel) on all exposed skin

surfaces. Prolonged or excessive applications of high concentrations can be toxic to young children. Long-sleeve shirts and long pants are essential wear in malarious or dengue areas. Spraying or soaking clothes, mosquito nets, and tents with permethrin (Duranon and Permanone) significantly reduce the number of bites and incidence of malaria. (*Chapter 9, Page* 65.)

2.21 Your patients are a young couple planning their first trip overseas. They ask about airline safety. The safest seats in an airplane are

   (A) in the first class section
   (B) at the back of the airplane
   (C) at the bulkhead in the coach section
   (D) off the aisle in the emergency exit row
   (E) in the cockpit

Answer: (D). The safest seats in an airliner are off the aisle at an emergency exit. (*Chapter 9, Page* 66.)

2.22 Which of the following vaccines is the only World Health Organization (WHO)-regulated vaccine currently required by some countries?

   (A) smallpox vaccine
   (B) yellow fever vaccine
   (C) Sabin oral polio vaccine
   (D) tetanus prophylaxis
   (E) plague vaccine

Answer: (B). The only WHO-regulated vaccine currently required by countries is yellow fever vaccine. These countries are listed in Health Information for International Travel (HIIT) with updates in Summary of HIIT. Physicians who infrequently advise travelers can find these resources immediately available on the Internet or by fax. Both cholera and meningococcal vaccines have been required in the past. Until a better cholera vaccine is available, cholera vaccine is unlikely to become officially required even in epidemic conditions. Nevertheless, an occasional border official demands evidence of vaccination but accepts a stamped cholera certificate or a statement of contraindication on a physician's letterhead. Meningococcal vaccine has been required by Saudi Arabia 10 days before the annual Hajji to Mecca. (*Chapter 9, Page* 66.)

2.23 Yellow fever vaccination for international travel

   (A) is available in the offices of most primary care providers
   (B) is an inactivated vaccine with a long shelf life

(C) comes in a multiple dose vial which can be used up to 12 hours following reconstitution

(D) can only be administered at an approved yellow fever vaccination center

(E) causes serious reaction in up to 20% of patients

Answer: (D). Only an approved yellow fever vaccination center can administer this vaccine. Some public health departments allow individual practitioners to be a designated center. It is a fastidious live viral vaccine that requires careful handling and use within 1 hour of reconstitution. Serious reactions are uncommon. (*Chapter 9, Page 66.*)

2.24 Which of the following is NOT a common cause of traveler's diarrhea (TD)?

(A) *Escherichia coli*
(B) *Shigella*
(C) *Campylobacter jejuni*
(D) *Salmonella*
(E) *Enterococcus*

Answer: (E). Bacterial etiologies account for 37 to 72+% of cases. The most common bacteria, in approximate order of frequency, are enterotoxigenic *Escherichia coli*, *Shigella, Campylobacter jejuni, Salmonella,* and *Vibrio* spp. The most common viral etiologies (responsible for up to 36% of cases of TD) are rotavirus and Norwalk viruses. Parasites, primarily *Giardia lamblia* and *Entamoeba histolytica*, cause up to 9% of cases. Frequently, more than one pathogen is found during a diarrheal illness, and 20 to 50% of cases of TD remain unexplained. (*Chapter 9, Page 70.*)

2.25 The first line of prevention for TD is

(A) doxycycline
(B) food and water safety and vaccination
(C) bismuth subsalicylate
(D) trimethoprim/sulfamethoxazole (TMP/SMX) prophylaxis
(E) norfloxacin

Answer: (B). Generally, antibiotic prophylaxis is avoided. The first line of prevention is food and water safety and vaccination. Prophylaxis is justified in special circumstances in which the risk of TD must be minimized and requires a short duration of antibiotic exposure. These situations might include an international sporting event, a honeymoon, or an intense, high-level business meeting. Agents with prophylactic efficacy include bismuth subsalicylate (PeptoBismol) 2 tablets q.i.d.; doxycycline (Vibramycin) 100 mg qd;

TMP/SMX-DS; Bactrim DS (Septra DS) 160 mg/800 mg qd; norfloxacin (Noroxin) 400 mg qd; and ciprofloxacin (Cipro) 500 mg qd. (*Chapter 9, Page 70.*)

2.26 The antibiotic with the broadest coverage against bacterial etiologies of TD is

(A) doxycycline
(B) TMP/SMX
(C) norfloxacin
(D) penicillin
(E) azithromycin

Answer: (C). Rapid treatment of adults can reduce the duration of TD to 1 day or less. The fluoroquinolones provide the broadest coverage against the bacterial etiologies of TD. Their cost limits widespread use in developing countries, resulting in infrequent resistance to this class of antibiotics. If there is no fever or bloody diarrhea, start with two loperamide (Imodium) capsules after the first loose stool and continue at the usual doses of loperamide. If the diarrhea continues, after the third loose stool, give two tablets of ciprofloxacin 500 mg or norfloxacin 400 mg. Most TD stops at this point, but if it continues longer than 24 hours continue with one tablet of the fluoroquinolone b.i.d. for 3 days. Distant second-line alternatives are bismuth subsalicylate 30 ml every half-hour for eight doses or doxycycline 100 mg or TMP/SMX-DS one tablet, either of the latter two b.i.d. for 3 days. Neither antibiotics nor antidiarrheal agents are recommended for children. (*Chapter 9, Page 70.*)

2.27 The best prophylaxis for high-altitude illness is

(A) adequate hydration
(B) acetazolamide
(C) slow ascent, less than about 300 m (1,000 feet) per day
(D) dexamethasone
(E) oxygen

Answer: (C). The best prophylaxis is slow ascent, less than about 300 m (1,000 ft) per day. For rapid ascents above 3,000 m (9,800 ft) lasting more than 12 hours, consider prophylaxis with 250 mg acetazolamide (Diamox) q hs, starting 24 hours before ascent and continuing during the first few days at high altitude. Over-the-counter analgesics are adequate for the headache. Acetazolamide can be reserved to treat mild cases of acute mountain sickness (AMS). Although dexamethasone (Decadron) 4 mg q6h can be used for prophylaxis, it is usually reserved for treatment of severe AMS, high-altitude pulmonary edema (HAPE), or high-altitude cerebral edema (HACE). Once dexamethasone is started, high-flow oxygen and descent should begin emergently. (*Chapter 9, Page 70.*)

2.28 Following a myocardial infarction, airline travel should be restricted for at least

    (A) 48 hours
    (B) 2 to 3 weeks
    (C) 4 to 8 weeks
    (D) 4 to 6 months
    (E) 1 year

Answer: (C). Airline travel should be restricted for 4 to 8 weeks after myocardial infarction and supplemental oxygen considered for the following 4 months. A general rule is that the cardiac patient should be able to walk 100 yards and climb 12 steps. (*Chapter 9, Page 71.*)

DIRECTIONS (Items 2.29 through 2.52): Each of the items in this section is a multiple true–false problem that consists of a stem and four lettered options. Indicate whether each of the four options is TRUE or FALSE.

2.29 The accuracy of a screening test is determined by its sensitivity and specificity. Which of the following is/are true?

    (A) Sensitivity is a measurement of the proportion of persons with a condition who test positive.
    (B) Specificity is a measurement of the proportion of persons without a condition who test positive.
    (C) If sensitivity is low or poor, there is a low percentage of false-negative test results.
    (D) An evaluation of a screening test includes the proportion of patients with a positive test result who have the disease.

Answer: (A-True, B-False, C-False, D-True). Sensitivity is a measurement of the proportion of persons with a condition who test positive. Conversely, specificity is a measurement of the proportion of persons without a condition who test negative. If sensitivity is low or poor, there is a high percentage of false-negative test results. If specificity is low or poor, there is a high percentage of false-positive test results. Additional evaluation of a screening test includes the proportion of patients with a positive test result who have the disease or the positive predictive value of the test. Conversely, the proportion of patients with negative test results who do not have a condition is known as the negative predictive value. (*Chapter 7, Page 38.*)

2.30 A 62-year-old white female restaurant worker asks about supplemental vitamins. Which of the following is/are true?

    (A) Low levels of selenium, vitamins A, C, and E, and beta-carotene may be associated with an increased risk of cancer mortality late in life.
    (B) High vitamin C intake is associated with an increased incidence of gastrointestinal cancer.
    (C) No vitamins have a protective effect on cataract formation.
    (D) Vitamin E may have a protective role in retarding atherosclerosis.

Answer: (A-True, B-False, C-False, D-True). Low plasma levels of selenium, vitamins A, C, and E, and beta-carotene may be associated with an increased risk of cancer mortality late in life. The evidence is particularly strong for men older than age 60. Low vitamin C intake is associated with increased gastrointestinal and stomach cancer. Vitamins A and E may inhibit cancer promotion. In addition, vitamins C and E and beta-carotene may protect older persons against cataract formation, and vitamin E may have a protective role as an antioxidant in reversing or retarding atherosclerosis. (*Chapter 7, Page 47.*)

2.31 Barriers to the delivery of clinical preventive services include

    (A) uncertainty about selecting preventive interventions
    (B) inadequate reimbursement
    (C) lack of patient understanding based on conflicting information
    (D) lack of office or clinic systems to integrate these services into routine patient care

Answer: (A-True, B-True, C-True, D-True). Barriers to the delivery of clinical preventive services most often cited by office-based clinicians include (1) uncertainty and confusion about selecting preventive interventions and their frequency of application; (2) inadequate or lack of reimbursement for the interventions and the time required to deliver them; (3) insufficient clinician knowledge about the importance of preventive services and how best to deliver them; (4) lack of patient understanding and confusion from conflicting information in the media; and (5) lack of office or clinic systems to integrate these services into routine patient care. (*Chapter 7, Page 51.*)

2.32 During a routine health maintenance examination, your 45-year-old white male patient asks about a health risk appraisal (HRA). Which of the following is/are true?

(A) The HRA is an instrument to determine an individual's risk from preventable death or chronic illness.
(B) The HRA is made on the basis of health history, lifestyle, physiologic test findings, age, and gender.
(C) The HRA can be used by physicians to help patients take greater responsibility for their health and make healthy life-style decisions.
(D) HRA are most appropriately used with patients with chronic illness, allowing them to avoid future complications and disabilities.

Answer: (A-True, B-True, C-True, D-False). HRAs can add impact to initial risk evaluation using flow sheets. These instruments determine an individual's risk from preventable death or chronic illness on the basis of health history, lifestyle, physiologic test findings, age, and gender. The patient's profile is compared with a database of epidemiologic and mortality statistics. HRAs can be used by physicians to motivate and educate patients, encourage them to take greater responsibility for their health, make healthy life-style decisions, and make appropriate use of medical services. They are intended to be used with persons who are free from chronic illnesses, and their use has been mostly with middle-class, middle-aged, white populations. HRAs should be used only in conjunction with risk reduction counseling or programs. (*Chapter 7, Pages 51–52.*)

2.33 True statements regarding the relationship of preventive health strategies and health insurance include which of the following?

(A) Preventive health stategies are generally not linked with health insurance.
(B) Poor women with Medicaid are more likely to be referred for mammography than more affluent women with private health insurance.
(C) Copayments and other methods requiring patients in health insurance plans to share costs have not been found to influence use of preventive services.
(D) There is significant variations in specific items covered on the various health plans.

Answer: (A-False, B-False, C-False, D-True). Use of preventive strategies has been strongly linked with insurance. For instance, poor women with Medicaid are less likely to be referred for mammography. Even enrollees in health insurance plans who are required to

share costs made significantly less use of preventive services than did those who received free care. In health maintenance organizations (HMO) and in settings where care is not billed to the patient, there is greater utilization of preventive services. There is significant variation in the specific items covered on various insurance plans. Point of service and HMO plans provide broader coverage than conventional indemnity and preferred provider organization plans. (*Chapter 7, Page 53.*)

2.34 Your office receives a call from your HMO, questioning some preventive practices and asking you to justify the cost-effectiveness of your emphasis on preventive clinical services. Which of the following is/are true?

(A) Prevention has been shown to be cost-effective in reducing medical expenditures over any 5-year period.
(B) Clinical prevention should be assessed according to how much health is obtained by spending money on medical care.
(C) Clinical prevention should be assessed according to how much money is saved by targeted expenditures for specific interventions.
(D) A potential cost of preventive services is the cost of diseases that the aged live to develop.

Answer: (A-False, B-True, C-False, D-True). Prevention may not save money; it usually adds to medical expenditures. Thus when assessing preventive interventions, a cost-effective analysis (how much health is obtained by spending money on medical care) is more appropriate than cost-benefit analysis (how much money is saved by spending some). The cost of success is often the price of longer life. Two potential "costs" to society are the cost of diseases that the aged live to develop and the added cost of old-age pensions, including Social Security payments. (*Chapter 7, Page 53.*)

2.35 A 46-year-old white male truck driver smokes two packs of cigarettes daily. He asks about the potential impact on his health of stopping tobacco use. Which of the following is/are true?

(A) Smoking cessation reduces all-cause mortality.
(B) Smoking cessation will reduce the risk of cancer, myocardial infarction, and stroke.
(C) Tobacco cessation at this patient's age will not lower the risk of his subsequently developing peripheral artery disease.
(D) With cessation of tobacco use, the risk of death from coronary heart disease is reduced by half in 1 year.

Answer: (A-True, B-True, C-False, D-True). Smoking cessation reduces all-cause mortality and the risk of cancer, myocardial infarction, stroke, chronic obstructive pulmonary disease mortality, peripheral artery disease, and low birth weight. The risk of death from coronary heart disease is reduced by half in 1 year, but it takes 10 years or more to halve the risk of lung, oral, or esophageal cancer. (*Chapter 8, Page 56.*)

2.36 You have been asked to speak to a high school class regarding tobacco and are preparing your talk. Tobacco dependence has some addictive components. These include

(A) habit cued by daily activities
(B) mild depression
(C) pleasure
(D) self-medication to reduce negative affect and withdrawal symptoms

Answer: (A-True, B-False, C-True, D-True). The addictive components of tobacco dependence include habit cued by daily activities, pleasure, and self-medication to reduce negative affect and withdrawal symptoms. Furthermore, nicotine produces euphoria similar to that from other addictive psychomotor stimulants and has addictive pharmacologic and behavioral properties that are similar to heroin and cocaine. (*Chapter 8, Page 56.*)

2.37 A 54-year-old bartender has failed to quit smoking on several attempts and asks for further help. You are considering referral to a smoking cessation program. True statements regarding tobacco cessation programs include which of the following?

(A) About one-fourth of smokers using tobacco cessation programs are likely to be successful.
(B) The most successful programs use both physician and nonphysician counselors and include face-to-face advice.
(C) Although setting a specific quit date is helpful with brief office advice, cessation programs that allow the patient to proceed at his or her own pace are more successful.
(D) A strong predictor of success is the number of months the patient is in contact with the program.

Answer: (A-True, B-True, C-False, D-True). Smokers who ask for further help or who have failed to quit previously, despite sincere efforts, are candidates for cessation programs. About one-fourth (23.6%) of smokers who attempted to quit since the early 1980s

by using a program were successful. Successful cessation programs include face-to-face advice, use of both physician and nonphysician counselors, reinforcing sessions, setting a specific quit date, and multiple modalities. A strong predictor of success is the number of months the patient is in contact with the program. (*Chapter 8, Page 57.*)

2.38 In working with patients on tobacco cessation, you have been aware that some smokers have high levels of nicotine dependence. True statements regarding these individuals includes which of the following?

(A) One characteristic is smoking within the first 30 minutes after waking.
(B) Such persons generally smoke more than 20 cigarettes per day and often more than 30.
(C) Higher doses of nicotine therapy may be needed.
(D) Clonidine may be especially effective in patients with high nicotine dependence.

Answer: (A-True, B-True, C-True, D-False). In smokers with high levels of nicotine dependence, high doses of nicotine replacement therapy are more effective. In particular, the 4-mg dose of gum is more effective than the 2-mg dose. One characteristic of persons with high nicotine dependence is smoking within the first 30 minutes after waking, especially within the first 5 minutes. Another characteristic of high nicotine dependence is smoking more than 20 cigarettes per day, particularly more than 30.

Prescription of clonidine resulted in statistically significant reductions in abstinence in only one of five studies; consequently, the USPSTF reported that the evidence was insufficient to recommend for or against prescription of clonidine. (*Chapter 8, Page 58.*)

2.39 The patient is a 27-year-old white female accountant who is slightly overweight. She asks about the benefits and risks of exercise. Which of the following statements is/are true?

(A) Exercise has not been shown to extend life expectancy.
(B) Exercise can eliminate one-third of the excess deaths due to coronary heart disease.
(C) Exercise increases the risk of hip fracture.
(D) Exercise may reduce the risk for developing diabetes mellitus (DM).

Answer: (A-False, B-True, C-False, D-True). Overall, exercise can add up to 2 years of life and eliminate one-third of the excess deaths due to coronary heart disease. Other benefits of exercise include better mental health, lower risk of hip fracture, and lower risk for adult-onset DM. In one cohort study, each 500-kcal increase in energy expended on leisure-time physical activity resulted in a 6% reduction in risk of developing DM. Despite the evidence about the benefits of exercise, more than half of the adults in the United States do not engage in regular physical activity. (*Chapter 8, Page 58.*)

2.40 True statements regarding the exercise prescription include which of the following?

(A) The exercise prescription should identify activity, frequency, duration, intensity, and program elements.
(B) The various aspects of the exercise prescription should be individualized according to the person's age and gender.
(C) Intensity is based on a set percentage of the maximal predicted heart rate (MPHR), which can be calculated by the formula "220 minus age."
(D) Sedentary persons may start an exercise program by achieving 90% of their MPHR.

Answer: (A-True, B-True, C-True, D-False). The exercise prescription should identify activity, frequency, duration, intensity, and program elements. These aspects of the exercise prescription should be individualized to the patient. Intensity is based on a set percentage of the MPHR, which can be determined by the formula "220 minus age." Sedentary persons may start by achieving 60% of MPHR and gradually progress to higher percentages; 90% is the maximum recommended. Program elements should include "warm-up" for 5 minutes with stretching exercises, the activity itself, and a 2- to 3-minute "cool-down" period. (*Chapter 8, Pages 60–61.*)

2.41 True statements regarding dietary fiber include which of the following?

(A) Dietary fiber can help replace calories from dietary fat.
(B) Water-soluble fiber can raise low-density lipoprotein levels.
(C) Dietary fiber tends to retard gastrointestinal function.
(D) Important sources of dietary fiber are fruits, vegetables, and grain products.

Answer: (A-True, B-False, C-False, D-True). Dietary fiber has several important properties. It is a means to replace calories from dietary fat; furthermore, apart from caloric replacement, water-soluble fiber can lower low-density lipoprotein levels. Dietary fiber also improves gastrointestinal function. Important sources of dietary fiber are fruits, vegetables, and grain products. (*Chapter 8, Page 61.*)

2.42 During international travel, which of the following statements is/are true concerning milk and food?

(A) Milk served in restaurants or homes may be unpasteurized.
(B) Cold buffets and chilled desserts should be avoided.
(C) Salads may be eaten safely if rinsed in "Clorox water."
(D) Peeling the intact skin of fruit before eating is not sufficient protection against infectious organisms.

Answer: (A-True, B-True, C-False, D-False). In developing countries, milk is often unpasteurized, as are dairy products. All meats and vegetables should be thoroughly cooked and served steaming hot. Avoid all cold buffets, chilled desserts, and salads. Peeling the intact skins of fruits before eating is safe. (*Chapter 9, Page 65.*)

2.43 Which of the following may be helpful in combating jet lag during travel?

(A) adjusting to the new time zone by 1 hour per 24-hour period before travel
(B) use of melatonin at bedtime for the first few days following arrival
(C) ingestion of 2 oz of alcohol during flight
(D) avoidance of hypnotic use during flight and for 2 days following arrival

Answer: (A-True, B-True, C-False, D-False). The best method to entrain circadian rhythms is unknown, although certain measures are helpful. Before travel, adjusting to the new time zone by 1 hour per 24-hour period is helpful. At the destination, taking 5 mg melatonin at bedtime for the first few days shortens the duration of jet lag. In the mornings at the destination, bright light is helpful, as is a high-protein breakfast. During travel, alcohol should be avoided and liberal hydration used. A prescription hypnotic such as zolpidem (Ambien) also promotes sleep at night. (*Chapter 9, Page 66.*)

2.44 Your patients are a middle-aged couple planning a vacation in South America in a rural area where there are several fresh lakes and streams. They inquire about bathing, wading, and even drinking such water in an emergency. Which of the following is/are true?

(A) In such a setting, all fresh water must be assumed to be fecally contaminated.
(B) Schistosomiasis is not present in moving water such as a stream.
(C) Schistosomiasis is only contracted after repeated prolonged exposure.
(D) After accidental tropical fresh water exposure, wiping with a towel may reduce the risk of schistosomiasis.

Answer: (A-True, B-False, C-False, D-True). All fresh water must be assumed to be fecally contaminated. After any accidental tropical or semitropical fresh water exposure, one should towel off quickly to minimize the risk of schistosomiasis and other waterborne diseases. (*Chapter 9, Page 66.*)

2.45 Your patient is a 21-year-old college student planning a trip to Nepal. He asks about protection against hepatitis A. Which of the following is/are true?

(A) This patient should receive ISG or hepatitis A vaccine unless there is evidence of immunity.
(B) Hepatitis A vaccine and ISG should never be given together.
(C) For trips of less than 5 months, ISG alone is more cost-effective.
(D) If the patient plans repeated trips to developing countries, hepatitis A vaccine is preferred.

Answer: (A-True, B-False, C-True, D-True). The prophylactic agent ISG before each trip or hepatitis A vaccine is recommended for every traveler to the developing world unless there is evidence of immunity. If departure is shorter than the 4 weeks it takes for adequate efficacy of the vaccine, ISG and the vaccine may be administered together with little effect on subsequent protection by the vaccine. A general rule of thumb for trips less than 5 months is that ISG alone is more cost-effective. If there will be three or more trips to developing countries within the next 10 years, use hepatitis A vaccine. (*Chapter 9, Page 67.*)

2.46 True statements regarding typhoid vaccination include which of the following?

(A) The current recommendation is a four-dose oral vaccine for routine use in travelers age 6 and older.
(B) The oral typhoid vaccine protection lasts only 18 to 24 months.

(C) Side effects of the oral typhoid vaccine are common and often severe, with headache, malaise, and fever.
(D) The oral typhoid vaccine contains live attenuated bacteria and so must be kept refrigerated.

Answer: (A-True, B-False, C-False, D-True). Typhoid vaccination is recommended when the risk of exposure during the protective duration of the vaccine totals more than 5 to 6 weeks. Ty21a, a four-dose oral vaccine, replaces injectable vaccine for routine use in travelers age 6 years and older. The efficacy (> 60%) of Ty21a is equal to that of injectable vaccine: Its protection lasts 5 years, and side effects are unusual and mild. Ty21a capsules contain live attenuated bacteria and so must be kept refrigerated and taken on an empty stomach with a cool or tepid beverage. The capsules are taken every other day and separated by several days from antibiotics and by 1 day from mefloquine and other vaccines. A new injectable typhoid vaccine called Vi CPS (Typhim) is useful for those 2 to 6 years old; it has few side effects, needs only one dose as a primary series, but lasts only 2 years. The old heat-phenol injectable vaccine is the only one approved for infants ages 6 months to 2 years old. Side effects to this vaccine are common and include local discomfort, headache, malaise, and an occasional high fever. (*Chapter 9, Page 67.*)

2.47 Meningococcus vaccine

(A) may be advised for travelers to selected areas including Nepal, Kenya, or Tanzania
(B) will probably continue to be required by Saudi Arabia for visitors to Mecca
(C) should be given within 48 hours of departure
(D) is often accompanied by troublesome side effects including nausea, headaches, and high fever

Answer: (A-True, B-True, C-False, D-False). Meningococcal meningitis is periodically epidemic in Nepal, Kenya, Tanzania, Rwanda, Burundi, Mongolia, and in a band across sub-Saharan Africa stretching from Mali to Ethiopia and Uganda and in the Delhi region of India. It will probably continue to be required by Saudi Arabia for pilgrims on Hajji to Mecca. Quadrivalent ACYW-135 should be administered at least 10 days before arrival; it has few side effects. (*Chapter 9, Page 67.*)

2.48 Hepatitis B vaccine is recommended for international travelers who

(A) plan a 3-week tour of the major capitals of Europe
(B) plan staying 6 month or longer in a developing country
(C) might be sexually exposed while abroad
(D) are medical personnel who will be providing local health care

Answer: (A-False, B-True, C-True, D-True). Seroconversion is common for those residing in the developing world. Therefore, hepatitis B vaccine is recommended for (1) travelers staying 6 months or longer, (2) pleasure seekers who might be sexually exposed, and (3) medical personnel. The primary series takes 6 months to complete, but a schedule with Energix-B given at days 0, 30, and 60 produces excellent seroprotection, with an additional booster suggested at 12 months if exposure continues. A more accelerated schedule of the same vaccine given on days 0, 7, and 21 or 28 has also resulted in good immunogenicity at 12 months. (Chapter 9, Page 69.)

2.49 The patient is a 36-year-old college professor planning a visit to South America that will include some jungle travel. He has asked for your recommendation regarding malaria prophylaxis; you have chosen to use mefloquine (Lariam). Which of the following statements is/are true?

(A) Mefloquine is effective only in chloroquine-sensitive areas.
(B) The drug is taken once weekly starting 1 to 2 weeks before arrival in the malarious area, taken once weekly during possible exposure, and continued for 4 weeks after the last possible exposure.
(C) Mefloquine has been known to cause visual disturbances and transient psychosis or seizures.
(D) The drug is safe to use during the first trimester of pregnancy.

Answer: (A-False, B-True, C-True, D-False). Probably the most prescribed antimalarial, mefloquine (Lariam) is effective in both chloroquine-resistant and chloroquine-sensitive areas. It is taken once weekly, starting 1 to 2 weeks before arrival in the malarious area, taken once weekly during possible exposure, and continued for 4 weeks after the last possible exposure. Most side effects, which are usually transient and occur during the first two doses, consist of dizziness or gastrointestinal upset. It has been reported to cause visual disturbances and transient psychosis or seizures in one of 13,000 individuals. It should not be used by airline pilots, travelers with previous psychiatric illness or epilepsy, and children weighing less than 5 kg. It is relatively contraindicated in those with cardiac conduction abnormalities, in the first trimester of pregnancy, and in persons who undertake dangerous tasks requiring fine coordination. Resistance is rare. (Chapter 9, Page 69.)

2.50 Your patient plans a trip to a forested area of Southeast Asia where chloroquine-resistant malaria is reported. Because he has epilepsy and cannot take mefloquine, you have decided to recommend doxycycline. True statements regarding doxycycline use include which of the following?

(A) Phototoxic side effects have not been a problem in individuals younger than age 40.
(B) Doxycycline use can be discontinued on the day after last possible exposure to malaria.
(C) Women should carry an antimonilial vaginal cream.
(D) The drug is safe for children in both liquid and capsule form.

Answer: (A-False, B-False, C-True, D-False). Effective against chloroquine-resistant malaria in lieu of mefloquine, possible phototoxic side effects limit general use of doxycycline in tropical areas. Start 1 day before possible malaria exposure, continuing daily during exposure and for 4 weeks after the last possible exposure. Its use requires meticulous application of a sunscreen (SPF >15) with ultraviolet A-blocking properties; women should carry an antimonilial vaginal cream. Doxycycline is contraindicated in children younger than 8 years old. (Chapter 9, Page 69.)

2.51 While planning a trekking vacation in Nepal, your patient, a 32-year-old high school teacher, asks about high-altitude illness. True statements include which of the following?

(A) High-altitude illness is most common with ascent above 3,000 m (9,800 ft).
(B) The most common symptom of acute mountain sickness is dyspnea.
(C) Severe acute mountain sickness can progress to ataxia and mental impairment.
(D) Vigorous exertion promotes tissue oxygenation and helps to prevent acute mountain sickness.

Answer: (A-True, B-False, C-True, D-False). The axiom is "climb high, but sleep low." The incidence of high-altitude illness increases with ascent above 3,000 meters (9,800 feet). Up to 80% of travelers experience some symptom of acute mountain sickness at 4,200 m

(12,700 ft). Common to the syndromes of AMS, HAPE, and HACE are rapid ascent and tissue hypoxia. The latter results from the lower partial pressure of oxygen at high altitudes. AMS ranges from a mild illness (headache being the most common symptom, followed by nausea or lassitude) to a severe illness (vomiting, dyspnea at rest, ataxia, mental impairment, or cyanosis). HAPE can develop after several days, usually during sleep, with symptoms of extreme dyspnea, cough, rales, mild fever, and cyanosis. HACE can develop after several days of mild AMS, presenting with progressively severe lassitude, decreasing alertness, psychosis, focal neurologic signs, and eventual coma. Predisposing factors to these syndromes are poorly understood but include increased exertion and prior residence at less than 3,000 ft. (*Chapter 9, Page 70.*)

2.52 Your patient is a 64-year-old white male executive planning a trip to Madrid. He is a heavy smoker and has chronic obstructive pulmonary disease (COPD). You are concerned about air travel. Which of the following is/are true?

(A) Aircraft maintain a cabin pressure equivalent to an elevation of up to 8,000 ft.
(B) In midflight, the PaO_2 in normal individuals falls to approximately 60 mm Hg.
(C) The use of oxygen supplementation during flight is not recommended for COPD patients because of pressurization concerns.
(D) With appropriate management, patients with all degrees of COPD can fly safely.

Answer: (A-True, B-True, C-False, D-False). Patients with COPD may require arterial blood gas determinations before travel. Aircraft maintain cabin pressure equivalent to 2,438 m (8,000 ft) or less. This altitude results in a fall of PaO_2 to approximately 60 mm Hg in healthy individuals. Although prediction of hypoxemia in the COPD patient is difficult, patients with a preflight PaO_2 of less than 70 mm Hg or oxygen saturation of less than 93% should receive supplemental oxygen from the airline during the flight. Individuals with preflight hypercapnia or vital capacity of less than 50% should travel by land or obtain specialty consultation. (*Chapter 9, Page 71.*)

3
Pregnancy, Childbirth, and Postpartum Care

The questions in this chapter constitute a review of the following chapters in *Family Medicine: Principles and Practice, Fifth Edition:*

Preconception Care (Chapter 10)
Normal Pregnancy, Labor, and Delivery (Chapter 11)
Medical Problems During Pregnancy (Chapter 12)
Obstetric Complications During Pregnancy (Chapter 13)
Problems During Labor and Delivery (Chapter 14)
Postpartum Care (Chapter 15)

DIRECTIONS (Items 3.1 through 3.39): Each of the questions or incomplete statements in this section is followed by five suggested answers or completions. Select the ONE that is BEST in each case.

3.1 Which of the following statements regarding rubella and pregnancy is true?

(A) A history of rubella during childhood is usually reliable.
(B) Women whose history is equivocal and have not received two doses of the measles/mumps/rubella (MMR) vaccine, and who are not pregnant, should receive the vaccine without testing.
(C) Women receiving the MMR vaccine may be advised that there is no risk to pregnancy.
(D) Pregnancy shortly following vaccination has a high risk of congenital defects.
(E) The MMR vaccine should be given to susceptible pregnant women at the first prenatal visit.

Answer: (B). A history of rubella during childhood is frequently inaccurate. Even with such a history, women who have not been tested previously, who have not received two doses of the MMR vaccine, and who by history are not pregnant should receive the vaccine without any testing. Women receiving the vaccination should be advised to avoid pregnancy for 3 months. Should conception occur soon after vaccination, the women can be reassured that she is not at appreciable risk regarding the vaccination. Several large series have identified no case of vaccination-related congenital defect. (*Chapter 10, Page 76.*)

3.2 Teratogenic drugs that should be avoided during early pregnancy include

(A) lithium
(B) isotretinoin
(C) anticonvulsants
(D) warfarin
(E) all of the above.

Answer: (E). Routine preconception modification of therapeutic regimens, including elimination of known teratogenic drugs such as gold, lithium, isotretinoin, folic acid antagonists, anticonvulsants, and warfarin can reduce anomalies. For example, isotretinoin (Accutane), a treatment for severe recalcitrant cystic acne, is highly teratogenic, causing craniofacial defects, malformations of the cardiovascular and central nervous systems (CNS), and defects of the thymus. (*Chapter 10, Page 77.*)

3.3 Women with idiopathic epilepsy who plan pregnancy and are seizure-free for 2 years or more and have a normal electroencephalogram should

(A) continue their current regimen throughout conception and pregnancy

(B) be switched to valproic acid
(C) add isoniazid hydrochloride to their regimen
(D) be offered a trial off the antiepileptic medicine before attempting pregnancy
(E) be advised not to have children

Answer: (D). Women with idiopathic epilepsy who are seizure-free for 2 years or more and have a normal electroencephalogram should be offered a trial off the antiepileptic medication before attempting pregnancy. Adequate time should be allowed to assess these results because hypoxic seizures early in pregnancy can have severe consequences. If anticonvulsant medications are required during pregnancy and if the woman plans to become pregnant, the least toxic medication should be initiated before pregnancy and the medication adjusted frequently to keep serum levels in the lowest effective range. (*Chapter 10, Page 78.*)

3.4 The ideal time for genetic investigation and counseling is

(A) before marriage
(B) before the couple attempts to conceive
(C) at 8 weeks of pregnancy
(D) at the beginning of the second trimester
(E) during the postpartum period

Answer: (B). The ideal time for genetic investigation and counseling is before a couple attempts to conceive. The identification of genetic risk can be accomplished by a careful genetic history. Patients with a specific indication such as advanced maternal age, a family history of genetic disease, or a previously affected pregnancy should be offered preconception genetic counseling. Carrier screening to determine if the parents are heterozygous for certain genetic conditions and therefore at increased risk for conceiving offspring with these disorders is of special significance because it allows relevant counseling before the first affected pregnancy. Common disorders for which genetic screening is recommended include Tay-Sachs disease for people of eastern European or French Canadian ancestry; beta-thalassemia for those of Mediterranean, Southwest Asian, Indian, Pakistani, or African ancestry; alpha-thalassemia for people of Southeast Asian ancestry; sickle cell anemia for people of African descent; and cystic fibrosis for those with a family history of the disease. The family history also might reveal other risks for genetic diseases such as fragile X disease or Down syndrome. (*Chapter 10, Page 78.*)

3.5 To prevent the development of neural tube defects (NTD), a preconception visit should include nutrition-al counseling to ensure that the pregnant woman consumes an adequate amount of

(A) folic acid
(B) nicotinic acid
(C) vitamin C
(D) vitamin D
(E) calcium

Answer: (A). The preconception visit should include nutritional counseling to ensure that the diet of any woman who might bear children contains an adequate amount of folic acid. It has been well demonstrated that a large portion of spina bifida and anencephaly can be prevented by using dietary folic acid supplementation when it is taken before conception and continued through the first trimester of pregnancy. In 1991 a large randomized trial of women who had a previous child with NTD conclusively demonstrated that 4-mg doses of folic acid before and during early pregnancy resulted in a 71% reduction of recurrence of NTDs. (*Chapter 10, Page 78.*)

3.6 The leading known cause of congenital mental retardation is

(A) Down syndrome
(B) spina bifida
(C) congenital human immunodeficiency virus (HIV) infection
(D) fetal alcohol syndrome
(E) congenital rubella

Answer: (D). Alcohol intake early in pregnancy can have devastating consequences for the fetus. Fetal alcohol syndrome (growth retardation, organ anomalies, neurosensory problems, and mental retardation) outranks Down syndrome and spina bifida in prevalence and is now the leading known cause of mental retardation. (*Chapter 10, Page 80.*)

3.7 The safe level of alcohol consumption during pregnancy is

(A) 1 to 2 drinks per day
(B) 1 to 2 drinks a week
(C) 1 to 2 drinks a month
(D) no more than 1 oz of alcohol daily
(E) has not been established

Answer: (E). A safe level of alcohol consumption during pregnancy has not been established. The adverse effects of alcohol might begin early in pregnancy, before a woman realizes she is pregnant. An estimated

11% of women who drink 1 to 2 oz of absolute alcohol a day during the first trimester have babies with features consistent with the prenatal effects of alcohol. All women of childbearing age should be given accurate information about the consequences of alcohol consumption during pregnancy, about the likelihood that effects begin early during the first trimester, and that no safe level of consumption has been established. (*Chapter 10, Page 80.*)

3.8 Which of the following laboratory tests is appropriate for *all* women at the time of preconception evaluation?

   (A) rubella titer
   (B) screening for gonorrhea and syphilis
   (C) screening for hemoglobinopathies
   (D) screening for Tay-Sachs disease
   (E) tuberculin skin test

Answer: (A). Laboratory tests offered to all women at a preconception evaluation include rubella titer, urine dipstick for protein and glucose, hemoglobin or hematocrit determination to detect iron deficiency anemia, hepatitis B surface antigen, HIV testing, and toxicology screening for illicit drugs. A Papanicolaou smear can be prepared, so if cervical dysplasia is detected, it can be treated before conception, which is safer than during pregnancy.

Women in high-risk groups can be offered other laboratory testing including tests for gonorrhea, syphilis, and *Chlamydia* and bacterial vaginosis screening so infection can be treated before conception. Laboratory assessment can also include titers for toxoplasmosis and screening for hemoglobinopathies, Tay-Sachs disease, and abnormal parental karyotypes for selected women. A purified protein derivative (PPD) test should be done in areas where tuberculosis is prevalent, so if treatment is necessary it can precede pregnancy. The Expert Panel on the Content of Prenatal Care noted that preconception testing of women for herpes simplex and cytomegalovirus can prove beneficial for some women. (*Chapter 10, Page 80.*)

3.9 What percentage of U.S. family physicians provide maternity care?

   (A) 20%
   (B) 30%
   (C) 40%
   (D) 50%
   (E) 60%

Answer: (B). Approximately 30% of U.S. family physicians provide maternity care. The current lack of access to prenatal care for many women in both rural and urban areas is a compelling reason for more family physicians to deliver these services. (*Chapter 11, Page 84.*)

3.10 Optimal weight gain during pregnancy

   (A) should be limited to 10 lb
   (B) should not exceed 25 lb
   (C) can cause harm to the fetus if greater than 25 lb
   (D) should vary depending on prepregnancy weight
   (E) should be between 25 and 30 lb for all patients

Answer: (D). Optimal weight gain during pregnancy varies depending on the prepregnancy weight. A thin woman may benefit from gaining 40 lb, whereas an obese woman might do well gaining 10 lb. The normal weight gain of 25 to 30 lb is often exceeded without harm to the fetus. Nutritional advice to pregnant women should focus on a high-quality, high-protein diet with a steady, gradual weight gain profiled to the woman's size and eating habits. (*Chapter 11, Page 86.*)

3.11 Universal screening tests appropriate for prenatal care for all women include all EXCEPT which of the following?

   (A) Papanicolaou smear
   (B) urinalysis
   (C) blood type and Rh factor
   (D) toxoplasmosis titer
   (E) indirect Coombs' test

Answer: (D). Medical conditions appropriate for prenatal screening can be divided into three groups: those that are universal, selective, and elective. Universal screening tests include the Papanicolaou smear, urinalysis, urine culture, complete blood count, blood type and Rh factor, indirect Coombs' test, and tests for syphilis, rubella immunity, *Chlamydia*, gonorrhea, hepatitis B surface antigen, and blood glucose. All these tests are appropriately performed at preconception or at the first prenatal visit, except that for blood glucose, which should be done at 24 to 28 weeks' gestation in low-risk patients. (*Chapter 11, Page 87.*)

3.12 During prenatal care, all Rh-negative patients should be screened for Rh antibodies at

   (A) the first prenatal visit
   (B) 6 weeks of gestation
   (C) 12 weeks of gestation

(D) 28 weeks of gestation
(E) 34 weeks of gestation

Answer: (D). Rh-negative patients should be screened for Rh antibodies at 28 weeks' gestation and given antenatal Rhogam if these tests are negative. (*Chapter 11, Page 87.*)

3.13 Elective screening for maternal serum alpha-feto-protein (MSAFP) is optimally performed at what time during gestation?

(A) During preconception care
(B) At first prenatal visit
(C) At 6 to 12 weeks of gestation
(D) At 16 to 18 weeks of gestation
(E) At the end of the first trimester

Answer: (D). Because MSAFP screening is widely available and is considered standard by some, the test should be discussed with all patients, with a mutual agreement of patient and practitioner regarding its use. The screening is done between 15 and 20 weeks' gestation, optimally at 16 to 18 weeks. (*Chapter 11, Page 87.*)

3.14 The patient is a 23-year-old gravida 2, para 1 black woman who asks when she will first feel the baby move. The correct response would be

(A) 6 to 8 weeks of pregnancy or earlier
(B) by the end of 12 weeks of pregnancy or earlier
(C) by 13 to 15 weeks of pregnancy or earlier
(D) by 16 to 20 weeks of pregnancy
(E) at 22 to 24 weeks of pregnancy

Answer: (D). Second-trimester prenatal care (14 to 28 weeks) includes confirmation of the estimated date of delivery by quickening at 18 to 20 weeks' gestation or earlier. (*Chapter 11, Page 89.*)

3.15 Which of the following statements about monitoring fetal heart rate (FHR) during labor is true?

(A) FHR should be monitored continuously in all patients.
(B) Intermittent fetal heart monitoring is unreliable and is no longer used.
(C) Continuous fetal monitoring provides the patient with a sense of freedom of movement.
(D) Continuous fetal monitoring has a low false-positive rate.
(E) Continuous fetal monitoring in low-risk patients has resulted in twice the frequency of cesarean sections without improving birth outcome.

Answer: (E). The HFR should be monitored during and immediately after a contraction every 30 minutes during the first stage by whatever method is most convenient (electronically, Doppler ultrasonography, or fetoscopic auscultation). Intermittent FHR monitoring is preferable to continuous monitoring in normal or low-risk patients, as continuous monitoring interferes with freedom of movement and has a high false-positive rate. Continuous electronic fetal monitoring (EFM) in low-risk patients has resulted in three times the diagnosis of fetal distress and twice the frequency of cesarean sections without improving birth outcome. (*Chapter 11, Page 90.*)

3.16 During the second stage of labor

(A) prolonged breath holding should be encouraged
(B) women push most effectively in the lithotomy position
(C) fatigued or hypotensive women may push best while lying supine with the legs extended
(D) the lithotomy position helps prevent inferior vena cava compression
(E) women may have less pain pushing when sitting or squatting

Answer: (E). Women succeed best during the second stage of labor (expulsion of the fetus) when they are allowed and encouraged to use their instincts about pushing. Prolonged breath holding and Valsalva maneuvers should be avoided, as they may result in decreased oxygenation of the placenta and fetal hypoxia. Women push more effectively and are in less pain when upright: sitting, squatting, kneeling, or standing. Fatigued or hypotensive women may push while lying on their side. Again, the lithotomy position should be avoided to prevent inferior vena cava compression and fetal distress. The FHR should be monitored every 15 minutes during the second stage in low-risk patients. (*Chapter 11, Page 90.*)

3.17 The most common medical complication of pregnancy is

(A) urinary tract infection (UTI)
(B) venous thromboembolic disease
(C) gestational diabetes mellitus
(D) anemia
(E) hypothyroidism

Answer: (A). UTI constitutes the most common medical complication of pregnancy. These infections usually occur as one or a combination of three distinct clinical presentations: (1) asymptomatic bacteriuria; (2) acute cystitis; or (3) pyelonephritis. (*Chapter 12, Page 93.*)

3.18 The diagnosis of uncomplicated cystitis in the pregnant woman is based primarily on finding

    (A) high fever
    (B) nausea and vomiting
    (C) positive urinalysis or urine culture
    (D) flank pain
    (E) chills

Answer: (C). Symptomatic lower UTI may be difficult to identify during pregnancy because these symptoms are also found frequently in pregnant women with sterile urine. Thus the diagnosis is based primarily on finding a positive urinalysis or urine culture in a pregnant woman with typical symptoms. Fever, nausea, vomiting, flank pain, and chills are usually absent in women with uncomplicated cystitis. The physical examination is normal except for suprapubic tenderness. In most cases, an adequate, clean-catch midstream urine sample is cloudy and malodorous, and it tests positive to nitrite. Microscopic examination of the urine usually discloses white and red blood cells (RBC), bacteria, and a positive nitrite test. (*Chapter 12, Page 94.*)

3.19 Appropriate therapy for uncomplicated lower UTI during pregnancy is any of the following EXCEPT

    (A) ampicillin
    (B) amoxicillin
    (C) tetracycline
    (D) cephalexin
    (E) nitrofurantoin

Answer: (C). A 7- to 10-day course of ampicillin, amoxicillin, cephalosporin, short-acting sulfa drug, or nitrofurantoin is effective, with cure rates between 50 and 90%. Single-dose antimicrobial therapy, using 3 g of amoxicillin or 2 g of cephalexin, may be just as effective. Urine cultures should be prepared 1 to 2 weeks after initial therapy and then monthly for the remainder of the pregnancy. If this therapy fails to eradicate the infection, the patient should be retreated with high-dose antimicrobial therapy (according to the sensitivity of the organism) for at least 3 weeks. (*Chapter 12, Page 94.*)

3.20 The major source of toxoplasmosis infection during pregnancy is

    (A) cats

    (B) dogs
    (C) parakeets
    (D) eggs
    (E) milk

Answer: (A). The key to managing toxoplasmosis during pregnancy is prevention. First, the major source of toxoplasma is cats, and therefore pregnant women with cats should be carefully counseled on preventive measures. Seronegative cats should be confined to the home. If the cat's toxoplasmosis status is unknown, care outside the home during pregnancy is recommended. If the cat does remain in the home, the litter box should be emptied daily, and the pregnant woman should avoid any contact with the cat box or cat feces. Second, because raw meat is a possible source, meat in the pregnant woman's home should always be stored at the proper temperatures and cooked thoroughly. It is also recommended that she avoid eating raw eggs or unpasteurized milk. (*Chapter 12, Page 97.*)

3.21 The major complication of immune thrombocytopenia purpura (ITP) during pregnancy is

    (A) DIC
    (B) hemorrhage
    (C) renal failure
    (D) septic shock
    (E) fetal demise

Answer: (B). The major complication of ITP during pregnancy is hemorrhage. Although hemorrhage is uncommon with platelet counts greater than 30,000/mm^3, close monitoring of all pregnant women with ITP is indicated. It has been recommended that treatment be instituted when bleeding time results are more than 20 minutes. Treatment modalities for this condition include glucocorticoids or, in severe cases, IgG or splenectomy. Platelet transfusions are of limited benefit because of the subsequent rapid destruction of the transfused platelets and therefore should be reserved for acute hemorrhagic events. (*Chapter 12, Page 99.*)

3.22 The patient is a 33-year-old gravida 3, para 2 white woman at 11 weeks' gestation with chronic hypertension during pregnancy. The currently recommended drug treatment for this patient is

    (A) methyldopa
    (B) atenolol
    (C) metoprolol
    (D) captopril
    (E) none of the above

Answer: (A). Treatment of chronic hypertension during pregnancy is controversial. Expert panel recommendations include treatment of pregnant women with diastolic blood pressures (BP) higher than 100 mm Hg, treating lower pressures only if there are other significant risk factors, such as renal disease or end-organ damage. Previous authors have reported no benefit of treating pregnant women with diastolic BPs less than 110 mm Hg. Most experts continue to recommend methyldopa as the drug of choice because of its long history of safety during pregnancy. Work evaluating beta-blockers in pregnant women have shown these agents to be efficacious for treatment of hypertension. However, atenolol and metoprolol have been associated with intrauterine growth retardation when treatment was started before midpregnancy. Labetolol has shown promise and is generally believed to be safe during pregnancy. Angiotensin-converting enzyme inhibitors are contraindicated, as they have been associated with fetal death. (*Chapter 12, Page 102.*)

3.23 Which of the following anticonvulsive medications is safe to use during pregnancy?

(A) trimethadione
(B) valproic acid
(C) phenytoin
(D) carbamazepine
(E) none of the above

Answer: (E). One major effect of seizure disorders on pregnancy stems from the effects of anticonvulsive medication. Much controversy remains regarding anticonvulsive medication during pregnancy. Trimethadione and valproic acid are contraindicated during pregnancy because of the high risk of adverse effects on the fetus. Phenytoin carries a relative risk of carcinogenesis, teratogenesis, and coagulopathy. Carbamazepine, although initially thought to be relatively safe for pregnancy, has been associated with craniofacial and NTDs. Phenobarbital is associated with possible teratogenesis, neonatal depression, and coagulopathy. It should also be noted that in approximately 10% of pregnant patients on antiseizure medications there is a hemorrhagic complication in either mother or neonate. Deficiency of vitamin K–dependent clotting factors has been particularly associated with phenytoin, primadone, and barbiturates. (*Chapter 12, Page 103.*)

3.24 The standard acute management of threatened abortion, if the bleeding is mild, is

(A) dilation and curettage
(B) vaginal administration of prostaglandin E_1

(C) sedation using diazepam 5 mg t.i.d.
(D) expectant, with activity restriction and abstinence from coitus until after the bleeding stops
(E) use of tocolytic medication for up to 3 months

Answer: (D). The standard acute management of threatened abortion, if bleeding is mild, is expectant. Many practitioners recommend activity restriction and abstinence from coitus until several days to 1 week after bleeding stops. There is no evidence, however, to support these recommendations. If ultrasonography demonstrates fetal life signs, especially with supporting laboratory evidence, the woman/couple can be reassured that the prognosis is good. The presence of intrauterine or subchorionic hematomas on ultrasound scans do not appear to adversely effect the pregnancy. In cases of incomplete abortion, with partial expulsion of the products of conception, the uterine contents are usually evacuated. (*Chapter 13, Page 107.*)

3.25 Ectopic pregnancy (EP)

(A) occurs in less than 1% of all pregnancies
(B) is becoming less common owing to effective antibiotic therapy of tubal disease
(C) has shown an increased death rate over the past few decades
(D) appears to have an increasing incidence over time, due in part to earlier diagnosis and higher reporting rates
(E) causes the greatest risk of death among elderly primigravidas

Answer: (D). EP is an increasingly common pregnancy complication, with an incidence of approximately 2% of pregnancies or 108,000 cases per year in the United States (1992 figures). This rate has increased four- to fivefold since the 1970s, the increase being attributed to a number of factors that affect tubal motility and to improved and earlier diagnosis and higher reporting rates. Despite this rapid increase in number of cases, death rates have decreased from 35.5 per 10,000 ectopic pregnancies in 1970 to 3.8 per 10,000 in 1989. The risk of death is highest among young and minority women. (*Chapter 13, Page 108.*)

3.26 The most common location of EP is

(A) in the distal third of the fallopian tube
(B) in the cervix
(C) on the ovary
(D) in the abdominal cavity
(E) in an endometrial cyst

Answer: (A). The word *ectopic* comes from the Greek word *ektopos,* meaning displaced. EPs can occur outside the uterus in any portion of the tube, in the cervix, on the ovary, or in the abdominal cavity. The most common location is the distal third of the fallopian tube. (*Chapter 13, Page 108.*)

3.27 The standard treatment of EP is

(A) unilateral salpingectomy
(B) linear salpingostomy
(C) unilateral salpingectomy and oophorectomy
(D) bilateral salpingectomy
(E) bilateral salpingectomy and abdominal hysterectomy

Answer: (B). It is estimated that 95% of women with EP can be successfully treated with conservative surgery; linear salpingostomy is the standard method. Women who have completed childbearing may be best treated by salpingectomy. Persistent EP is a complication of conservative surgical treatment and occurs in approximately 5 to 15% of cases. For this reason, women undergoing conservative surgery should have weekly human chorionic gonadotropen (hCG) levels. Serum hCG should steadily decline over 6 weeks. Subsequent pregnancy rates of 41 to 64% (average, 56%; n = 806) have been reported following laparoscopic surgery for EP, with repeat EP, rates of 0 to 29% (average, 17%). (*Chapter 13, Page 109.*)

3.28 The HELLP syndrome (hemolysis, elevated liver enzymes, low platelet count)

(A) occurs in about 10% of women with severe preeclampsia
(B) is more common in African American women
(C) is especially prevalent in young primigravidas
(D) generally is first noted following the onset of labor
(E) is most often seen during first pregnancies

Answer: (A). The HELLP syndrome typically presents during the early third trimester: 70% of cases occur before and 30% after the onset of labor. The syndrome is seen in approximately 10% of women with severe preeclampsia and is increased among whites, older and multiparous women with preeclampsia, and in cases with late diagnosis. (*Chapter 13, Page 112.*)

3.29 The best treatment of preeclampsia for the mother is

(A) delivery
(B) salt restriction
(C) diuretics
(D) fluid restriction
(E) bed rest

Answer: (A). The best treatment of preeclampsia for the mother is delivery, but this may not be true for the fetus. Salt restriction and diuretics are contraindicated because these measures may lead to worsening renal function and aggravation of the hypovolemia already present. Volume expansion with colloids or crystalloids has been associated with maternal pulmonary edema but might be considered as a single bolus during labor in cases of severe preeclampsia with evidence of volume reduction. Finally, bed rest may confer some benefit to the fetus and is a standard part of therapy despite inadequate evidence of benefit. (*Chapter 13, Page 114.*)

3.30 The patient is a 23-year-old primigravida at 34 weeks' gestation with painful uterine contractions every 5 minutes and intact membranes with cervical effacement of 90%. She has

(A) Braxton-Hicks contractions
(B) preterm labor (PTL)
(C) normal third-trimester findings
(D) fetal malposition
(E) false labor

Answer: (B). PTL is diagnosed by using the following criteria: (1) gestational age of 20 to 36 weeks; plus (2) documented uterine contractions (four per 20 minutes or eight per 60 minutes); plus (3) ruptured membranes or intact membranes and cervical dilation greater than 2 cm or intact membranes and cervical effacement of more than 80% or intact membranes and cervical change during observation. (*Chapter 13, Page 116.*)

3.31 Currently used tocolytic agents include all EXCEPT

(A) beta-adrenergic agonists
(B) magnesium sulfate
(C) prostaglandin synthetase inhibitors
(D) angiotensin converting enzyme inhibitors
(E) calcium channel blockers

Answer: (D). The choice of a tocolytic agent depends on the familiarity and comfort of the treating clinician, the institutional preference, side effects profile, and cost considerations. Medications include beta-adrenergic agonists, direct muscle relaxants such as magnesium sulfate, prostaglandin synthetase inhibitors, and calcium channel blockers. Differences in cost, frequency, and severity of side effects have been demonstrated, but most randomized controlled trials comparing these agents have found no significant differences in successful labor cessation (approximately 75%), duration of gestation, or neonatal outcome. None of the current tocolytic agents used for long-term treatment have been demonstrated to improve neonatal survival. (*Chapter 13, Page 118.*)

3.32 The patient is a 22-year-old white woman at 31 weeks in her first pregnancy. Her mother suffered a severe pelvic infection following a cesarean section, and she is very worried about the possibility of needing a cesarean section. She asks, "What would be the most likely cause of my needing a cesarean section?" What should be your answer to this question?

(A) herpes infection of the birth canal
(B) dystocia
(C) placenta abruption
(D) preeclampsia
(E) fetal malposition

Answer: (B). Dystocia, or difficult labor, is a particularly vexing problem for the primigravida patient and her provider. It accounts for nearly half of the cesarean sections nulliparas have undergone during the cesarean "epidemic" of the past 25 years. (*Chapter 14, Page 123.*)

3.33 Fetal scalp pH monitoring sometimes helps resolve concern raised by EFM. A fetal scalp blood pH of what range is reassuring?

(A) 7.25 or greater
(B) 7.20 to 7.24
(C) 7.20 or less
(D) 6.4 to 6.8
(E) No single level could be considered reassuring, and repeated sampling is necessary to document a direction of change.

Answer: (A). Fetal scalp sampling to determine the presence of fetal acidosis has been shown to lower the false-positive rate of continuous EFM, thereby lowering the rate of both forceps and cesarean deliveries. A fetal pH of 7.25 or above is reassuring. An intermediate result of 7.20 to 7.24 should be repeated. pH less than 7.20 warrants expeditious delivery. As a clinical alternative to scalp pH testing, numerous studies have demonstrated a correlation between spontaneous or inducible FHR accelerations with nonacidotic fetuses. (*Chapter 14, Page 126.*)

3.34 Placental abruption is a dangerous bleeding complication during labor. Of women experiencing placental abruption, about half have which ONE of the following risk factors?

(A) abdominal trauma
(B) grand multiparity
(C) uterine anomalies
(D) short umbilical cord
(E) hypertension

Answer: (E). Placental abruption occurs when there is premature separation of the placenta prior to birth. It is thought to occur because of disease of the decidua and uterine blood vessels. This theory is supported by the strong association between hypertension (both preexisting and pregnancy-induced) and placental abruption. Among women experiencing a placental abruption, about half have hypertension. Other associated risk factors for placental abruption include abdominal trauma, grand multiparity, uterine anomalies, nutritional (folate) deficiencies, short umbilical cord, cigarette smoking, cocaine use, a history of abruption, and advanced maternal age. (*Chapter 14, Page 128.*)

3.35 In a gravida 2, para 1 white woman in the early second trimester, a placenta previa can be visualized via ultrasonography. In such patients, partial placenta previa during the second trimester

(A) rarely resolves
(B) should be treated with cesarean section at 32 weeks' gestation
(C) tends to resolve in 95% of cases if partial or marginal
(D) should be followed with weekly sonography
(E) is likely to be associated with placental abruption

Answer: (C). During the early second trimester, a placenta previa can be visualized via ultrasonography 5 to 8% of the time. If partial or marginal, it tends to resolve in 95% of cases with upward migration of the placenta and 10-fold lengthening of the lower uterine segment. Placenta previa is associated with increased perinatal morbidity and mortality, particularly when a woman presents with active bleeding secondary to a placenta previa during the second trimester. (*Chapter 14, Page 129.*)

3.36 Which of the following drugs is safe to use when breast-feeding?

(A) tetracycline
(B) bromocriptine
(C) lithium

(D) ergotamine
(E) none of the above

Answer: (E). Prescription of drugs to nursing mothers requires careful consideration of their effect on the newborn. Drugs contraindicated during breast-feeding include tetracycline, chloramphenical, bromocriptine, cyclophosphamide, cyclosporine, doxorubicin, ergotamine, lithium, methotrexate, phenindione, recreational drugs, and radiopharmaceuticals. Other drugs that should be used with caution include sulfonamides, metronidazole, salicylates, antihistamines, psychotropic agents, phenobarbital, and large amounts of caffeine. (*Chapter 15, Page 131.*)

3.37 Following delivery, women with D-negative blood who have not been sensitized to the D antigen, and who have delivered D-positive infants, should

(A) have no further therapy
(B) receive immunoglobulin prophylaxis within 72 hours of delivery
(C) receive prednisone, beginning at 80 mg daily tapered over 1 week
(D) receive transfusion with one unit of D-positive packed RBC
(E) be reassured that there is little risk during future pregnancies

Answer: (B). Women with D-negative blood who have not been sensitized to the D antigen and who have delivered D-positive infants should receive immunoglobulin prophylaxis within 72 hours of delivery to prevent hemolytic disease in future pregnancies. Many hospitals have routine protocols for screening mothers' and infants' blood and for administering immunoglobulin when indicated so this important procedure is not overlooked. (*Chapter 15, Page 132.*)

3.38 The most common cause of postpartum hemorrhage is

(A) use of aspirin during the third trimester
(B) cervical laceration
(C) vaginal laceration
(D) uterine atony
(E) twin gestation

Answer: (D). Critical to the management of postpartum hemorrhage is early determination of the source of bleeding. Uterine atony, the most common cause of postpartum hemorrhage, should be suspected with the clinical finding of a large boggy uterus. (*Chapter 15, Page 132.*)

3.39 Common problems during the first 2 to 4 weeks postpartum include all the following EXCEPT

(A) emotional tension
(B) fatigue
(C) decreased appetite
(D) hemoptysis
(E) hot flashes and sweating

Answer: (D). At 1 month postpartum, most women suffer emotional tension, fatigue, and concerns about their sexual or marital relationship. Other symptoms prevalent during the first few weeks after delivery include breast and vaginal discomfort, constipation and hemorrhoids, decreased appetite, hot flashes and sweating, acne, dizziness, and hand numbness. Several of these problems (breast and vaginal symptoms, constipation and hemorrhoids, fatigue, and dizziness) may continue for months. (*Chapter 15, Page 133.*)

DIRECTIONS (Items 3.40 through 3.96): Each of the items in this section is a multiple true–false problem that consists of a stem and four lettered options. Indicate whether each of the options is TRUE or FALSE.

3.40 Your patient is a 22-year-old white female waitress. She married a year ago, and she and her husband are planning a family. She is worried about a past history of multiple sexual partners and asks specifically about HIV. Which of the following statements regarding HIV is/are true?

(A) Even without treatment, the risk of perinatal transmission of HIV is negligible.
(B) Therapy during pregnancy and labor can reduce the risk of perinatal HIV transmission.
(C) Perinatal transmission of HIV is a major cause of death among children in the United States.
(D) Perinatal transmission of HIV varies with maternal factors including CD4+ lymphocyte counts and placental membrane inflammation.

Answer: (A-False, B-True, C-True, D-True). Perinatal transmission of HIV has become a major cause of illness and death among children in the United States, having infected more than 15,000 children and having claimed more than 3,000 lives. In the absence of treatment, the risk of perinatal transmission is 15 to 40% and varies with maternal factors such as p24 antigenemia, CD8+ and CD4+ lymphocyte counts, and placental membrane inflammation. An important turning point occurred in 1994 when the AIDS Clinical Trial Group demonstrated that zidovudine administered to a group of HIV-infected women during pregnancy and labor and to their newborns reduced the risk of perinatal HIV infection by two-thirds, from 25.5 to 8.3%. (*Chapter 10, Page 75.*)

3.41 True statements regarding HIV testing before pregnancy include which of the following?

  (A) HIV testing should only be offered to patients in high-risk groups.
  (B) Women who test negative for HIV require no further counseling.
  (C) Women testing positive for HIV must be counseled regarding the risk of perinatal transmission to the infant.
  (D) Offering contraception to women who test positive for HIV compromises the woman's autonomy and is considered unethical.

Answer: (A-False, B-False, C-True, D-False). All women should be offered HIV testing before pregnancy. Women who test negative for HIV should be counseled about safe sexual practices. Those women testing positive must be informed of the risks of vertical transmission to the infant and the associated morbidity and mortality. These women should be offered contraception. Those choosing pregnancy are counseled about the availability of treatment to prevent vertical transmission and the importance of early prenatal care. (*Chapter 10, Page 76.*)

3.42 Which of the following women should be tested for hepatitis B virus (HBV) and if susceptible, should be vaccinated before they become pregnant?

  (A) sexual contacts of HBV persons
  (B) recent immigrants from Mexico and Central America
  (C) women in military service
  (D) women who have recently migrated from Southeast Asia

Answer: (A-True, B-False, C-False, D-True). Women at ongoing risk for HBV (sexual contacts of HBV-infected persons, users of illicit injectable drugs, prostitutes, institutionalized women, and Southeast Asians) can be tested for evidence of previous or ongoing HBV infection and, if susceptible, should be vaccinated before they become pregnant. (*Chapter 10, Page 76.*)

3.43 Your patient is a 26-year-old college teacher whose hobby is breeding cats. She is planning her first pregnancy and is worried about toxoplasmosis. Which of the following statements is/are true?

  (A) Antibodies to toxoplasmosis are rare in adult women in the United States.
  (B) Congenital toxoplasmosis occurs in approximately 1.1 of 1,000 live births.
  (C) Children of mothers who had toxoplasmosis during pregnancy are rarely affected at birth.
  (D) Fetal effects are more common with toxoplasmosis infection contracted during the first or second trimester.

Answer: (A-False, B-True, C-False, D-True). About one-third of adult women in the United States have antibodies to toxoplasmosis; the remainder may be at risk for a primary maternal infection during pregnancy that can result in congenital infection. Prospective studies performed in the United States have established an incidence of congenital toxoplasmosis of 1.1 per 1,000 live births. Of children born to mothers who had toxoplasmosis during pregnancy, approximately 8% are severely affected at birth. The remainder are affected with mild disease or subclinical infection but are at risk for late sequelae such as chorioretinitis, mental retardation, and sensorineural hearing loss. Severe fetal effects are more likely if infection is acquired during the first or second trimester. (*Chapter 10, Page 76.*)

3.44 Your patient is a 22-year-old woman with insulin-dependent diabetes mellitus (IDDM). She and her husband are planning their first pregnancy. Which of the following statements regarding IDDM during pregnancy is/are true?

  (A) The chief risk is a major congenital malformation.
  (B) Congenital malformations associated with gestational diabetes can affect almost any organ system.
  (C) Malformations occur during the period of fetal organ development, at about the end of the first trimester.
  (D) Excellent blood glucose control early in pregnancy reduces the rate of congenital malformations.

Answer: (A-True, B-True, C-False, D-True). Improved control of maternal glucose and antepartum fetal surveillance has led to a significant reduction in the perinatal mortality rate seen during pregnancies complicated by IDDM. Today, the leading causes of perinatal mortality during pregnancies complicated by IDDM are major congenital malformations. Whereas the risk of major malformations in the general population is 2 to 3%, these malformations are observed in approximately 10% of pregnancies complicated by

IDDM. Although virtually any organ system can be affected, the most characteristic abnormalities include sacral agenesis, complex cardiac defects, spina bifida, and anencephaly. These malformations occur during the critical period of fetal organogenesis, approximately 5 to 8 weeks after the last menstrual period. The increased rate of congenital malformations in infants born to mothers with IDDM is significantly reduced when these women maintain excellent blood glucose control during organogenesis. *(Chapter 10, Page 77.)*

3.45 Your patients are a couple in their mid-20s planning their first pregnancy. They are concerned about genetic disease in the family, and they are asking about genetic counseling. Which of the following statements is/are true?

(A) If either member of the couple is affected by a genetic disease or has an affected relative, the couple should be referred for genetic counseling at the time of the first prenatal visit.
(B) Testing during pregnancy may include chorionic villous sampling and amniocentesis early in pregnancy.
(C) For fetuses identified to be at high risk for genetic defects, there are a variety of management options available.
(D) Genetic testing done before conception allows consideration of options that include not bearing children and artificial insemination.

Answer: (A-False, B-True, C-False, D-True). If either member of a couple is affected by genetic disease or has an affected relative, the couple should be referred for genetic counseling and possible genetic testing. Genetic counseling allows the couple to understand their risk and, if necessary, to arrange for diagnostic tests such as chorionic villous sampling or amniocentesis early in pregnancy. Such determinations could influence a couple's decision to conceive or adopt and could alter the clinical management of the pregnancy and newborn. Preconception screening not only provides a couple more time to consider their options and make plans, it also adds to the number of options available. For fetuses identified to be at high risk during pregnancy, confirmatory testing only provides the management option of induced abortion. When testing is done before conception, additional options include not bearing children, artificial insemination, in vitro fertilization, surrogate pregnancy, and adoption. *(Chapter 10, Page 78.)*

3.46 Marked obesity in pregnancy may be associated with which of the following?

(A) gestational diabetes
(B) rapid labor and delivery
(C) hypertension
(D) macrosomic infants

Answer: (A-True, B-False, C-True, D-True). Preconception assessment of nutrition status should identify women who are underweight or overweight. Women who are underweight and subsequently gain little weight during pregnancy are at high risk of fetal and neonatal morbidity and mortality. At the other extreme, marked obesity is associated with gestational diabetes, NTDs, hypertension, macrosomic infants, and resultant prolonged labor and shoulder dystocia. Thus treatment for both underweight and obese women is best before pregnancy. *(Chapter 10, Page 79.)*

3.47 During preconception care, which of the following statements is/are true regarding vitamin A?

(A) The recommended dietary allowance for women is 2,700 IU of vitamin A per day.
(B) Women considering pregnancy should increase their vitamin A intake to 15,000 IU daily.
(C) High doses of vitamin A can be teratogenic.
(D) To achieve adequate doses of vitamin A, pregnant women should be advised to consume a diet high in liver products.

Answer: (A-True, B-False, C-True, D-False). The recommended dietary allowance for women is 2,700 IU of vitamin A per day. Currently, about 1 to 2% of women average more than 10,000 IU of vitamin A from supplements. Evidence in humans suggests that more than 10,000 IU of vitamin A per day is teratogenic, resulting in cranial/neural crest defects. Women in the reproductive age group are advised to avoid consuming vitamin A at these levels and should consume liver products only in moderation, as they contain large amounts of vitamin A. Women with a history of a previous pregnancy resulting in a fetus with NTDs should be advised not to attempt to achieve high doses of folic acid (i.e., 4 mg) by taking multivitamins because of the possibility of ingesting harmful levels of vitamin A. *(Chapter 10, Page 79.)*

3.48 Which of the following statements is/are true regarding infants born to women with classic phenylketonuria (PKU) and a maternal blood phenylalanine level of more than 20 mg/dl?

(A) Infants may have microcephaly.
(B) Infants may have mental retardation.

(C) Infants are at no increased risk of congenital heart disease.

(D) Infants are at increased risk of intrauterine growth retardation.

Answer: (A-True, B-True, C-False, D-True). Infants born to women with classic PKU and a maternal blood phenylalanine level of more than 20 mg/dl are likely to have microcephaly and mental retardation and are at increased risk of congenital heart disease and intra-uterine growth retardation. Dietary restrictions that result in lowered levels of maternal phenylalanine during the earliest weeks of gestation appear to reduce the risk of fetal malformation. (*Chapter 10, Page 79.*)

3.49 True statements regarding domestic violence during pregnancy include which of the following?

(A) Victims of domestic violence are not likely to be abused during pregnancy.

(B) Up to 25% of obstetric patients are abused during pregnancy.

(C) Physical assault can lead to placental separation, antepartum hemorrhage, and preterm labor.

(D) Physical assault has not been shown to cause fetal fractures because the infant is protected by amniotic fluid.

Answer: (A-False, B-True, C-True, D-False). Victims of domestic violence should be identified preconceptionally, as they are likely to be abused during pregnancy. Up to 25% of obstetric patients are physically abused while pregnant. Such assaults can result in placental separation; antepartum hemorrhage; fetal fractures; rupture of the uterus, liver, or spleen; and preterm labor. Information about available community, social, and legal resources, and a plan for dealing with the abusive partner should be made available to abused women. (*Chapter 10, Page 79.*)

3.50 The patient is a 20-year-old black woman at 6 weeks of pregnancy. She has smoked a pack of cigarettes daily since the age of 16. She asks for your advice regarding smoking. Which of the following is/are true?

(A) Tobacco use during pregnancy can cause a low-birth-weight infant.

(B) Abruptio placentae has not been shown to be related to smoking.

(C) Smoking may contribute to intrauterine growth retardation.

(D) There is no relation between smoking and sudden infant death syndrome.

Answer: (A-True, B-False, C-True, D-False). Smoking contributes to many obstetric problems such as pre-term delivery, intrauterine growth retardation, abruptio placentae, placenta previa, and spontaneous abortion. Each year tobacco-related products are responsible for an estimated 32,000 to 61,000 infants born with low birth weight (representing 11 to 21% of low-birth-weight births) and 14,000 to 26,000 infants who require admission to a neonatal intensive care unit. Tobacco use is also responsible for an estimated 1,900 to 4,800 infant deaths resulting from perinatal disorders and 1,200 to 2,200 deaths from sudden infant death syndrome. (*Chapter 10, Page 80.*)

3.51 Which of the following statements is/are true regarding the use of cocaine during the first trimester of pregnancy?

(A) Use may occur before the woman is aware that she is pregnant.

(B) Occasional use of cocaine during pregnancy has not been shown to cause problems with the pregnancy.

(C) Subsequent use may be associated with placental abruption.

(D) There is no risk of congenital defects if the woman does not continue to use cocaine later during the pregnancy.

Answer: (A-True, B-False, C-True, D-False). Use of cocaine, heroin, and other substances during pregnancy may lead to spontaneous abortion, premature delivery, abruptio placentae, fetal growth retardation, congenital anomalies, and fetal or neonatal death. An estimated 10 to 15% of women use cocaine, heroin, methadone, amphetamines, PCP, or marijuana during pregnancy. A careful history to identify use of illegal substances should be obtained as part of the preconception risk assessment. Occasional recreational use may not be considered by the woman to be a problem, nor may she be aware of the dangers of such occasional use during early pregnancy. Use of cocaine during the first trimester, possibly before the woman is aware that she is pregnant, is associated with abruption and with congenital defects even if the woman does not continue to use it later during the pregnancy. (*Chapter 10, Page 80.*)

3.52 Which of the statements is/are true regarding family support during pregnancy?

(A) Detection and intervention in family supports improve maternal sense of well-being but has not been shown to improve perinatal outcome.

(B) Issues may include a history of maternal deprivation, physical abuse, or substance use by significant others.
(C) Pregnant women generally mention family problems to the physician during early prenatal visits.
(D) Public social service programs are often important in dealing with the pregnant patient and family support problems.

Answer: (A-False, B-True, C-False, D-True). Pregnancy is an opportunity to assess family supports and liabilities and to intervene with the potential of an improved perinatal outcome. If there is a history of maternal deprivation, postpartum depression, physical abuse, or substance use by significant others, interventions can be begun during pregnancy and continued during care of the parent(s) and child. The physician must ask explicitly about these issues, which often are not spontaneously mentioned by women. Finally, physicians should be knowledgeable and able to recommend the public social service programs available to aid and support the pregnant patient and family. (*Chapter 11, Page 86.*)

3.53 An elevated level of msAFP may be found in patients with

(A) chromosomal trisomy (e.g., Down syndrome)
(B) molar pregnancy
(C) multiple gestation
(D) normal pregnancy

Answer: (A-False, B-False, C-True, D-True). An elevated msAFP level may be found in patients with inaccurate dates, multiple gestation, neural tube defects, abdominal wall defects, congenital nephrotic syndrome, fetal demise, fetomaternal hemorrhage, and normal pregnancy. A low level may be found with inaccurate dates, chromosomal trisomy (e.g., Down syndrome), fetal demise, molar pregnancy, and normal pregnancy. (*Chapter 11, Page 87.*)

3.54 Tests appropriate during third-trimester prenatal care include screening for

(A) anemia
(B) gestational diabetes
(C) msAFP
(D) culture for group B *Streptococcus*

Answer: (A-True, B-True, C-False, D-True). Third-trimester prenatal care includes screening for anemia, gestational diabetes, and sexually transmitted diseases (STD) if risk is present. Culture for group B *Streptococ-

cus* is also done during this time (34 to 36 weeks). Screening for msAFP is done between 15 and 20 weeks' gestation. (*Chapter 11, Page 89.*)

3.55 Methods to assess the fetal well-being during pregnancy include

(A) pelvimetry
(B) fetal movement counting
(C) nonstress test (NST)
(D) ultrasonography for amniotic fluid evaluation

Answer: (A-False, B-True, C-True, D-True). Methods have been developed to assess the well-being of the fetus during pregnancy, including fetal movement counting, NST, nipple stimulation or oxytocin contraction stress test, and ultrasonography for amniotic fluid evaluation. (*Chapter 11, Page 89.*)

3.56 Which of the following statements regarding labor is/are true?

(A) Progress during the early (latent) stage of labor is often slow because of the time needed for effacement of the cervix.
(B) With regular frequent contractions, the average rate of cervix dilation is 2 to 3 cm/hour.
(C) Although there is considerable individual variation, the active stage of labor is more rapid and predictable than the early (latent) phase.
(D) Arrest of labor occurs when there has been no cervical dilation for 2 hours during the active phase of labor.

Answer: (A-True, B-False, C-True, D-True). Labor in the first stage is defined as progressive dilation of the cervix with uterine contractions. The early (latent) stage of labor occurs up to 4 cm dilation and is variable in duration. Progress during this stage is often slow because of the time needed for effacement of the cervix. The active stage of labor is more rapid and predictable, yet there is still considerable individual variation. With frequent, regular contractions, the average is 1.2 cm dilation/hour in primigravidas and 1.5 cm/hour in multigravidas, but flexibility is important. Friedman attempted to describe labor, not to define parameters women must follow. Arrest of labor is present where there has been no cervical dilation for 2 hours during the active stage. (*Chapter 11, Page 89.*)

3.57 Early in labor your patient asks about an episiotomy. You might respond that

(A) episiotomy is recommended routinely because it shortens the second stage of labor
(B) routine episiotomy would be avoided
(C) episiotomy may be used to deliver a large infant
(D) episiotomy may be necessary when delivery must occur rapidly

Answer: (A-False, B-True, C-True, D-True). Normal delivery of the infant should occur in whatever position is comfortable for the woman, and the physician should be as flexible as possible with birth positions. The infant's head should remain flexed during delivery to lessen the diameter presenting to the perineum. An episiotomy is avoided unless the infant is large or delivery must occur quickly. (*Chapter 11, Page 90.*)

3.58 The patient is a 22-year-old white female clerical worker, and this is her first pregnancy. She asks about epidural anesthesia. True statements about epidural anesthesia include which of the following?

(A) Elective use of epidural anesthesia during labor may increase the need for oxytocin augmentation.
(B) Elective use of epidural anesthesia during labor may decrease the need for cesarean section.
(C) Epidural anesthesia has not been found to prolong the first stage of labor.
(D) Epidural anesthesia may relax the pelvic diaphragm, predisposing to minor malpresentation.

Answer: (A-True, B-False, C-False, D-True). Lumbar epidural anesthesia has become increasingly common and provides effective pain relief. It has a place in the management of dystocia and is of benefit for cesarean section. Its use during labor should be carefully considered, not elective. Studies in Europe and North America have shown that elective use of epidural anesthesia during labor increases the need for oxytocin augmentation and may increase the cesarean rate. Documented effects of epidural anesthesia on labor include decreased uterine activity, prolongation of the first stage of labor, relaxation of the pelvic diaphragm predisposing to minor malpresentation, decreased maternal urge and ability to push, prolonged second stage of labor, and increased use of instrumental vaginal delivery. (*Chapter 11, Page 90.*)

3.59 Delivery of the placenta (third stage of labor)

(A) is likely when there is a sudden gush of blood, and the uterus becomes globular or firm
(B) is facilitated by vigorous traction on the cord
(C) is not facilitated by suprapubic pressure

(D) is considered to be prolonged if the placenta has not been delivered by 20 minutes following the end of the second stage of the labor

Answer: (A-True, B-False, C-False, D-False). Delivery of the placenta (third stage of labor) should not be attempted until separation has occurred from the uterus (up to 20 minutes). Placental separation is likely when there is a sudden gush of blood, the uterus becomes globular or firm and rises in the abdomen, and the cord protrudes farther out of the vagina. Gentle traction on the cord and suprapubic pressure to avoid uterine inversion spontaneously delivers the placenta. The placenta is examined for completeness, number of vessels, and abnormalities. (*Chapter 11, Page 91.*)

3.60 UTI during pregnancy may result in

(A) postdates pregnancy
(B) septic shock
(C) bacteremia
(D) PTL

Answer: (A-False, B-True, C-True, D-True). If infection occurs in the urinary tract, the physiologic changes of pregnancy may result in serious infectious complications such as septic shock, bacteremia, and even death. Other obstetric complications such as PTL, premature delivery (PTD), and pregnancy-induced hypertension have also been associated with UTIs. (*Chapter 12, Page 93.*)

3.61 The patient is a 25-year-old gravida 3, para 2, white woman at 10 weeks' gestation. Routine screening has detected asymptomatic bacteriuria (ASB). The patient asks about the significance of this finding. Which of the following is/are true?

(A) ASB occurs in less than 1% of pregnant women.
(B) Criteria for the diagnosis for ASB on a catheterized specimen in the absence of the usual symptoms of a lower UTI is 1,000 to 10,000 colonies/per ml of one organism.
(C) Treatment is unnecessary because ASB during pregnancy generally subsides without antibiotic therapy.
(D) Screening and treatment have been shown to reduce morbidity due to ASB.

Answer: (A-False, B-True, C-False, D-True). ASB is defined as 100,000 colonies or more/ml of one organism from a midstream, clean-catch urine culture or 1,000 to 10,000 colonies/ml of one organism on a catheterized specimen in a woman without traditional symptoms of a lower UTI, such as dysuria, urinary frequency, and urgency or suprapubic pain. The prevalence of ASB during pregnancy is about 2 to 10% in pregnant women, similar to that in the nonpregnant state. The most common organisms identified in ASB, accounting for 85 to 90% of all organisms isolated, are *Escherichia coli, Klebsiella, Enterobacter, Streptococcus, Staphylococcus, Proteus, Pseudomonas,* and *Citrobactor.* The significance of ASB during pregnancy is that, if untreated, 20 to 30% of affected women develop acute pyelonephritis during the third trimester. Screening and treatment have been shown to reduce the rate to 3%. (*Chapter 12, Page 93.*)

3.62 The patient is a 28-year-old gravida 2, para 1 white woman at 28 weeks' gestation. She has nausea, vomiting, fever, chills, right-sided flank pain, and tenderness. Microscopic examination reveals pyuria and bacteriuria. This patient should be

(A) hospitalized for intravenous (IV) antimicrobial therapy
(B) should have a short course of external fetal monitoring early in therapy
(C) should be treated with large (IV) doses of ampicillin
(D) should be monitored carefully for signs of septic shock

Answer: (A-True, B-True, C-False, D-True). All pregnant women presenting with pyelonephritis should be hospitalized for IV antimicrobial therapy. Because of the potential risk of preterm labor and fetal distress, the initial evaluation should also include a short course of external fetal monitoring. Frequent assessment of vital signs and urine output with careful evaluation of fluid status is crucial to look for signs of septic shock. Increasing resistance to ampicillin by *Enterobacteriaceae* calls for initial therapy with a second- or third-generation cephalosporin or an aminoglycoside such as gentamicin. (*Chapter 12, Page 94.*)

3.63 Which of the following statements regarding screening high-risk pregnant women for tuberculosis is/are true?

(A) Tuberculin testing should rarely be used because its safety during pregnancy is uncertain.
(B) The multipuncture test (e.g., Mono-Vacc or Tine) is preferred during pregnancy.
(C) A positive PPD test requires exclusion of active disease, including a chest radiograph.

(D) If the chest radiograph suggests active disease or symptoms are present, sputum smears and cultures are obtained.

Answer: (A-False, B-False, C-True, D-True). All high-risk pregnant women should be screened for tuberculosis using the 5 TU Mantoux intradermal test (PPD). Tuberculin skin testing has been found to be safe during pregnancy. Providers should question each woman to ensure she has not had a previous positive test. Multipuncture tests (e.g., Mono-Vacc or Tine) have been shown to produce a high false-negative rate, thereby limiting their usefulness as a screening study. A positive PPD test requires exclusion of active disease through a complete history and physical examination and with a posteroanterior chest radiograph (the lateral view adds little to the evaluation) using abdominal shielding. If the chest radiograph is suggestive of active disease or symptoms are present, sputum smears and cultures are obtained. (*Chapter 12, Page 96.*)

3.64 The patient is a 27-year-old black woman at 20 weeks' gestation. For the past 2 to 3 days, her left calf area has had pain and swelling. There is local tenderness and a positive Homan sign. Which of the following is/are true regarding confirmatory tests?

(A) The test of choice is radioactive iodine fibrinogen scanning.
(B) Single impedance plethysmography is a sensitive and useful test.
(C) Duplex ultrasound scanning is especially sensitive for proximal lower extremity thrombosis.
(D) Magnetic resonance imaging (MRI) has proved useful for diagnosing deep vein thrombosis (DVT) in pregnant women.

Answer: (A-False, B-False, C-True, D-True). Most pregnancy-associated venous thromboses originate in the distal venous system but can extend into the iliac or femoral veins, where the potential for embolization is higher. During pregnancy, the use of noninvasive diagnostic testing is limited because radioactive iodine used for fibrinogen scanning is contraindicated and single impedance plethysmography has a comparably low sensitivity. Although venography has been called the "gold standard," many experts cite concern about the high rate of ionizing radiation, the technical difficulties, and the possibility that the procedure itself may predispose to thrombosis as reasons not to use venography routinely to diagnose DVT. Duplex ultrasound scanning and color Doppler ultrasonography with compression have higher diagnostic sensitivity for proximal lower extremity thrombosis especially during the first and second trimesters but are inferior for identifying DVT of the calf veins. Both these tests are subjective and highly dependent on the skill of the examiner. MRI has proved useful for diagnosing DVT in pregnant women. (*Chapter 12, Page 98.*)

3.65 Pulmonary embolism (PE) during pregnancy

   (A) continues to be a major cause of maternal mortality in the United States

   (B) typically occurs early in labor

   (C) begins with bradypnea as an early sign

   (D) is usually associated with an electrocardiogram (ECG) and chest radiographs that are diagnostic

Answer: (A-True, B-False, C-False, D-False). PE during pregnancy continues to be a major cause of maternal mortality in the United States. Typically, the patient is in the puerperium but may be postpartum by several weeks. Tachypnea, dyspnea, and chest pain in a pregnant woman should immediately alert the physicians to the possibility of PE, especially in patients at high risk. Hypoxemia is usually present with an arterial PO_2 less than 85 mm Hg and accompanying hypocarbia and respiratory alkalosis. Unless the embolus is massive, the ECG and chest radiographs are typically nonspecific. (*Chapter 12, Page 98.*)

3.66 The patient is a 32-year-old businesswoman who has had two spontaneous abortions (SA). She is worried about her fertility. Which of the following statements that you might use in counseling is/are true?

   (A) Approximately 12 to 14% of clinically recognized pregnancies end in SA.

   (B) Most clinically recognized SAs occur between 4 and 7 weeks' gestation.

   (C) Fetal death occurs very shortly before the onset of SA.

   (D) SA following 16 weeks' gestation occurs in about 1% of pregnancies.

Answer: (A-True, B-False, C-False, D-True). SA is defined as expulsion of the embryo or fetus before viability is achieved (500 g or less or prior to 20 to 22 weeks' gestation). The incidence varies depending on whether preclinical losses (loss prior to clinical recognition of pregnancy) are considered. Studies testing for early pregnancy with hCG report preclinical losses of between 8 and 57%. Estimates of loss for clinically recognized pregnancy are 12 to 14%, resulting in an overall incidence of SA (preclinical and clinical) of 43% on average. Although most clinically recognized SAs

occur between 7 and 15 weeks' gestation, most fetal deaths occur earlier in pregnancy. Studies using early prenatal ultrasonography report loss rates of about 3% after 8 weeks' and 1% after 16 weeks' gestation. (*Chapter 13, Page 106.*)

3.67 The patient is a 30-year-old gravida 2, para 1 white woman at 30 weeks' gestation. You have just made a diagnosis of gestational diabetes. Which of the following is/are true regarding management?

   (A) The recommended weight gain is 11 to 16 kg (24 to 35 lb).

   (B) The diet should consist of 40 kcal/kg body weight, not to exceed 3,500 kcal/day.

   (C) The fasting plasma or glucose level should be maintained at 140 mg/dl or less.

   (D) Fetal ultrasonography is recommended during the third trimester.

Answer: (A-True, B-False, C-False, D-True). Once the diagnosis is made, maternal education and dietary consults are critical. Recommended weight gain is 11 to 16 kg (24 to 35 lb), with a diet consisting of 30 kcal/kg body weight, not to exceed 2,500 kcal/day. Careful monitoring of the plasma or capillary glucose is recommended, keeping the fasting level less than 105 mg/dl and the 1-hour level less than 140 mg/dl. Fetal ultrasonography is recommended during the third trimester to evaluate fetal growth, amniotic fluid volume, and malformations. (*Chapter 12, Page 100.*)

3.68 Hyperthyroidism during pregnancy

   (A) requires no treatment until the pregnancy is over

   (B) is often treated with propylthiouracil (PTU)

   (C) is best treated with methimazole

   (D) should be treated surgically during the pregnancy

Answer: (A-False, B-True, C-False, D-False). Hyperthyroidism represents most of the thyroid disease that occurs during pregnancy. The most common cause of this condition is Graves' disease. Hyperthyroidism during pregnancy must be treated because of the risks of neonatal thyrotoxicosis, premature birth, and abortion. Thyroid-stimulating immunoglobulin crosses the placenta, resulting in stimulation of the fetal thyroid gland. Antithyroid medications such as PTU and methimazole also cross the placenta, affecting fetal thyroid function. Optimal management for the hyperthyroid pregnant patient achieves high normal free thyroid hormone levels using as little medication as possible. PTU is the drug of choice as it has low rates of placental transfer and because methimazole has a questionable association with congenital malformations of the scalp. Frequent monitoring of the pregnant patient on PTU is necessary to minimize the amount of drug required to keep the patient in the euthyroid state. Studies have demonstrated that the intelligent quotients of infants of mothers treated with antithyroid drugs during pregnancy did not suffer compared with controls. Surgical treatment has little place in the treatment of the pregnant hyperthyroid patient. (*Chapter 12, Page 100.*)

3.69 The patient is a 34-year-old gravida 2, para 1 white woman. She comes today for her first prenatal visit at 14 weeks' gestation. Her BP is 152/96. She has not seen a physician for several years but believes that she was told that she had high BP in the past and also seems to remember an elevated BP during her first pregnancy 5 years ago. Two years ago, a physician prescribed a diuretic for her high BP, but she stopped this medication after several months because of leg cramps. She has no proteinuria or edema, and her uric acid level is 4.8 mg/dl. Which of the following is/are true?

(A) This patient probably has transient hypertension of pregnancy.
(B) This patient probably has preeclampsia of pregnancy.
(C) This patient probably has chronic hypertension that existed prior to pregnancy.
(D) This patient may become normotensive during the second trimester, with a return of the hypertensive state during the third trimester.

Answer: (A-False, B-False, C-True, D-True). In patients without an established diagnosis of chronic hypertension but who are found to be hypertensive during pregnancy, it is sometimes difficult to determine whether the hypertension was caused by pregnancy or was preexisting hypertension discovered during pregnancy. Determining the etiology of hypertension is particularly a problem when women without previous BP measurements are not seen until the second trimester. Chronically hypertensive patients often are normotensive during the midtrimester, with a return of their BP to its hypertensive state during the third trimester, leading to a misdiagnosis of preeclampsia. Chronic hypertension is less likely to be associated with proteinuria or nondependent edema. Also, a uric acid level of less than 5 mg/dl is more likely found with chronic hypertension, as an elevated uric acid level is a sensitive marker of preeclampsia. (*Chapter 12, Page 102.*)

3.70 The patient is a 22-year-old primigravida woman with a history of migraine headaches. Which of the following is/are safe to use during pregnancy?

(A) acetaminophen
(B) antiemetics
(C) ergotamine alkaloids
(D) isometheptene mucate (Midrin)

Answer: (A-True, B-True, C-False, D-False). Treatment of migraine consists of rest, removal from noxious stimuli, occasional acetaminophen use, and if necessary, antiemetics. Ergotamine alkaloids and isometheptene mucate (Midrin) should be avoided during pregnancy. Narcotic use should be judiciously reserved for the recalcitrant severe cases along with consideration of prophylaxis using propranolol. (*Chapter 12, Page 104.*)

3.71 The patient is a 26-year-old black woman at 8 weeks' gestation of her first pregnancy. She has had a few days of slight vaginal bleeding. Which of the following is/are true?

(A) Threatened abortion occurs in 20 to 25% of all pregnancies.
(B) Half of all women with vaginal bleeding during the first half of pregnancy will abort.
(C) No pelvic examination should be performed because of the risk of causing further bleeding.
(D) The demonstration of fetal life during weeks 6 to 9 is followed by a successful pregnancy in at least 90% of cases.

Answer: (A-True, B-True, C-False, D-True). Threatened abortion (vaginal bleeding during the first half of pregnancy) occurs in 20 to 25% of pregnancies, and half of these women abort. Evaluation includes the hematocrit and an examination for the source of bleeding and any evidence of cervical dilation or expulsion of the products of conception. The ability to differentiate a viable from a nonviable fetus depends on the gestational age and available equipment. Using transvaginal ultrasonography, the gestational sac can be seen at 4 weeks', the yolk sac at 5 weeks', and fetal cardiac activity at 6 weeks' gestation—approximately 1 week earlier for each parameter than when using transabdominal ultrasonography. The demonstration of fetal life during weeks 6 to 9 is followed by a successful outcome in 90 to 100% of cases. (*Chapter 13, Page 107.*)

3.72 Following SA, women who are Rh-negative should

(A) receive $Rh_o(D)$ immunoglobulin to prevent sensitization
(B) receive $Rh_o(D)$ immunoglobulin if there is a positive antibody titer
(C) require no further therapy at this time and should have testing done early in the next pregnancy
(D) receive prednisone 40 to 60 mg/day for 1 week to reduce the risk of sensitization

Answer: (A-True, B-False, C-False, D-False). Following SA, women who are Rh-negative should receive $Rh_o(D)$ immunoglobulin to prevent sensitization. The need for $Rh_o(D)$ in cases of threatened abortion is unclear. If the patient is already sensitized to Rh, $Rh_o(D)$ immunoglobulin will not benefit this patient in subsequent pregnancies. (*Chapter 13, Page 107.*)

3.73 A monoclonal antibody urine pregnancy test is sometimes used in the setting of suspected EP. True statements regarding such use include which of the following?

(A) The test sensitivity is 200 mIU hCG/ml.
(B) The test detects pregnancy within 3 days following conception.
(C) A negative test virtually excludes the diagnosis of EP.
(D) The false-negative rate for detection of pregnancy using this test is approximately 20%.

Answer: (A-True, B-False, C-True, D-False). Once an EP is suspected, laboratory investigation should proceed with a rapid sensitive monoclonal antibody urine pregnancy test. The sensitivity of this hCG assay is 20 mIU/ml, which detects pregnancy at or just prior to the time of expected menses. A negative test virtually excludes the diagnosis of EP, as the false-negative rate for detection of pregnancy using this screening test is approximately 1%. (*Chapter 13, Page 109.*)

3.74 The best primary prevention method(s) to prevent EP is/are to

(A) perform a pelvic examination with tubal insufflation prior to pregnancy
(B) reduce the incidence of STDs and pelvic infection
(C) treat high-risk patients with penicillin during the first 4 weeks of pregnancy
(D) advise patients against becoming pregnant if there is a past history of pelvic inflammatory disease

Answer: (A-False, B-True, C-False, D-False). The most promising avenue for primary prevention of EP is to

reduce the incidence of STDs and pelvic infection. Strategies include patient education and access to condoms, with strong encouragement of their use. Early screening with hCG assays and transvaginal sonography should be performed for women with a history of EP, pelvic infection, pelvic or tubal surgery, or treatment for infertility and current users of intrauterine devices as soon as pregnancy is suspected. (*Chapter 13, Page 109.*)

3.75 Preeclampsia is a pregnancy-specific condition with which of the following characteristics?

(A) increased BP
(B) proteinuria
(C) edema
(D) seizures

Answer: (A-True, B-True, C-True, D-False). Preeclampsia is a pregnancy-specific condition of increased BP accompanied by proteinuria (0.3 g or more during a 24-hour period), edema (clinically evident swelling), or both. BP criteria are either an increase in systolic BP of 30 mm Hg or more or an increase in diastolic BP of 15 mm Hg or more over early values (prepregnancy BP or averaged values obtained before 20 weeks' gestation). If the prior BP is not known, readings of 140/90 mm Hg or higher are considered sufficient to meet the BP criteria for preeclampsia. For women with chronic hypertension, the diagnosis of superimposed preeclampsia is based on the same increase in systolic or diastolic BP plus proteinuria or edema. (*Chapter 13, Page 111.*)

3.76 Risk factors for preeclampsia include

(A) being an African American
(B) twin pregnancy
(C) being an elderly primigravida
(D) previous preeclampsia

Answer: (A-False, B-True, C-False, D-True). The incidence of preeclampsia has been reported at 2.6 to 7.0% of all deliveries. Risk factors for the development of preeclampsia include young age (two- to threefold higher for girls younger than 15 years old), single marital status, previous preeclampsia (especially if the prior episode of preeclampsia was accompanied by the birth of an infant of low birth weight), twin pregnancy (fivefold increased risk), chronic hypertension, pregestational diabetes mellitus, collagen-vascular diseases, large and rapidly growing hydatidiform mole (10-fold increased risk), and a current pregnancy complicated by fetal hydrops. There is also evidence of the tendency for preeclampsia to be inherited. For eclampsia, a maternal age of younger than 20 years was associated with a nearly fivefold greater risk; race and marital status are not associated with increased risk. (*Chapter 13, Page 111.*)

3.77 The HELLP syndrome (intravascular hemolysis, elevated liver enzymes, low platelet count)

  (A) can cause abdominal pain, malaise, and headache
  (B) is associated with a drop in BP during the third trimester or early in labor
  (C) is usually associated with proteinuria
  (D) can cause perinatal mortality of 30 to 40%

Answer: (A-True, B-False, C-True, D-True). Symptoms include epigastric or right upper quadrant pain (90%), malaise (90%), headache (50%), and nausea and vomiting (45 to 86%). Physical findings include diastolic BP greater than 110 mm Hg (68%), edema (55 to 67%), right upper quadrant tenderness (86%), and occasionally hepatosplenomegaly. Urinalysis usually shows proteinuria of more than 2+ (85 to 95%). The importance of early recognition of this syndrome cannot be overemphasized. Maternal mortality is 3.3%, often (38%) associated with DIC. Perinatal mortality is 37%, with 40% of newborns delivered prior to 30 weeks' gestation. (*Chapter 13, Page 112.*)

3.78 In a 17-year-old primigravida woman with preeclampsia, which of the following are worrisome findings?

  (A) proteinuria of 2 g or more in 24 hours
  (B) serum creatine of 1.1 mg/dl
  (C) platelet count of 350,000/ml
  (D) epigastric pain

Answer: (A-True, B-False, C-False, D-True). Although preeclampsia should always be considered a potentially dangerous condition, the following signs are particularly worrisome: (1) systolic BP 160 mm Hg or greater or diastolic BP 110 mm Hg or greater; (2) proteinuria 2 g or more in 24 hours; (3) serum creatinine greater than 1.2 mg/dl; (4) platelet count less than 100,000/ml; (5) elevated liver enzymes; (6) headache or other cerebral or visual disturbance; (7) epigastric pain; (8) retinal hemorrhage or papilledema; and (9) PE. (*Chapter 13, Page 113.*)

3.79 Which of the following are risk factors for PTD and low birth weight?

  (A) maternal age older than 30
  (B) diabetes mellitus
  (C) occupational fatigue and long work hours
  (D) hematocrit greater than 38%

Answer: (A-False, B-True, C-True, D-False). Risk factors associated with PTD and low birth weight include demographic factors such as race (black), age (younger than 19 years), single marital status, and low socioeconomic status; preexisting medical risk factors, including uterine anomalies, incompetent cervix, exposure to DES, low prepregnancy weight for height, more than two induced abortions, and diabetes mellitus; behavioral and psychosocial risk factors, particularly cigarette smoking, poor nutritional status, absent or inadequate prenatal care, a short interpregnancy interval, heavy physical labor, occupational fatigue and long (more than 36 hours/week) work hours, alcohol, illicit drug use (cocaine in particular), and psychological stress; and current pregnancy risk factors such as multiple gestation, severe preeclampsia, infections (particularly of the genital and urinary tract), placenta previa, abruptio placentae, poor third trimester weight gain (less than 0.38 kg/week), fetal malformation, and hematocrit value less than 34%. Among multiparous women, prior PTD carries a recurrence risk of 17 to 37%. (*Chapter 13, Page 115.*)

3.80 The patient is a 28-year-old gravida 3, para 2 black woman in preterm labor (PTL) at 30 weeks' gestation. She will be a candidate for tocolytic therapy if she has which of the following?

  (A) a healthy fetus
  (B) a history of significant vaginal bleeding over the past week
  (C) severe preeclampsia
  (D) cervical dilation of 6 to 7 cm

Answer: (A-True, B-False, C-False, D-False). Women in PTL who are candidates for tocolytic therapy include (1) gestational age between 20 and 34 to 36 weeks; (2) a healthy fetus; (3) no significant vaginal bleeding; (4) no contraindications to prolongation of pregnancy (e.g., severe preeclampsia); (5) no contraindications to the medication; and (6) cervical dilation of less than 4 cm. Gestational age criteria are somewhat controversial, and many institutions do not use tocolysis beyond 34 weeks' gestation. (*Chapter 13, Page 118.*)

3.81 The postdates pregnancy

  (A) is one that lasts more than 42 weeks after the onset of the last menstrual period

(B) occurs in less than 2% of pregnancies
(C) rarely persists beyond 43 weeks of pregnancy
(D) is generally, in reality, a pregnancy that has incorrect dating

Answer: (A-True, B-False, C-False, D-True). The postdates, or postterm, pregnancy is one that lasts more than 42 weeks (294 days) after the onset of the last menstrual period. The postdates pregnancy occurs 3.5 to 12.0% of the time, with one-fourth of these pregnancies lasting beyond 43 weeks. The prolonged pregnancy is one lasting between 41 and 42 weeks. The variation noted in the incidence of the postdates pregnancy is related to inaccurate gestational age dating and irregular ovulation. Studies that have used basal body temperature curves to identify ovulation or routine dating by ultrasound scans at 17 weeks' gestation have found the incidence of the postdates pregnancy to be about 4%. It is clear that most postdates pregnancies are, in reality, pregnancies that have incorrect dating. (*Chapter 14, Page 122.*)

3.82 The patient is a 29-year-old white female college professor who is at 42 weeks' gestation. She has carefully conducted a search on the Internet to seek information regarding her pregnancy. In postdates pregnancy, there is an increased risk of

(A) postmaturity syndrome
(B) fetal malformations
(C) fetal macrosomia
(D) meconium aspiration syndrome

Answer: (A-True, B-True, C-True, D-True). Although studies from the 1960s indicated a twofold increase in the perinatal mortality rate beginning at 42 weeks' and a fourfold increase by 44 weeks' gestation, more recent evidence suggests that the risk of fetal death in the postdates pregnancy monitored by serial NSTs is about two in 1,000. Nevertheless, the postdates pregnancy is associated with an increased rate of postmaturity syndrome, fetal malformations, fetal macrosomia, and meconium aspiration syndrome. (*Chapter 14, Page 122.*)

3.83 The patient is a 22-year-old nulliparous woman at term, who is having protracted active-phase labor and back pain. Examination reveals the infant in an occiput posterior (OP) position. Which of the following statements is/are true regarding management of this condition?

(A) The patient should remain in a supine position until the end of the second stage of labor.
(B) Ambulation may be helpful.

(C) The knee–hands position may be helpful.
(D) Assisted vaginal delivery with the neonate in a persistent OP position should never be attempted.

Answer: (A-False, B-True, C-True, D-False). The nulliparous patient who is experiencing protracted active-phase labor and back pain often has an OP-positioned fetus. If patients are able to tolerate this back pain, ambulation is encouraged. There is preliminary evidence that assuming the knee–hands position may help effect a spontaneous rotation. If the OP persists, an attempt at manual rotation to occiput anterior can be attempted early in stage 2 before significant caput forms. If the fetal vertex descends to a +2 or lower station and appropriate indications arise, an assisted vaginal delivery, keeping the neonate in a persistent OP position, may be attempted. The potential for a "failed" attempt is greater in this situation. (*Chapter 14, Page 124.*)

3.84 Shoulder dystocia during obstetric delivery

(A) is a common occurrence
(B) should be referred to a neonatologist for management
(C) is defined as impaction of the posterior shoulder against the sacrum
(D) is unrelated to fetal weight

Answer: (A-False, B-False, C-False, D-False). Although shoulder dystocia is an uncommon obstetric emergency (occurring in 0.15 to 0.60% of all deliveries), all practitioners should be prepared to manage this potentially devastating delivery complication. Shoulder dystocia is defined as impaction of the anterior shoulder against the symphysis pubis after the fetal head has delivered. The incidence increases with fetal weight, but prediction of macrosomia is of limited assistance for avoiding shoulder dystocia, as more than 50% of cases occur with fetuses weighing less than 4,000 g. Antepartum risk factors include maternal diabetes, maternal obesity and excessive weight gain, narrow anteroposterior diameter on clinical pelvimetry, and a history of previous shoulder dystocia. This complication frequently occurs in low-risk patients. (*Chapter 14, Page 124.*)

3.85 When shoulder dystocia occurs during obstetric delivery,

(A) the response should be made cautiously following obstetric consultation
(B) an institutional protocol should be followed

(C) extra personnel should be notified

(D) newborn resuscitation is unlikely to be needed

Answer: (A-False, B-True, C-True, D-False). Response to this obstetric emergency must be expeditious and deliberate. It is helpful to prepare in advance and develop and practice an institutional protocol. The protocol should include notification of extra personnel, recording the timing and sequence of maneuvers used to resolve the dystocia, and preparation for newborn resuscitation. (*Chapter 14, Page 125.*)

3.86 Which of the following statements is/are true regarding FHR monitoring during labor?

(A) The FHR is under CNS control.

(B) The FHR changes can indicate decreased CNS oxygenation.

(C) Normal FHR varies from 80 to 120 beats per minute (bpm).

(D) FHR variability represents the difference in rate from beat to beat, normally greater than 6 bpm.

Answer: (A-True, B-True, C-False, D-True). The fetal CNS is susceptible to hypoxia. Because the FHR is under CNS control through sympathetic and parasympathetic reflexes, FHR pattern changes can indicate decreased CNS oxygenation or reflex responses. Normally, the baseline FHR can vary from 120 to 160 bpm. Tachycardia (greater than 160 bpm) or bradycardia (less than 120 bpm) can indicate CNS hypoxia. A more important baseline pattern, however, is the variability of the FHR, which represents the difference in rate from beat to beat. Normal FHR variability (greater than 6 bpm) implies that the CNS is adequately oxygenated at the time of observation. (*Chapter 14, Page 125.*)

3.87 During FHR monitoring, the accelerations and decelerations of the FHR can be evaluated by

(A) DeLee stethoscope

(B) Doppler sonography

(C) external electronic monitoring

(D) internal electronic monitoring

Answer: (A-True, B-True, C-True, D-True). These FHR patterns can be evaluated by auscultation (DeLee stethoscope or Doppler sonography) or by electronic monitoring (external or internal). With the advent of liberal use of continuous EFM during the 1970s, there was great hope that intrapartum fetal death and morbidity associated with intrapartum asphyxia could be virtually eliminated. Large retrospective studies using

historical controls were encouraging. It was simply assumed that continuous EFM would be more effective than intermittent auscultation. Numerous prospective randomized controlled trials, however, have not confirmed the original hopes for improved newborn outcomes. (*Chapter 14, Page 126.*)

3.88 Up to 13% of patients who present in PTL have infected amniotic fluid. Which of the following statements is/are true regarding preterm chorioamnionitis?

(A) Labor should be stopped immediately with tocolytic agents.

(B) Broad-spectrum antibiotics should be administered intravenously.

(C) Clindamycin may be used if anaerobic coverage is necessary.

(D) Known carriers of group B *Streptococcus* PTL should have prophylactic administration of penicillin G.

Answer: (A-False, B-True, C-True, D-False). If preterm chorioamnionitis has been diagnosed based on clinical or microbiologic grounds, labor should be allowed to progress. Prompt administration of broad-spectrum antibiotics is recommended, generally ampicillin 2 g IV bolus followed by 1 g q6h and gentamicin 120 to 140 mg loading dose followed by 1.0 to 1.5 mg/kg IV q8h. If anaerobic coverage is deemed necessary, clindamycin 500 to 750 mg q6h can be used. If atypical coverage for *Ureaplasma* or Chlamydia is indicated, erythromycin 1 g IV q6h is administered. The American College of Obstetrician-Gynecologists recommends prophylactic administration of ampicillin in patients with PTL if they are known carriers of group B *Streptococcus* and consideration of empiric treatment if the carrier status is unknown. (*Chapter 14, Page 128.*)

3.89 Chorioamnionitis at term

(A) occurs in about 10% of all term labors

(B) may be associated with colonization with *Neisseria gonorrhoeae* or group B *Streptococcus*

(C) has not been found to be related to repeated vaginal examinations

(D) may be followed by postpartum endometritis

Answer: (A-False, B-True, C-False, D-True). Chorioamnionitis at term occurs in about 1% of all term labors. The following factors are associated with an increased incidence of this condition: colonization with *Neisseria gonorrhoeae* or group B *Streptococcus*, prolonged labor with rupture of membranes, and repetitive vaginal examinations. The microbiologic agents responsible for infection are the same as noted above. This condition is also associated with an increased incidence of dystocia and the need for oxytocin administration. There is an increased incidence of postpartum endometritis, particularly if cesarean intervention is required. (*Chapter 14, Page 128.*)

3.90 Which of the following statements is/are true regarding placental abruption during labor?

(A) Blood products should be immediately available.
(B) Emergency cesarean section should be performed immediately on the diagnosis of placental abruption.
(C) DIC is uncommon in the presence of a viable fetus.
(D) Following delivery, the patient should receive an IV infusion of cryoprecipitate.

Answer: (A-True, B-False, C-True, D-False). The maternal and fetal status must be carefully and continually assessed. Patients are often hemodynamically unstable, and IV access (peripheral and central) is critical to correct hypotension. Blood products should be immediately available. With mild (grade I) abruption without fetal distress, half of the patients safely deliver vaginally. When a nonreassuring FHR tracing is present, an emergency cesarean section is usually necessary, keeping in mind that DIC is uncommon in the presence of a viable fetus. This operative approach results in a lower perinatal mortality rate. In the presence of DIC, expeditious delivery of fetus and placenta should be accompanied by use of blood products and fresh-frozen plasma. Cryoprecipitate is used sparingly because of its potential to carry blood-borne infections. Heparin has not been found to be of use for this form of DIC. (*Chapter 14, Page 129.*)

3.91 Factors associated with placenta previa include

(A) first pregnancy
(B) past history of dilation and curettage
(C) maternal age 19 years and younger
(D) abnormal fetal lie during the third trimester

Answer: (A-False, B-True, C-False, D-True). Placenta previa occurs when the mature placenta covers or is proximate to the internal cervical os. It is seen with 0.4 to 0.6% of all births. It is more common in multiparas and has a recurrence rate of 4 to 8%. One case-control study showed a significant relation between placenta previa and a history of cesarean section, dilation and curettage, SA, and evacuation of retained products of

conception. This point supports the theory that a major reason for a blastocyst implantation situated low in the uterine segment is previous endometrial or myometrial disruption. Other predisposing factors associated with placenta previa include increased maternal age, multiple pregnancy, and abnormal fetal lie during the third trimester. (*Chapter 14, Page 129.*)

3.92 Which of the following is/are true regarding the management of placenta previa?

(A) If bleeding is minimal, bed rest until 37 to 38 weeks' gestation is desirable.
(B) Many women with placenta previa are delivered by 36 weeks' gestation.
(C) The usual mode of delivery is per vagina.
(D) Blood products for transfusion must be readily available.

Answer: (A-True, B-True, C-False, D-True). Once diagnosed, management of this disorder is usually conservative: bed rest until 37 to 38 weeks' gestation so long as there is not enough bleeding to pose a threat to the mother and fetus. Women with a placenta previa are delivered by 36 weeks' gestation 50% of the time. The usual mode of delivery is cesarean section. Marginal and partial previa can sometimes be managed expectantly for a vaginal delivery if preparations are made for an immediate cesarean. The availability of blood products for transfusion is essential for safe management of this condition. (*Chapter 14, Page 129.*)

3.93 During the postpartum period, your patient complains of painful hemorrhoids. Measures to relieve postpartum hemorrhoids include

(A) stool softeners
(B) topical steroids
(C) oxycodone
(D) increased activity

Answer: (A-True, B-True, C-False, D-True). Several measures may help to alleviate early postpartum discomfort. Analgesics ease pain due to uterine cramps or surgical wounds. Perineal pain often responds to such local measures as ice packs, witch hazel, tub baths, or topical anesthesia. Painful hemorrhoids are also relieved by these measures, as well as by stool softeners, topical steroids, dietary fiber, fluids, and increased activity. Severe hemorrhoids that do not improve over time may require surgical excision. (*Chapter 15, Page 131.*)

3.94 Following delivery, women who have had cesarean sections

(A) require additional postoperative care
(B) are at increased risk for endometritis, UTI, and paralytic ileus
(C) are less likely to have postpartum hemorrhage than women who have had a vaginal delivery
(D) should be kept at bed rest for 5 days postpartum

Answer: (A-True, B-True, C-False, D-False). Women who have had cesarean sections require additional postoperative observation and care. They are at increased risk for several problems including endometritis, parametritis, peritonitis, superficial wound infection, UTI, sepsis, pneumonia, paralytic ileus, hemorrhage, PE, and DVT. Measures commonly used to prevent thromboembolic and hemorrhagic complications include early ambulation and postoperative use of oxytocic agents. (*Chapter 15, Page 132.*)

3.95 The patient is a 30-year-old man whose wife delivered their first child 1 month ago. He believes he is experiencing some depressive symptoms. During the first month of the postpartum period, *fathers*

(A) have not been shown to experience noteworthy physical or emotional changes after the arrival of a baby
(B) may exhibit fatigue, irritability, and insomnia
(C) have not been shown to have an increased risk of depression or psychosis
(D) may exhibit fear of death, feelings of rage, and somatic delusions

Answer: (A-False, B-True, C-False, D-True). Although most of the literature on postpartum disorders focuses on problems experienced by mothers, fathers and other children in the family may also wrestle with "postpartum" disturbances. Fathers, like mothers, not uncommonly experience physical and emotional changes after the arrival of a baby. When fathers with newborns are compared with men who do not have newborns, fathers with infants show a greater prevalence of the following symptoms: fatigue, irritability, headaches, difficulty concentrating, insomnia, nervousness, and restlessness. Mental disorders such as depression and psychosis have also been observed in fathers around the time of childbirth, and although symptoms occasionally begin during pregnancy, most childbirth-related psychiatric disturbances in fathers begin or climax after delivery. Other psychological problems that may be experienced by new fathers include impulsive behavioral disturbances, psychosomatic problems, sexual deviance, and borderline syndromes, such as fear of death, feelings of rage, and somatic delusions. (*Chapter 15, Page 136.*)

3.96 The patient is a 23-year-old white woman who is 9 weeks' postpartum. She is concerned by a decrease in sexual activity. Which of the following is/are true regarding her concerns?

(A) A decrease in sexual activity is uncommon during the postpartum period.
(B) A decline in sexual activity during the postpartum period is most commonly related to her partner's disinterest.
(C) Episiotomy discomfort and dyspareunia may be factors.
(D) A useful inquiry may be whether the patient has a decreased sense of attractiveness.

Answer: (A-False, B-False, C-True, D-True). The postpartum period is also characterized by a decrease in sexual activity, which often persists for 1 year or more. Such a decline appears to be related more to the mothers' than to the fathers' disinterest, and this disinterest, in turn, is caused by factors such as episiotomy discomfort, fatigue, vaginal bleeding or discharge, dyspareunia, insufficient lubrication, fears of waking or not hearing the baby, fear of injury, and a decreased sense of attractiveness. (*Chapter 15, Page 136.*)

4

Care of the Infant and Child

The questions in this chapter constitute a review of the following chapters in *Family Medicine: Principles and Practice, Fifth Edition:*

    Genetic Disorders (Chapter 16)
    Problems of the Newborn and Infant (Chapter 17)
    Communicable Diseases of Children (Chapter 18)
    Behavioral Problems of Children (Chapter 19)
    Musculoskeletal Problems in Children (Chapter 20)
    Selected Problems of Infancy and Childhood (Chapter 21)

DIRECTIONS (Items 4.1 through 4.42): Each of the questions or incomplete statements in this section is followed by five suggested answers or completions. Select the ONE that is BEST in each case.

4.1 The most frequent chromosomal disorder is the one associated with

    (A) Down syndrome
    (B) Turner syndrome
    (C) Klinefelter syndrome
    (D) trisomy 18
    (E) cri du chat

Answer: (A). The most frequent chromosome disorder (one of 800 births in the United States) is the one associated with Down syndrome. Down syndrome is caused primarily by nondisjunction during development of the egg, with failure of a chromosome 21 pair to segregate during meiosis. The event is random. Another cause (3 to 4% of cases) is a robertsonian translocation, in which chromosome 21 attaches to another chromosome. Although the amount of genetic material is normal, the number of chromosomes is 45 instead of 46. (*Chapter 16, Page 138.*)

4.2 The most common cause of hypogonadism in males is

    (A) trauma
    (B) undescended testicles
    (C) Klinefelter syndrome
    (D) Turner syndrome
    (E) mumps orchitis

Answer: (C). Klinefelter syndrome is characterized by a 47,XXY karyotype. It has an incidence of 1.7 of 1,000 male infants. The disorder usually is diagnosed at puberty or during an infertility evaluation. In adolescents, its characteristics include gynecomastia (40%), small testicles (less than 2.5 cm long), tall stature, and an arm span that is greater than the person's height. Klinefelter syndrome is the most common cause of hypogonadism in males, with testosterone levels about half the normal value. (*Chapter 16, Page 140.*)

4.3 All the following are dominant genetic disorders EXCEPT

    (A) Marfan syndrome
    (B) Huntington's disease
    (C) neurofibromatosis
    (D) familial hypercholesterolemia
    (E) phenylketonuria

Answer: (E). With classic dominant inheritance, the affected person has a parent with the disorder. The parent usually mates with someone without the genetic disorder, and the offspring have a 50% chance of having the disorder. Typically, predisposition for the disorder is carried on one chromosome, and expression of the disorder is modified by the chromosomal makeup of the other parent. The dominant condition usually does not alter the ability to reproduce but tends to alter materials that provide structure to a body. Examples of dominant disorders include Marfan syndrome, Huntington's disease, neurofibromatosis, achondroplasia, and familial hypercholesterolemia. (*Chapter 16, Page 141.*)

4.4 Some cancer families have a defective gene that is inherited. One example of an inherited defective gene involves

(A) Tay-Sachs disease
(B) Down syndrome
(C) Wegener's granulomatosis
(D) retinoblastoma
(E) prostate cancer

Answer: (D). Certain families have an increased risk for specific cancers. Many of these families have an identifiable gene associated with the disorder. Possession of the gene does not automatically mean that cancer will develop in the patient. Most genes can be altered by environmental factors and by other genes. In some families, a defective gene is inherited, such as for retinoblastoma. (*Chapter 16, Page 143.*)

4.5 Prematurity is associated with all the following EXCEPT

(A) polycythemia of the newborn
(B) hyaline membrane disease (HMD)
(D) apnea of the newborn
(D) jaundice of the infant
(E) intracranial hemorrhage of the infant

Answer: (A). Prematurity is associated with hyaline membrane disease, apnea, jaundice, and intracranial hemorrhage. (*Chapter 17, Page 148.*)

4.6 The empiric initial treatment for neonatal sepsis is

(A) ampicillin plus gentamicin
(B) aqueous penicillin
(C) chloramphenicol
(D) cefixime
(E) sulfamethoxazole plus erythromycin

Answer: (A). Antibiotics should be initiated quickly with a combination of ampicillin (200 mg/kg/day intravenous (IV) or intramuscularly divided b.i.d. for infants during the first week of life, t.i.d. thereafter)

plus gentamicin (2.5 mg/kg per dose b.i.d. for the first week, t.i.d. thereafter). Dosages are reduced for low birth-weight infants or if meningitis is excluded. Antibiotics can be stopped at 48 hours with sterile cultures unless the suspicion for infection was high; treatment is then continued by IV at least 7 days, while monitoring gentamicin levels. If the latter assay is not available, cefotaxime can be used instead of gentamicin. Methicillin should replace ampicillin when starting antibiotics after 3 days of life. Bacteremia is treated for 7 to 10 days depending on the response. Meningitis requires at least 14 days of therapy. (*Chapter 17, Page 148.*)

4.7 The patient is a neonate born preterm and small for gestational age (SGA). The infant has tachypnea, retractions, and cyanosis. Physical examination and testing reveals hypercarbia, hypoxia, and a "ground-glass" radiograph with air bronchograms. The most likely diagnosis is

(A) sepsis
(B) pneumococcal pneumonia
(C) HMD
(D) patent ductus arteriosus
(E) tracheoesophageal fistula

Answer: (C). HMD affects preterm newborns, who manifest "stiff" lungs, hypercarbia, hypoxia, and a "ground-glass" radiograph with air bronchograms. Rapid stabilization and early surfactant therapy improves outcome. Meconium aspiration usually occurs after 34 weeks, causing airway obstruction and edema. Radiography reveals hyperinflation and possibly pneumothorax. After resuscitation, aggressive support with ventilation and oxygen should maintain the PO_2 above 80 mm Hg. Sepsis workup and antibiotic coverage are indicated for HMD and meconium aspiration because the risk of pneumonia is increased. (*Chapter 17, Page 148.*)

4.8 A loud murmur during the first 24 hours of life

(A) is a normal finding in up to half of all newborns
(B) is considered benign
(C) should be evaluated only if accompanied by cyanosis or respiratory distress
(D) suggests valvular stenosis or regurgitation
(E) is characteristic of HMD

Answer: (D). Soft benign murmurs are common during the first 24 hours of life, but loud murmurs suggest valvular stenosis or regurgitation. Murmurs of cardiac shunts may be heard at 72 hours but more often at 2 to 3 weeks. Loud murmurs, abnormal heart sounds, or findings suggesting cardiac disease (i.e., cyanosis, poor color or feeding, tachycardia, bradycardia, abnormal blood pressure, respiratory distress, or hepatomegaly) necessitate a prompt electrocardiogram, chest radiograph, and if pathology is suspected, cardiology consultation. All neonates require careful auscultation at the 2-week visit. (*Chapter 17, Page 149.*)

4.9 Jaundice in the newborn during the first 24 hours of life

(A) should be rechecked on day 2
(B) is found in 40% of normal newborns
(C) requires prompt evaluation
(D) should be evaluated with a serum bilirubin level ordered for the routine blood draw the following morning
(E) is usually due to breast-feeding

Answer: (C). Jaundice during the first 24 hours of life requires prompt evaluation and consideration for exchange transfusion if hemolysis is found. (*Chapter 17, Page 149.*)

4.10 A central venous hematocrit value less than 45% in the neonate delivered at 34 weeks is most likely due to

(A) hemolysis
(B) blood loss
(C) congenital anemia
(D) hypoglycemia
(E) postmaturity

Answer: (B). A central venous hematocrit value less than 45% in newborns delivered after 34 weeks' gestation is often caused by blood loss and less often by hemolysis or congenital anemias. Careful review of the history, physical examination, red blood cell indices, and peripheral smear can guide further evaluation. Coombs' test, reticulocyte count, and Kleihauer-Betke stain of maternal blood to look for fetomaternal transfusion may be needed. Shock requires repeated 5-ml/kg infusions over 5 minutes of cross-matched or O-negative blood until symptoms are alleviated. Severe hemolysis may require exchange transfusion. (*Chapter 17, Page 150.*)

4.11 The patient is a 6-week-old female infant born to a mother who is human immunodeficiency virus (HIV)-positive. This infant should

(A) be followed with serial HIV tests
(B) be placed in an isolation nursery
(C) be treated with trimethoprim plus sulfamethoxazole to prevent *Pneumocystis carinii* pneumonia (PCP)

(D) be treated with zidovudine for 1 year
(E) be observed and reevaluated next at 12 weeks of age

Answer: (C). Prevention of PCP is one of the most important goals of HIV management. Thus all infants 6 weeks to 1 year of age born to HIV-positive mothers or who prove to be HIV infected themselves should receive prophylaxis with 150 mg of trimethoprim plus 750 mg sulfamethoxazole/m² body surface/day divided twice daily and given 3 days weekly. If HIV infection can later be reasonably excluded, PCP prophylaxis can be discontinued. (*Chapter 17, Page 151.*)

4.12 Breast milk feeding of the infant

(A) is no longer the preferred form of infant feeding
(B) is less digestible than infant formula
(C) allows the infant to share the mother's immunity to pathogens
(D) causes an increased incidence of gastrointestinal reactions
(E) has been associated with an increased risk of otitis media in the infant

Answer: (C). Breast milk is the preferred form of sustenance for newborns and young infants because of its better digestibility and enhancement of infant immunity. Breast-feeding allows the infant to share the mother's immunity to the pathogens present in the community at any given time. It also results in significant reductions in the incidence of gastrointestinal infections and otitis media as well as perhaps other respiratory infections. Although two of the principal immunologic factors have their highest concentrations in the colostrum, the immunologic protection increases with the duration of breast-feeding and is greatest for serious and persistent infections. (*Chapter 17, Page 154.*)

4.13 Failure to thrive (FTT) during infancy

(A) is defined as failure to achieve three or more developmental milestones
(B) may lead to permanent cognitive defects
(C) has a low incidence in rural areas
(D) has not been found to be associated with later behavioral disorders
(E) is not associated with short stature later in life

Answer: (B). FTT can be defined as failure to grow at an appropriate rate, with weight crossing two major channels on the National Center for Health Statistics (NCHS) growth curve or falling below the 5th percentile for age and sex after correcting for parents' stature, prematurity, or growth retardation at birth. Because of a high prevalence of FTT in urban and rural areas (5 to 10%) and significant morbidity (developmental delay, permanent cognitive deficits, behavioral disorders, short stature, chronic physical problems, and medical illness), it is advisable to begin following any child whose weight declines across one NCHS channel or if a parent suspects a growth problem. (*Chapter 17, Page 156.*)

4.14 The leading cause of infant death past the neonatal period and peaking at age 2 months is

(A) sudden infant death syndrome (SIDS)
(B) bronchiolitis
(C) croup
(D) accidental injury
(E) retinoblastoma

Answer: (A). SIDS is the leading cause of death for infants past the neonatal period, peaking at age 2 months. Characterized by being unexpected and without an apparent cause, despite thorough postmortem examination, it represents a collection of etiologies involving an abnormality of cardiorespiratory regulation. (*Chapter 17, Page 159.*)

4.15 The major cause of bronchiolitis and pneumonia in young children is

(A) respiratory syncytial virus (RSV)
(B) *Streptococcus pneumoniae*
(C) group A beta-hemolytic *Streptococcus*
(D) ECHO virus
(E) *Haemophilus influenzae*

Answer: (A). RSV is the major cause of bronchiolitis and pneumonia in young children, with outbreaks occurring yearly during the winter and early spring. When an outbreak occurs, RSV tends to dominate infant and small child illnesses in a community, seeming to brush aside the activity of other respiratory viruses. An abrupt increase in bronchiolitis and pediatric pneumonia in a community suggests RSV infection, which may be confirmed by performing viral cultures or rapid diagnostic tests in initial cases. Naturally acquired immunity to RSV is incomplete, and repeated infections are common, although the primary encounter generally results in the most severe illness. (*Chapter 18, Page 166.*)

4.16 Kawasaki disease (mucocutaneous lymph node syndrome)

(A) is an acute gastroenteritis
(B) primarily affects middle-aged adults

(C) occurs most commonly in patients of lower socioeconomic class
(D) occurs most commonly during the winter months
(E) has shown no evidence of person-to-person spread

Answer: (E). Kawasaki disease (mucocutaneous lymph node syndrome) is an acute vasculitis that primarily affects infants and young children. It must be included in the differential diagnosis of fever, cervical adenitis, acute exanthems, and other mucocutaneous diseases. The etiology is unknown; but infectious, antigenic, and environmental agents are suggested as primary causes or cofactors. There are no known socioeconomic or climatic risk factors and no evidence of person-to-person spread. Most cases occur in children younger than 5 years; it is rare under 6 months, and the male/female ratio is 1.5:1.0. It is worldwide and most prevalent in persons of Asian descent. The recurrence rate is 3%, and the rate of disease in siblings is 1 to 2%. (*Chapter 18, Page 167.*)

4.17 The most common identifiable cause of acute childhood diarrhea in the United States is

(A) viral gastroenteritis
(B) giardiasis
(C) milk-borne toxins
(D) *Escherichia coli*
(E) lactose intolerance

Answer: (A). Viral gastroenteritis is the most common identifiable cause of acute childhood diarrhea in the United States, with rotavirus the most frequent agent in young children. Annual rotavirus epidemics begin in Mexico during late fall and progress systematically across the continent, reaching the Northeast by spring. Nosocomial and daycare outbreaks are common. (*Chapter 18, Page 168.*)

4.18 The natural host of the pinworm *Enterobius vermicularis* is

(A) clothing containing particles of feces
(B) cats
(C) humans
(D) pigs
(E) dogs

Answer: (C). Humans are the only natural host of the pinworm *Enterobius vermicularis*, a 1-cm white, threadlike helminth responsible for millions of infections in the United States. It is most common in school-age children, regardless of socioeconomic status, and is most prevalent among family members, in institutions, and in areas of crowding. (*Chapter 18, Page 169.*)

4.19 In the management of attention deficit/hyperactivity disorder (AD/HD), psychostimulant medications

- (A) are beneficial in up to 25% of patients
- (B) are risky and should be used with caution
- (C) cause numerous side effects in the majority of patients
- (D) are postulated to cause increased arousal in the areas of the brain that control impulses and attention
- (E) work by decreasing availability of dopamine and norepinephrine

Answer: (D). The psychostimulant medications are beneficial in 70 to 80% of patients with AD/HD. Stimulants are remarkably safe, have few side effects, and have not been shown to result in persisting adverse effects. The mechanism of action is postulated to be increased arousal in the areas of the brain that control impulses and attention. Increased availability of dopamine and norepinephrine normalizes the patients' behavior while the medication is in the circulation. (*Chapter 19, Page 175.*)

4.20 The patient is an 8-year-old child who has recently been found to have AD/HD. His behavior in class and at home is highly disruptive. You and the family have decided to use a treatment plan that includes medication. An appropriate initial prescription would be

- (A) dextroamphetamine (Dexedrine) 10 g t.i.d.
- (B) propranolol (Inderal) 20 mg t.i.d.
- (C) imipramine (Tofranil) 100 mg at bedtime
- (D) methylphenidate (Ritalin) 5 mg twice daily
- (E) pemoline (Cylert) 75 mg twice daily

Answer: (D). The stimulant medication used most often is methylphenidate (Ritalin), which has a duration of action of 3 to 5 hours. The methylphenidate dose is usually initiated at 5 mg twice each day, before breakfast and before lunch. The child's behavior is closely monitored; if problems continue, the dose is increased slowly up to a maximum daily dose of 0.6 mg/kg. Many children require a dose of 10 or 20 mg twice each day. This second dose is usually given after lunch, but it can be problematic for teachers and administrators or cause a stigma to the student. The sustained release form of methylphenidate may be helpful for children who need higher doses but have difficulty taking medication at school. This long-acting formulation has the same bioavailability as the regular tablet, with slower absorption. (*Chapter 19, Page 175.*)

4.21 Children with conduct disorders may exhibit all EXCEPT which one of the following?

- (A) respect for the rights of others
- (B) aggression toward people or animals
- (C) property destruction
- (D) lying
- (E) running away from home

Answer: (A). Conduct disorders are some of the most common behavioral problems of children. Up to 50% of patients younger than 18 receiving outpatient psychiatric care have a conduct disorder diagnosis. The defining feature is a persistent behavior pattern involving violation of others' rights and the failure to abide by socially accepted rules. Conduct disordered children and adolescents usually exhibit at least one of the following symptom clusters: (1) aggression toward people or animals (or both); (2) property destruction (i.e., vandalism); (3) lying ("conning" others or theft); (4) serious violations of rules such as multiple school truancies or running away from home overnight. (*Chapter 19, Page 177.*)

4.22 A young couple bring their 9-year-old daughter with a recurrent "tic" involving the muscles around the right eye. The symptoms have been present for about 6 weeks. Which of the following is true regarding transient tic disorder?

- (A) Transient tic disorder is an early stage of Tourette syndrome.
- (B) These disorders occur at some time in about 25% of children.
- (C) The tics rarely subside without therapy.
- (D) Behavior modification is ineffective in therapy.
- (E) The cornerstone of treatment of transient tic disorder is muscle relaxant medication.

Answer: (B). Transient tic disorders occur at some time in about 25% of children. Some parents are upset or aggravated by these nervous habits, but the tics often fade if ignored. When treatment is required, the principles of behavior modification are important. Relaxation training, self-monitoring, and habit reversal have all been studied for transient tic disorder, with varying success. (*Chapter 19, Page 179.*)

4.23 You are finishing the examination of a 5-year-old child whose mother complains that he has severe temper tantrums. For the parents, the key to management of this problems is

(A) recognition that temper tantrums represent deliberate misbehavior
(B) firm physical discipline when misbehavior occurs
(C) reliance on techniques based on the parents' own upbringing
(D) understanding and practicing consistency
(E) maintaining flexibility while avoiding setting limits for the child

Answer: (D). These stages of behavioral development are important for the child and the parent to weather. Parents must learn that temper tantrums are not deliberate misbehavior but the way children test their limits. The children must be given rules and discipline, but the parents must avoid emotionally demeaning actions and harsh physical discipline. Child-rearing practices are rarely formally taught. Parents often rely on techniques based on their own upbringing. The family physician's office often permits direct observation of inappropriate discipline. The parents' goal is, of course, to change the child's behavior, which is done by explaining behavior modification in terms appropriate to the parent. The most important practice for parents is to understand consistency. They must set and maintain limits for the child and have clear consequences for any misbehavior. (*Chapter 19, Page 180.*)

4.24 The most common cause of significant sleep disturbance during the first year of life is

(A) colic
(B) reaction to immunizations
(C) food allergies
(D) common cold
(E) a room that is too hot or too cold

Answer: (A). Colic is probably the most common cause of significant sleep disturbance during the first year of life. Frequently, the colicky infant is overly sensitive to the surroundings or stimulation. Chaos in their environment is unpleasant, and they respond by crying. (*Chapter 19, Page 181.*)

4.25 The most common orthopedic condition in the pediatric age group is

(A) rotational problems resulting in gait abnormalities
(B) fractures of long bones

(C) dislocations, especially of the elbow
(D) subluxations of the patella
(E) idiopathic scoliosis

Answer: (A). Rotational problems resulting in gait abnormalities are the most common orthopedic conditions in the pediatric age group. Parents are frequently concerned that their child will grow up deformed or be unable to play sports as they observe in-toeing or out-toeing and seek medical attention. (*Chapter 20, Page 183.*)

4.26 At the 6-week visit, you notice that the infant has flexible metatarsus adductus (MA). You should recommend which of the following treatment to the parents?

(A) passively correcting the range of deformity with each diaper change
(B) casting
(C) Pavlik harness
(D) surgery
(E) corrective shoes with metarsal pads

Answer: (A). Treatment for flexible MA involves having the parents passively correct the range of deformity (as described above) with each diaper change. Straight shoes do not correct a deformed foot but are sometimes used along with passive stretching by the parents as a sort of "milieu therapy" for mild cases. Rushforths reported that 86% of flexible MA feet normalize or have a mild residual deformity after 7 years, and 10% are moderately deformed but asymptomatic. (*Chapter 20, Page 184.*)

4.27 The preferred management for internal tibial torsion is usually

(A) braces
(B) reassurance
(C) splints
(D) twister cables
(E) orthopedic shoes

Answer: (B). Correction is almost always spontaneous. Bracing, splints, twister cables, and shoe modifications have not been shown to be effective and are not recommended, as most of these deformities correct spontaneously by 3 to 4 years of age. (*Chapter 20, Page 185.*)

4.28 Clinical characteristics of clubfoot include all but which of the following?

(A) talar plantar flexion
(B) pes planus

(C) hindfoot varus
(D) forefoot adduction
(E) soft tissue contractures

Answer: (B). Talipes equinovarus (clubfoot), which occurs in approximately one per 1,000 births, is characterized by talar planter flexion, hindfoot varus, forefoot adduction, and soft tissue contractures, resulting in a cavus foot deformity. (*Chapter 20, Page 187.*)

4.29 The initial treatment of clubfoot in the infant is

(A) observation
(B) passive stretching
(C) casting
(D) Pavlik harness
(E) corrective shoes

Answer: (C). Proper intervention involves reduction of the displaced navicular on the head of the talus and mobilization of tight capsules and tendons through manipulation followed by placement in a series of carefully molded corrective casts. The need for extensive surgery is reduced if casting is early and effective. Operative intervention is indicated if complete correction cannot be obtained or maintained. Recognition and treatment of clubfoot deformity should be initiated in the newborn nursery; therefore recognition and referral of this entity are imperative. (*Chapter 20, Page 187.*)

4.30 The patient is a 3-year-old child who has been in the care of a 12-year-old baby-sitter who plays vigorously with the child. There is no history of trauma and no complaints of pain, yet the child refuses to use the left arm. She holds her arm at the side with the elbow slightly flexed and the forearm is pronated. The most likely diagnosis is

(A) radial head subluxation at the elbow
(B) fracture of the clavicle
(C) torus fracture of the distal tibia
(D) supracondylar fracture of the humerus
(E) dislocation of the shoulder

Answer: (A). The child with a radial head subluxation presents by refusing to use the affected limb but may not complain of pain. Often the shoulder is suspected to be the culprit. At presentation, the arm is held at the side with elbow partially flexed and the forearm pro-rated. Clinical findings include tenderness to palpation over the radial head and decreased range of motion at the elbow. Radiographs may show soft tissue swelling but are usually negative. Although the elbow is a com-monly injured joint in children, interpretation of the radiograph may be difficult owing to joint anatomy. Because the radial epiphysis is not ossified, subluxation is diagnosed on clinical grounds. (*Chapter 20, Page 188.*)

4.31 The treatment of radial head subluxation of the elbow in a young child is

(A) casting in the position of function
(B) reduction with the child sitting in the parent's lap
(C) observation
(D) surgery
(E) use of a sling to rest the injured extremity

Answer: (B). Reduction of the radial head is possible if the proximal edge of the annular ligament does not extend beyond the widest part of the radial head. Reduction of the annular ligaments is achieved by supination of the forearm, flexion of the elbow, and simultaneous pressure over the radial head. This maneuver is also achieved when manipulating the elbow to obtain an anteroposterior roentgenogram. An audible click may be heard with reduction, associated with significant relief. Often the arm can be used immediately after reduction. Immobilization is not necessary. (*Chapter 20, Page 188.*)

4.32 The most common disorder causing a limp in children is

(A) Legg-Calvé-Perthes disease (LCPD)
(B) Osgood-Schlatter disease
(C) transient synovitis of the hip (TSH)
(D) trauma
(E) apophysitis of the hip

Answer: (C). TSH, a self-limited unilateral disease of unknown etiology, is the most common disorder causing a limp in children. TSH is most common between the ages of 2 and 10 years (average, 6 years) and occurs more frequently in boys. The condition often parallels or follows a viral upper respiratory infection and has been considered by some to represent a viral or perhaps "viral-immune response" disorder affecting the hip. The few biopsies reported for this benign transitory disease have revealed only nonspecific inflammatory congestion and hypertrophy of the synovial membrane. (*Chapter 20, Page 189.*)

4.33 The patient is a 10-month-old infant with a temperature of 102°F. He holds the thigh in a position of flexion, abduction and external rotation, and cries

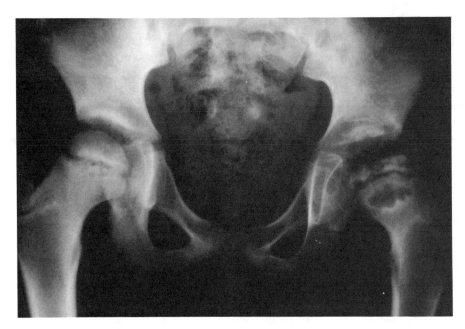

Fig. 4.1. Question 4.37. (From Lillegard W, Kruse R. In Taylor RB, editor. *Family Medicine: Principles and Practice.* 4th ed. New York: Springer-Verlag, 1993. With permission.)

vigorously with any attempt of movement with the right hip. The mother describes a recent history of middle ear infection treated a week ago; she stopped the antibiotic therapy after 2 days when the child appeared improved. The mostly like diagnosis is

(A) reoccurrence of the ear infection
(B) septic hip
(C) cellulitis of the thigh
(D) congenital dislocation of the hip
(E) sciatic nerve palsy

Answer: (B). A septic hip is considered a medical emergency, as surgical drainage of pus soon after onset of symptoms prevents destruction of the femoral head and neck. Accumulating fluid and pus containing destructive enzymes rapidly elevate the intra-articular pressure and permanently injure vessels and articular cartilage. Microorganisms usually enter the hip joint by bacteremia, the result of distant infection (skin or subcutaneous abscess, otitis media, pharyngitis, pneumonia, or umbilical infection). In neonates, nosocomial infection may occur via catheters or venipuncture. (*Chapter 20, Page 189.*)

4.34 The most common serious disorder of the hip in adolescents is

(A) hip pointer
(B) slipped capital femoral epiphysis (SCFE)
(C) LCPD

(D) developmental dysplasia of the hip
(E) TSH

Answer: (B). SCFE is the most common serious disorder of the hip in adolescents. The peak age incidence is 11 years for girls and 14 years for boys; the incidence in the general population is approximately two per 100,000. SCFE is characterized by sudden or gradual anterior displacement of the femoral neck from the capital femoral epiphysis. The epiphysis remains in the acetabulum, resulting in a retroversion deformity of the femoral neck. The goals of treatment for a patient with an SCFE are to stabilize the slip and prevent further displacement while avoiding the complications of avascular necrosis, chondrolysis, and early osteoarthritis. (*Chapter 20, Page 190.*)

4.35 The patient is a newborn found on physical examination to have positive Barlow and Ortolani tests. This patient might reasonably be treated with

(A) parental instructions regarding stretching exercises
(B) Pavlik-type harness
(C) spica cast
(D) orthopedic shoes
(E) observation with repeat examination in 6 weeks

Answer: (B). Neonatal hip instability or dislocation can be treated with a Pavlik-type harness, with 85 to 90% success in infants up to 6 to 8 months of age. This harness holds the infant's hips in a flexed and abducted position, directing the femoral head into the developing acetabulum. Pavlik harness use requires close ultrasound or radiographic monitoring and frequent clinical follow-up. Most hips stabilize after 2 to 3 months. Dislocated hips diagnosed at 6 to 18 months of age require closed or open surgical reduction under anesthesia, followed by spica cast immobilization. (*Chapter 20, Page 191.*)

4.36 LCPD is

(A) avascular necrosis of the femoral head
(B) subluxation of the patella
(C) synonymous with SCFE
(D) a common sports injury
(E) a reducible subluxation of the hip

Answer: (A). LCPD is avascular necrosis of the femoral head in otherwise clinically normal children. LCPD typically presents between 4 and 8 years of age, with the boy/girl ratio approximately 5:1. Interesting parallels exist between LCPD and "constitutional delay of growth." Children with LCPD are often small for age, thin, and hyperactive, with bone age that is delayed by 1 to 2 years. Age at onset is an important indicator of outcome; children younger than 5 years of age often do well without specific treatment, whereas children more than 10 years develop more severe avascular necrosis and do poorly no matter how well they are treated. (*Chapter 20, Page 191.*)

4.37 The child whose radiograph is shown above has

(A) subluxation of the hip
(B) fracture of the left hip
(C) LCPD
(D) osteomyelitis of the hip
(E) congenital dislocation of the hip

Answer: (C). The radiograph shows severe changes of the left femoral head due to LCPD. (*Chapter 20, Page 192.*)

4.38 Eighty percent of cases of osteochondritis dissecans occur

(A) in the capital femoral epiphysis
(B) at the calcaneal-talar joint
(C) on the lateral aspect of the medial femoral condyle
(D) on the tibial tubercle
(E) on the posterior fibular condyle

Answer: (C). Osteochondritis dissecans is characterized by separation of a fragment of bone with overlying articular cartilage from the surrounding normal bone. More than 80% of cases occur on the lateral aspect of the medial femoral condyle (*Chapter 20, Page 194.*)

4.39 The most common autosomal chromosomal disorder causing mental retardation is

(A) Down syndrome
(B) trisomy 13
(C) Huntington's disease
(D) Tay-Sachs disease
(E) neural tube defect

Answer: (A). Down syndrome is the most common autosomal chromosomal disorder causing mental retardation. (*Chapter 21, Page 199.*)

4.40 Screening for lead poisoning is done by

(A) blood lead levels
(B) urinary lead levels
(C) cerebrospinal fluid lead levels
(D) screening radiography
(E) serial stool specimens

Answer: (A). Screening is done by determining blood lead levels. Children who regularly reside in houses built before 1960, have siblings with a history of lead poisoning, or live with adults whose jobs or hobbies involve exposure to lead are considered at high risk. They should have their initial screening done at 6 months of age, and children at low risk should begin at 12 months of age. (*Chapter 21, Page 201.*)

4.41 The major cause of death in children 0 to 19 years of age is

(A) acquired immunodeficiency syndrome
(B) motor vehicle accidents
(C) meningitis
(D) cancer
(E) croup

Answer: (B). Injuries to motor vehicle occupants are the major cause of death in children up to 19 years old. (*Chapter 21, Page 202.*)

4.42 The patient is a 7-year-old boy who has passed his feces into his underwear once every 2 to 3 days for about 12 months. This patient mostly likely

(A) has encopresis

(B) has Hirschsprung's disease
(C) has a congenital neurologic defect
(D) has hyperthyroidism
(E) meets DSM IV criteria for a type of conduct disorder

Answer: (A). Encopresis is the regular, voluntary or involuntary passage of feces into inappropriate places (e.g., underwear) by a child who is developmentally 4 years of age or older. *Primary* encopresis occurs when the child has not been continent of stool for at least 1 year. *Secondary* encopresis is present when fecal incontinence occurs after the child has been continent for at least 1 year. Encopresis is four to five times more common among boys, and secondary encopresis accounts for 50 to 60% of cases. Organic causes of soiling, such as inflammatory bowel disease, hypothyroidism, hypercalcemia, and aganglionic megacolon, should be excluded. (*Chapter 21, Page 205.*)

DIRECTIONS (Items 4.43 through 4.91): Each of the items in this section is a multiple true–false problem that consists of a stem and four lettered options. Indicate whether each of the four options is TRUE or FALSE.

4.43 The patient is a 41-year-old white primigravida woman who is concerned about the possibility of Down syndrome. She asks for more information about the syndrome. Which of the following is/are true?

(A) Cardiac abnormalities occur in up to 5% of Down syndrome patients.
(B) Other congenital conditions are often present.
(C) Intellectual development usually plateaus at the level of the first or second grade.
(D) Most children are able to leave home and live independently as adults.

Answer: (A-False, B-True, C-False, D-True). During a discussion about children with Down syndrome, important points that should be made include the 33% chance of cardiac abnormalities, the presence of other congenital conditions, intellectual development to the level of the third to ninth grade, and the ability of most children to leave home and live independently as adults. (*Chapter 16, Page 139.*)

4.44 You have just delivered a newborn infant of a 43-year-old mother. This is her second child. Her first delivery 10 years ago was normal and produced a healthy infant. Because of her age you are worried about the possibility of Down syndrome. You should examine the infant for which of the following findings?

(A) hypotonia
(B) epicanthal folds
(C) narrow nasal bridge
(D) a wide space between the first two toes

Answer: (A-True, B-True, C-False, D-True). At birth, a child with Down syndrome is identified on the basis of the following physical examination findings: hypotonia, craniofacial features of brachycephaly, oblique palpebral fissures, epicanthal folds, broad nasal bridge, protruding tongue, and low-set ears. The children may display Brushfield's spots, short broad fingers, a single flexion crease in the hand (the so-called simian crease, which 30% of children with Down syndrome and about 5% of normal children have), and a wide space between the first two toes. (*Chapter 16, Page 139.*)

4.45 Turner syndrome

(A) involves errors in one of the Y chromosomes
(B) involves errors in one of the X chromosomes
(C) may be associated with a webbed neck
(D) is characterized by tall stature

Answer: (A-False, B-True, C-True, D-False). Turner syndrome has an incidence of about one per 2,000 births. The syndrome involves errors in one of the X chromosomes, such as the absence of one X chromosome (60% of cases), a structural abnormality of an X chromosome (20% of cases), or mosaicism involving the X chromosome of at least one cell line (20% of cases). Fetal lymphedema may cause a webbing of the neck, a low posterior hair line, and auricular malrotation. Failure of growth occurs in virtually all patients with Turner syndrome. (*Chapter 16, Page 140.*)

4.46 Cystic fibrosis

(A) is a recessive disorder affecting nearly 30,000 persons in the United States
(B) carriers generally have a strong family history of the disease
(C) is diagnosed during the first year of life in the majority of patients
(D) is diagnosed based on the concentration of chloride in serum

Answer: (A-True, B-False, C-True, D-False). A recessive disorder currently discussed widely is cystic fibrosis. Nearly 30,000 people in the United States have this disorder. It is carried by about one in 25 whites in the United States, and these carriers often do not have a family history of cystic fibrosis. The clinical characteristics of cystic fibrosis include pancreatic insufficiency (85% of patients), pulmonary disease characterized by recurrent infections and bronchiectasis, and failure to grow. In more than 60% of patients, the diagnosis is made during the first year of life. It is of interest that the diagnosis is made in 5% of patients after age 15. The diagnosis is based on the concentration of chloride in sweat being greater than 60 mEq/L and clinical suspicion of the disease. (*Chapter 16, Page 142.*)

4.47 Genetic screening for cystic fibrosis is

(A) not effective in detecting carriers
(B) recommended in preconception care for patients with a family history of cystic fibrosis
(C) recommended in preconception care for partners of patients with a family history of cystic fibrosis
(D) can detect 85% of cystic fibrosis carriers

Answer: (A-False, B-True, C-True, D-True). Testing is recommended for patients with a family history of cystic fibrosis and their partners. There are more than 150 mutations of the cystic fibrosis gene, and testing can detect 85% of the carriers. (*Chapter 16, Page 142.*)

4.48 BRCA1, a tumor suppressor gene,

(A) accounts for up to 10% of all cases of breast cancer
(B) accounts for at least 50% of all cases of colorectal cancer
(C) is an autosomal dominant gene
(D) cannot be detected by current tests

Answer: (A-True, B-False, C-True, D-False). BRCA1, a tumor suppressor gene, accounts for 5 to 10% of all cases of breast cancer. It is autosomal dominant. A woman from a family prone to breast or ovarian cancer who carries certain mutations of BRCA1 has about an 80% chance that breast cancer will develop and a 40 to 60% chance of ovarian cancer. Members of a family with multiple cases of breast or ovarian cancer can be tested to determine if they have a genetic alteration in BRCA1. (*Chapter 16, Page 143.*)

4.49 Basic resuscitation skills for a depressed newborn include

(A) controlling the thermal environment
(B) positioning, suctioning, and tactile stimulation
(C) umbilical vein catheterization
(D) suctioning of meconium through an endotracheal tube

Answer: (A-True, B-True, C-False, D-True). Basic resuscitation skills for a depressed newborn include (1) con-

trolling the thermal environment with proper use of a radiant warmer and rapid thorough drying; (2) positioning, suctioning, and gentle tactile stimulation; (3) catheter suctioning of meconium from the airway on the perineum followed by gentle bulb syringe suctioning after delivery, as well as tracheal suctioning of thick or particulate meconium through an endotracheal tube (repeat until clear unless the neonate is overly distressed); and (4) providing immediate bag and mask ventilation for newborns with apnea or poor respiratory effort. (*Chapter 17, Page 146.*)

4.50 Following newborn resuscitation, postresuscitation priorities include

(A) assessment for emergent anomalies
(B) pulse oximetry and cardiorespiratory monitoring
(C) maintaining oxygen saturation at 60 to 70%
(D) breast- or bottle-feeding initiated within 2 hours to maintain nutrition

Answer: (A-True, B-True, C-False, D-False). Postresuscitation priorities include assessment for emergent anomalies, maintenance of basic needs, effective communication with and support of the family, and deciding on the level of care required. Pulse oximetry and a cardiorespiratory monitor are used to monitor ongoing success. Oxygen saturations should be kept at 88 to 92% for preterm newborns and 92 to 95% for term newborns. Baseline tests for unstable newborns include a chest radiograph, complete blood count, glucose, and blood gases (arterial if possible, otherwise capillary). A sepsis workup and other laboratory tests may then be considered. Ventilatory support is needed for persistent respiratory distress, apnea, or deteriorating blood gases (especially PCO_2 greater than 60 with acidosis). Feedings should then be avoided and a nasogastric tube placed. IV fluids are started with 10% dextrose in water (slow) at 65 to 80 ml/kg/day for the first 24 hours. Timely transport of unstable or high-risk neonates for tertiary care enhances outcome (e.g., early surfactant therapy for HMD). (*Chapter 17, Pages 146–147.*)

4.51 The patient is a 23-year-old white woman at 41.5 weeks' gestation. She is concerned that her infant will be post-term and wants to know what the effect might be on the infant. Post-term infants may have which of the following?

(A) abundant lanugo and vernix
(B) scaly skin
(C) decreased alertness

4. Care of the Infant and Child 55

(D) small for gestational age (SGA)

Answer: (A-False, B-True, C-False, D-True). After 42 weeks' gestation, there may be absent lanugo and vernix, long nails, scaly skin, abundant scalp hair, and increased alertness. Some are large and at risk for birth trauma and asphyxia; others are SGA due to placental insufficiency with risks as described above. (*Chapter 17, Page 148.*)

4.52 Neonatal sepsis

(A) is often accompanied by nonspecific signs and symptoms
(B) is a diagnosis that is apparent to experienced observers
(C) occurs more commonly following preterm labor and premature rupture of the membranes
(D) is accompanied by a temperature elevation greater than 37.8°C in at least 90% of instances

Answer: (A-True, B-False, C-True, D-False). Sepsis is often accompanied by nonspecific signs and symptoms, making early detection difficult: two per 1,000 neonates have bacterial sepsis. Risk increases with preterm labor, premature rupture of membranes, or intrapartum fever. Group B *Streptococcus* and *Escherichia coli* are responsible for 70% of the infections and *Listeria monocytogenes*, enterococcus, *Staphylococcus aureus*, and *Haemophilus influenzae* for the rest. Early manifestations include temperature instability, lethargy, and poor feeding. Only about 50% have a temperature higher than 37.8°C (100°F) axillary. (*Chapter 17, Page 148.*)

4.53 The patient is a newborn girl who is 48 hours old. The parents have noticed that the child appears "yellow." Which of the following statements is/are true regarding neonatal jaundice?

(A) Jaundice is noted in at least half of white newborns.
(B) The total serum bilirubin (TSB) threshold for kernicterus seems to be 15 to 18 mg/dl.
(C) The TSB threshold level leading to kernicterus is lower in sick premature neonates.
(D) Earlier discharge of mothers and neonates has lowered the risk of kernicterus.

Answer: (A-True, B-False, C-True, D-False). Jaundice is noted in at least 50% of white newborns, with 6% having TSB levels more than 12.9 mg/dl. Higher levels are noted in Asian and Native American newborns. Kernicterus leading to death or severe neurologic handicap is pre-

ventable if bilirubin levels do not exceed 25 to 30 mg/dl (lower in sick premature neonates). Early discharge may contribute to delayed recognition of high TSB levels and a resurgence of kernicterus. (*Chapter 17, Page 149.*)

4.54 Physiologic jaundice of the newborn

(A) is uncommon
(B) typically represents unconjugated hyperbilirubinemia
(C) reaches an average peak of 14 mg/dl by day 3
(D) resolves within 1 week in term infants

Answer: (A-False, B-True, C-False, D-True). Physiologic jaundice is common with a typical pattern of unconjugated hyperbilirubinemia, reaching an average peak of 6 mg/dl by day 3 and resolution within 1 week in term infants and within 2 weeks in preterm infants. (*Chapter 17, Page 149.*)

4.55 Blood glucose levels in the neonate

(A) should be greater than 40 mg/dl
(B) may be low without risk factors
(C) if low, will generally be accompanied by physical findings characteristic of hypoglycemia
(D) if low, may cause apathy, poor feeding, or convulsions

Answer: (A-True, B-True, C-False, D-True). Blood glucose levels should be greater than 40 mg/dl for all newborns. Hypoglycemia can occur without risk factors and be asymptomatic. The most common symptoms are "jitteriness," cyanosis, convulsions, apnea, apathy, abnormal cry, limpness, and poor feeding. A capillary glucose strip from a warmed heel allows screening of high-risk or symptomatic infants. Any value less than 45 mg/dl must be confirmed by venipuncture. (*Chapter 17, Page 150.*)

4.56 Erb's palsy of the neonate

(A) is caused by birth injury
(B) causes arm adduction and internal rotation
(C) may be accompanied by diaphragm paralysis
(D) results in complete recovery in 3 to 6 weeks

Answer: (A-True, B-True, C-True, D-False). Erb's palsy (neuritis of C5–C6 roots due to delivery trauma) causes arm adduction and internal rotation, elbow extension and pronation, and wrist flexion ("waiter's tip" posture). Five to nine percent have diaphragm paralysis. Early improvement or hand grasp suggests a favorable prognosis. Recovery is complete within 3 to 6 months. If no shoulder, arm, or clavicle fractures exist, the infant's sleeve can be pinned in a functional position for 1 week followed by gentle passive exercises. (*Chapter 17, Page 150.*)

4.57 The patient is a 19-year-old primigravida woman who delivered in a bus station a few hours ago. She admits to being an IV heroin user and having multiple sexual partners. You are concerned about HIV infection. You should

(A) screen only the mother for HIV
(B) screen only the infant for HIV
(C) screen both mother and infant for HIV
(D) screen neither mother nor infant for HIV

Answer: (A-False, B-False, C-True, D-False). If a woman at high risk for acquiring HIV delivers with an unknown HIV status, the Center for Disease Control recommends that both mother and infant should be screened for HIV. (*Chapter 17, Page 151.*)

4.58 The patient is the first child of a 23-year-old mother. Both mother and father are significantly overweight. The parents are concerned that their child may become obese, even though he is not overweight at his current age of 6 weeks. The following interventions may lower the risk of developing obesity later in childhood and adult life.

(A) bottle-feeding
(B) early introduction of solids
(C) not using the bottle as a pacifier
(D) using only a small spoon to feed solids

Answer: (A-False, B-False, C-True, D-True). The significance of being overweight as an infant is unclear, with up to three-fourths of such infants becoming normal-weight adults and most obese adults not being obese as infants. However, when there is a genetic predisposition to obesity, especially if associated with a strong family history of cardiovascular disease, hypercholesterolemia, and diabetes, it is reasonable to encourage primary prevention. It can include breast-feeding and delayed introduction of solids, avoiding overfeeding by not using the bottle as a pacifier, and using only a small spoon to feed solids. (*Chapter 17, Page 155.*)

4.59 The patient is a 5-month-old infant, the first child of young high school teachers. They complain that the child seems to have colic, with recurrent crying as though in pain. Which of the following is/are true?

(A) Colic episodes typically last for a total of 3 hours in a day.
(B) Colic generally occurs daily.
(C) Colic is most common between the ages of 2 weeks and 4 months.
(D) Parental behavior is a major factor in the cause of colic.

Answer: (A-True, B-False, C-True, D-False). The syndrome of colic is most commonly defined as paroxysms of irritability, fussing, or crying, with the infant seeming to be in pain and difficult to console without apparent cause. Episodes typically last for a total of more than 3 hours a day but rarely occur daily. They most often appear in the afternoon or evening between the ages of 2 weeks and 4 months. Because up to 49% of all infants can present with this picture, the other factor that seems to define these babies is that one or both parents have difficulty in dealing with this facet of the infant's behavior. Parental behavior does not seem to be a cause of the colic, however, only a response. (*Chapter 17, Page 155.*)

4.60 Risk factors for SIDS include

(A) maternal smoking
(B) maternal drug use
(C) poor prenatal care
(D) supine sleeping position

Answer: (A-True, B-True, C-True, D-False). At this time, the greatest impact on reducing the incidence of SIDS has involved targeting the risk factors known to be associated with a two- to threefold increase in the risk of SIDS. These factors include maternal smoking or drug use, poor prenatal care, complications of delivery and prematurity, and prone (stomach) sleeping position. To address the last risk factor, infants who have no medical contraindications should be placed for sleep in the supine (back) or side position, although there are no controlled studies demonstrating efficacy. (*Chapter 17, Page 159.*)

4.61 Parents of an 11-month-old child are planning to interview facilities offering child care. They ask for your advice. Which of the following is/are true?

(A) The optimal adult/child ratio before 1 year of age is 1:3.
(B) Staff should have training in child development.
(C) Staff should ignore a child that is upset because this tends to reinforce bad behavior.
(D) Staff should wash their hands after each instance of diapering.

Answer: (A-True, B-True, C-False, D-True). Parents can compare several programs by making scheduled and unscheduled visits to observe the emotional atmosphere and sanitation. The optimal adult/child ratio before 1 year is 1:3 and should not exceed 1:4. Staff should be (1) trained in child development; (2) be paid sufficiently to minimize turnover; (3) enjoy their interactions with children, respond positively to children's accomplishments, and attend quickly when a child is upset; and (4) wash their hands after diapering and before food preparation, use disposable tissue for wiping running noses, and routinely wash changing tables. (*Chapter 17, Page 159.*)

4.62 The patient is a 15-year-old primigravida girl at 32 weeks' gestation. She is single and accompanied by her mother. The mother is especially concerned regarding the fact that her daughter will soon become an adolescent parent. You might appropriately tell her that

(A) even with access to appropriate prenatal care, adolescent mothers usually give birth to infants that are SGA and often suffer from congenital diseases
(B) the children of adolescent mothers typically are not well adjusted
(C) the true risk factors for adolescent parents include poverty, family violence, and substance abuse
(D) lack of access to appropriate resources including pre- and postnatal care may be a greater risk than being an adolescent parent

Answer: (A-False, B-False, C-True, D-True). Adolescent parents are often perceived as high risk, when, in fact, adolescent girls who have access to appropriate resources, including pre- and postnatal care, give birth to healthy infants and raise children who are well adjusted. True risk factors are poverty, lack of access to health care, family violence, and substance abuse. Adolescents who grow up in a family with violence, sexual abuse, or chemical dependence initiate sexual intercourse at an earlier age than the general population and experience a higher rate of pregnancy. (*Chapter 17, Page 161.*)

4.63 Which of the following is/are true concerning croup?

(A) Croup is caused by a specific RSV.
(B) Croup is characterized by varying degrees of inspiratory stridor.
(C) Cough is uncommon in croup.
(D) Hoarseness in croup is due to laryngeal-region obstruction.

Answer: (A-False, B-True, C-False, D-True). Croup is a spectrum of viral respiratory syndromes characterized by varying degrees of inspiratory stridor, cough, and hoarseness due to laryngeal-region obstruction. These syndromes include laryngitis (older children and adults) and nonrecurrent and spasmodic croup (diseases of young children caused predominantly by parainfluenza 1 viruses). Prompt diagnosis and assessment of the severity of crouplike illnesses are essential. (*Chapter 18, Page 163.*)

4.64 You have received a telephone call from one of your patient families. Staying with them is a 13-year-old male exchange student from the People's Republic of China. The family has no information regarding his immunization status, and there is a concern that he may have been exposed to mumps. As you consider what to tell this family, which of the following is/are true?

(A) Mumps is a local illness of the parotid glands.
(B) The spread of mumps is primarily by fingers to feces to food to mouth and thus to the parotid gland.
(C) The incubation period is 16 to 18 days.
(D) The period of communicability is 7 days before swelling and up to 9 days after.

Answer: (A-False, B-False, C-True, D-True). Mumps virus infects only humans and causes a systemic illness, which may serve as a prototype for other systemic viral illnesses. It is spread primarily by respiratory droplets. The usual incubation period is 16 to 18 days (range, 12 to 25 days). The period of communicability ranges from 7 days before swelling to 9 days after. The disease is most common during late winter and spring in North America, where a few thousand cases still occur each year. Mumps is predominantly a disease of school-age children. (*Chapter 18, Page 166.*)

4.65 The management of Kawaski disease may include the use of

(A) calcium antagonists
(B) intravenous gamma-globulin
(C) dipyridamole (Persantine)
(D) aspirin

Answer: (A-False, B-True, C-True, D-True). Goals of management are control of the acute inflammatory process and prevention of coronary artery involvement. Aspirin (100 mg/kg/day in four divided doses) is initiated once the diagnosis is tentatively made. A single infusion of IV gamma-globulin (2 g/kg) is given. After resolution of fever and other inflammatory signs, aspirin is continued at a single daily dose of 3 to 5 mg/kg/day for its antiplatelet effect. It may be discontinued at 6 to 8 weeks if no coronary involvement is present. Aspirin is continued at 3 to 5 mg/kg/day long term if coronary involvement is present (indefinitely if aneurysms persist). Dipyridamole (Persantine) (36 mg/kg/day in three divided doses) is used if the patient is aspirin-intolerant. (*Chapter 18, Page 168.*)

4.66 The parents of a 5-year-old girl have reported that the child has a low-grade fever, nausea, and five to six loose bowel movements daily over the past 2 days. This appears to be a viral diarrhea. Appropriate management includes ingestion of

(A) oral rehydration solutions
(B) undiluted apple juice
(C) plain water used as necessary to reduce thirst
(D) chicken broth

Answer: (A-True, B-False, C-False, D-False). Oral rehydration is the mainstay of outpatient treatment of viral diarrhea, and vomiting is not a contraindication (use small frequent administrations). Breast-fed infants may be managed by continuing breast-feeding and supplementing with oral rehydration solutions. Rehydration with clear liquids such as soft drinks, gelatin water, and apple juice is not recommended owing to the high-carbohydrate, high-osmolality, and low-electrolyte composition of these fluids. Diluting small amounts of such items into commercial solutions, however, may be required so older infants and children can accept the rehydration solution. Caffeine, plain water, and excessive use of soups (high-sodium content) must be avoided. (*Chapter 18, Page 169.*)

4.67 Patients with pinworms

(A) may be asymptomatic
(B) generally have eosinophilia on a routine blood count
(C) may present with vulvovaginitis-urethritis
(D) may present with perianal itching, restless sleep, and irritability

Answer: (A-True, B-False, C-True, D-True). A large proportion of patients are asymptomatic; and the classic symptoms of perianal itching, restless sleep, and irritability may be no more common among infected than uninfected children. Occasionally, the parasite migrates to cause vulvovaginitis-urethritis (most common), salpingitis, prostatitis, and bowel, liver, and other organ system disease. Anorexia, weight loss, and

personality changes (due to the misconceived stigmata associated with having pinworms) are sometimes seen. Unless peritoneal invasion occurs, eosinophilia is not present. (*Chapter 18, Page 169.*)

4.68 The patient is a 7-year-old child found to have pinworms. You should treat

(A) the patient
(B) all family members
(C) all school classmates
(D) children who attended a birthday party at your patient's home 5 days ago

Answer: (A-True, B-True, C-False, D-False). Because pinworm infection spreads within families and may be asymptomatic, initial treatment of all family members is best. The medication kills only adult worms so retreatment of symptomatic individuals 2 weeks after the initial treatment may improve cure rates. (*Chapter 18, Page 170.*)

4.69 Appropriate treatment for pinworms might include which of the following?

(A) mebendazole (Vermox)
(B) ketoconazole (Nizoral)
(C) pyrantel pamoate (Antiminth)
(D) avoidance of thumb sucking

Answer: (A-True, B-False, C-True, D-True). Mebendazole 100 mg (Vermox chewable tablets) in a single dose for adults and children produces the fewest side effects (rarely abdominal pain and diarrhea) but should not be used during pregnancy. Pyrantel pamoate (Antiminth) suspension, 11 mg/kg in a single dose (maximum, 1 g), is an effective alternative but may have significant gastrointestinal side effects. Preventive measures such as frequent hand and fingernail washing, avoidance of digit sucking, and decontamination of clothing, sleeping quarters, and toilet seats may decrease infection but may not justify the associated increased psychological trauma and stigmata associated with pinworms. (*Chapter 18, Page 171.*)

4.70 The management of AD/HD may include which of the following?

(A) medication
(B) behavioral skills such as list-making
(C) family therapy
(D) support groups

Answer: (A-True, B-True, C-True, D-True). Once the diagnosis of AD/HD is secure, treatment usually begins in several areas. The parent or teacher is often expecting pills, but the physician also should emphasize skills. Instruction about developing behavioral skills is crucial to help the parent and student understand that medication may be used for only a short period (months) if the student is diligent in gaining organizational skills while better able to focus. For instance, students can be taught list-making to allow them to concentrate on one task at a time. Behavior modification, psychotherapy, family therapy, and support groups are indicated for many AD/HD children and their families. Treatment with medication is often initiated at the first office visit or later if the behavior modifications take first priority. (*Chapter 19, Page 175.*)

4.71 The patient is a 9-year-old child here for an annual examination. Her mother reports that the school has found that she has a learning disability, and she would like to discuss the meaning of this diagnosis. Which of the following is/are true?

(A) When the child exhibits a learning disability in one or more academic skill areas, the child's global level of intellectual functioning is generally below average.
(B) The child's hearing and vision should be evaluated before a learning disability diagnosis is considered.
(C) The possibility of lead poisoning should be considered.
(D) The diagnosis of a learning disability is generally evident by the end of the first grade.

Answer: (A-False, B-True, C-True, D-False). Learning disabilities tend to occur in one or more of several key areas, including reading, spelling, numerical calculation, or written expression. A child may exhibit evidence of a learning disability in more than one academic skill area, although the child's global level of intellectual functioning is assumed to be at least average. Additionally, the family physician should be sure to establish that the child's hearing and vision are not impaired before a learning disability is seriously considered. Environmental health factors, such as elevated lead levels, should also be ruled out. It is assumed that the learning disabled child has had adequate exposure to formal education; thus the diagnosis is often not assigned until at least the second grade. (*Chapter 19, Page 176.*)

4.72 Oppositional defiant disorder is characterized by

(A) frequent arguments
(B) depression

(C) temper tantrums
(D) refusal to comply with adult requests

Answer: (A-True, B-False, C-True, D-True). Oppositional defiant disorder is characterized by frequent argumentative and negativistic verbalizations, temper tantrums, and refusal to comply with adult requests. Oppositional defiant children, like those with conduct disorder, often are reared in families with inconsistent discipline, although the parents are more likely to be depressed than overtly antisocial. Conduct disorder is distinguished from AD/HD and oppositional defiant disorder by an emphasis on aggressive, illegal, and overtly destructive acts. (*Chapter 19, Page 177.*)

4.73 The family environments of children with conduct disorder

(A) are generally not significantly different from other family environments other than the need to cope with the conduct disorder within the household
(B) are often single family households with an absent father
(C) are often characterized by overprotective parenting with "smothering" parental warmth
(D) often fail to monitor children's activities

Answer: (A-False, B-True, C-False, D-True). The family environments of conduct-disordered children are often chaotic, with supervision and discipline either nonexistent or sporadic. Fathers are often absent or exhibit antisocial behavior. Direct observation of these families has shown little parental warmth, few positive verbalizations toward their children, and failure to monitor childrens' activities. (*Chapter 19, Page 177.*)

4.74 Following several sessions with a local counselor, a young couple in your care has just been told that their 7-year-old son has a "phobia." Which of the following is/are true regarding pediatric phobias?

(A) These are synonymous with childhood fears of the dark or of animals.
(B) The phobic situation is avoided or tolerated with great discomfort.
(C) The diagnosis requires impaired social, academic, or family functioning.
(D) The phobic reaction occurs unexpectedly without anticipatory anxiety.

Answer: (A-False, B-True, C-True, D-False). Phobias are common in both children and adults. The overall lifetime prevalence for specific phobias is about 10%.

Pediatric phobias are distinct from common childhood fears of the dark, strangers, and animals. The degree of fear is disproportionate, and the phobic situation is avoided or tolerated with great discomfort. For a child to be diagnosed as phobic, the distress or avoidance should result in impaired social, academic, or family functioning. Preoccupation and anticipatory anxiety about the phobic object or situation is also common. The treatment of choice is relaxation training (deep breathing with the possible addition of systematic tensing and relaxation of muscle groups) coupled with graded exposure to the phobic stimulus. (*Chapter 19, Page 179.*)

4.75 Obsessive-compulsive disorder (OCD) in children and adolescents

    (A) is readily apparent to primary care physicians because of the distinct symptoms of the patient
    (B) has an average age of onset at about 13 years
    (C) is more common in girls than boys
    (D) has a prevalence of about 10%

Answer: (A-False, B-True, C-False, D-False). OCD in children and adolescents appears to be underdiagnosed. Until recently, the disorder was often not recognized in children. However, retrospective studies of adults with OCD indicated that about 40% of these patients reported onset during childhood and adolescence. The average age of onset appears to be about 13 years. Whereas adult-onset OCD occurs about equally across genders, childhood onset appears to be more common in boys. The prevalence in children and adolescents appears to be about 1%. (*Chapter 19, Page 179.*)

4.76 Sucking of the thumb

    (A) is seldom seen because young parents have usually been taught ways to prevent this activity
    (B) rarely occurs after age 6
    (C) may have a psychological benefit in toddlers
    (D) has not been shown to effect the child's dental health

Answer: (A-False, B-False, C-True, D-False). Sucking of the thumb is a relatively common activity among young children, with an incidence of 30 to 40% among preschoolers and 10 to 20% in children older than age 6. Thumb sucking may have a psychological benefit in toddlers. This substitute form of nurturing allows them to consolidate emotions and handle their stresses. The habit can adversely affect a child's dental health, however, and has been associated with an anterior open bite, malocclusion, narrowing of the dental arches, mucosal trauma, and deformity of the thumb. (*Chapter 19, Page 179.*)

4.77 Stuttering during childhood

    (A) disrupts both the fluency and temporal patterning of speech
    (B) is unrelated to external stress
    (C) is often more intense when speaking to an authority figure
    (D) rarely ceases in the absence of active therapy

Answer: (A-True, B-False, C-True, D-False). Both the fluency and temporal patterning of speech is disrupted with stuttering. There is currently debate about whether stuttering is primarily a language disorder or a motor skill deficit. The apparent increase in stuttering with school attendance suggests that external stress may be contributory. Additional support for the role of stress is that stuttering is more pronounced during public speaking, while talking on the phone, or when interacting with authority figures. Stuttering may disappear when singing or reading aloud. Up to 70% of young children stop stuttering on their own. (*Chapter 19, Page 180.*)

4.78 Your patient is a 10-year-old girl who is having nightmares and bad dreams. Which of the following statements is/are true?

    (A) These complaints are uncommon during childhood.
    (B) They occur only during rapid eye movement (REM) sleep.
    (C) The patient is in danger of physically harming herself during the bad dream.
    (D) The dream, if recalled, may explain itself.

Answer: (A-False, B-True, C-False, D-True). Nightmares and bad dreams are common and occur only during REM sleep, when all dreams occur. During REM sleep, the body cannot move, so only the memories of the dreams are harmful. When children wake up from a nightmare, they are truly frightened and need full reassurance and support. These episodes are most common in children ages 3 to 6 but can occur at any age. They may represent deep-seated issues for the child to discuss, but mostly the dream explains itself. (*Chapter 19, Page 181.*)

4.79 In-toeing (metatarsus adductus, MA)

    (A) occurs when the forefoot bones are deviated medially at the tarsal-metatarsal junction
    (B) causes a "bean-shaped" foot
    (C) is unrelated to intrauterine position or genetic predisposition
    (D) may be associated with hip dysplasis

Answer: (A-True, B-True, C-False, D-True). The terms *metatarsus adductus* and *metatarsus varus* are used interchangeably. MA occurs when the forefoot bones are deviated medially at the tarsal-metatarsal junction, causing the foot to appear to curve inward at the midfoot (bean-shaped foot). It is probably caused by a combination of intrauterine position and genetic predisposition and can be either flexible or rigid. The incidence of hip dysplasia is higher among patients with metatarsus varus than in the general population. (*Chapter 20, Page 184.*)

4.80 You are examining a 6-year-old for the first time and notice bowlegs with a tibial-femoral angle of approximately 28 degrees. Diagnostic considerations include

  (A) renal disease
  (B) intrauterine positioning
  (C) rickets
  (D) Blount's disease

Answer: (A-True, B-False, C-True, D-True). Excessive genu varus deformities with a tibial-femoral angle of more than 20 degrees should be investigated if they have not started correcting by 2 years of age. Growth charts should be carefully reviewed and consideration given to renal disease, abnormal calcium and phosphorus metabolism, rickets, and Blount's disease. Appropriate laboratory and standing radiographic studies should be ordered. The posteroanterior (PA) standing radiographs must be taken with the child's feet together or shoulder width apart and both feet pointing straight forward. The physis should be carefully examined. (*Chapter 20, Page 186.*)

4.81 True statements regarding knock-knees include which of the following?

  (A) One-fifth of 3-year-olds have more than 15 degrees of valgus.
  (B) The tibial-femoral angle is documented on standing PA radiographs with the feet pointing straight ahead.
  (C) Young children with knock-knees tend to progress to a more serious problem.
  (D) Older children with knock-knees should be reassured that the condition will correct spontaneously during the teen years.

Answer: (A-True, B-True, C-False, D-False). Most children have a slight genu valgus by 3 to 5 years of age, with 20% of 3-year-olds having more than 15 degrees valgus. It can become excessive later during childhood or early adolescence when the normal val-

gus fails to resolve; it may represent an acceleration of normal angulation caused by abnormal forces across the knee. Standing PA radiographs with the feet pointing straight ahead may be obtained to document the tibiofemoral angle and to rule out underlying disease. Young children with this problem tend toward spontaneous resolution. With older children, knock-knees is less likely to correct completely. (*Chapter 20, Page 186.*)

4.82 Pes cavus in the infant may be caused by which of the following?

  (A) spina bifida
  (B) amyotrophic lateral scoliosis
  (C) Charcot-Marie-Tooth disease
  (D) Friedreich's ataxia

Answer: (A-True, B-False, C-True, D-True). Pes cavus, or cavus foot, is a fixed equinus and pronation deformity of the forefoot in relation to the hindfoot, usually resulting from an underlying neuromuscular condition: spinal dysraphism (spina bifida, lipoma, tethered cord, diastematomyelia), Charcot-Marie-Tooth disease, Friedreich's ataxia, or cord tumor. Occasionally, cases are familial or idiopathic. (*Chapter 20, Page 187.*)

4.83 The patient is a 1-year-old white boy whose father is concerned that the child has flat feet. You can reassure the parents that all children have flat feet at birth and that the normal foot may appear flat until the child is 2 to 3 years of age. The reasons include

  (A) ligament laxity
  (B) intrauterine positioning
  (C) the presence of subcutaneous fat that occupies space in the arch
  (D) hindfoot varus

Answer: (A-True, B-False, C-True, D-False). Reasons include ligament laxity, flexibility of cartilage, neuromuscular development, and the presence of subcutaneous fat that occupies space in the arch. The support ligaments gradually tighten to give the longitudinal arch increasing definition with normal growth. As a result, the true flexible flat foot is difficult to diagnose clinically before the child is 2 years old. (*Chapter 20, Page 187.*)

4.84 Techniques for diagnosing LCPD include which of the following?

  (A) radiography
  (B) laboratory testing
  (C) magnetic resonance imaging (MRI)
  (D) arthrography

Answer: (A-True, B-False, C-True, D-True). Techniques for diagnosing LCPD and determining its prognosis include radiography, technetium scanning, MRI, arthrography, and computed tomography (CT) scans. They are all equally useful, and each has its advantages and disadvantages. Laboratory evaluation is normal. (*Chapter 20, Page 191.*)

4.85 Osgood-Schlatter disease

(A) is the most common apophyseal disorder
(B) occurs at an earlier age in boys than in girls
(C) is rarely bilateral
(D) causes prominence and tenderness over the anterior tibial tubercle

Answer: (A-True, B-False, C-False, D-True). Osgood-Schlatter disease, the most common apophyseal disorder, was independently described in 1903. The condition is found most commonly in boys age 10 to 15 years and in girls 2 years earlier; it is often bilateral (20 to 30% of cases). On examination, exquisite tenderness may be noted over the anterior tibial tubercle, with prominence and swelling at that location. (*Chapter 20, Page 193.*)

4.86 The initial treatment of Osgood-Schlatter disease might include which of the following?

(A) bed rest
(B) ice and anti-inflammatory medication
(C) a contoured knee pad
(D) surgery

Answer: (A-False, B-True, C-True, D-False). The patient and family must understand that 12 to 18 months may be required to allow spontaneous resolution by physiologic epiphysiodesis. Treatment with ice, anti-inflammatory medication, and an appropriately contoured knee pad relieves symptoms. The level of sporting activity is balanced with tolerance and severity of symptoms. If symptoms progress to disability with activities of daily living, a brief course (7 to 10 days) of knee immobilization usually resolves the discomfort. Steroid injections into the tibial tubercle should never be done. Rare persistent cases that fail to respond to a lengthy trial of conservative therapy may resolve with surgical removal of the bony ossicle overlying the tibial tubercle. (*Chapter 20, Page 193.*)

4.87 Sever's disease

(A) involves the calcaneal apophysis
(B) is common in adolescents who engage in soccer and running

(C) presents with tenderness at the insertion of the Achilles tendon on the talus
(D) is often associated with a stress fracture of the calcaneus

Answer: (A-True, B-True, C-False, D-False). In 1912, Sever described a benign inflammatory condition to the calcaneal apophysis in active adolescents. The sports most commonly associated with Sever's disease are soccer and running. The disease presents with unilateral or bilateral (60%) posterior heel pain in the 8- to 13-year-old athlete. It is associated with accelerated growth, tight heel cords, and other bio-mechanical abnormalities. Patients present with tenderness at the insertion of the Achilles tendon on the calcaneus. Radiographs may show partial fragmentation and increased density of the os calcis, thereby ruling out other rare causes of heel pain, such as unicameral bone cyst or a stress fracture. (*Chapter 20, Page 193.*)

4.88 The patient is a 12-year-old girl found on school screening examination to have scoliosis of the spine. She and her parents are worried about this finding. Which of the following is/are true?

(A) Scoliosis is typically associated with congenital anomalies of the vertebrae.
(B) It is inherited in an autosomal dominant manner.
(C) It occurs in approximately 2% of the population.
(D) At least half of all individuals with idiopathic scoliosis require treatment.

Answer: (A-False, B-True, C-True, D-False). Idiopathic scoliosis is defined as lateral deviation of the spine of more than 10 degrees (measured by the Cobb method), with structural change and without congenital anomalies of the vertebrae. It is inherited in an autosomal dominant manner with variable penetrance or a multifactorial condition. It occurs in approximately 2% of the population. Normally, only about one-fifth to one-sixth of this group require treatment. (*Chapter 20, Page 195.*)

4.89 Scheuermann's disease

(A) is synonymous with juvenile kyphosis
(B) must be distinguished from postural round back
(C) may show a familial incidence
(D) is more common in girls than boys

Answer: (A-True, B-True, C-True, D-False). Scheuermann's disease (juvenile kyphosis) is defined as an abnormal increase in thoracic kyphosis (normal, 20 to 40 degrees) during puberty with at least 5 degrees of anterior wedging of at least three or more adjacent vertebrae. It is to be distinguished from postural round back, which is more flexible and lacks radiographic changes in the vertebrae. The etiology is unclear, but a familial incidence is noted in 30 to 48% of cases. It occurs in about 1% of the population and is more common in boys. (*Chapter 20, Page 196.*)

4.90 Lead poisoning should be considered in children in which of the following settings?

(A) young minority children in urban settings
(B) older children with developmental delays
(C) children with recurrent abdominal pain
(D) autistic children

Answer: (A-True, B-True, C-True, D-True). Young, male, minority children residing in central cities accounted for a disproportionate share of these 1.7 million children. In most communities, all children aged 6 to 72 months should be screened for lead intoxications. Older children with developmental delays should be screened as well, as they may exhibit pica or increased hand-to-mouth activity. Lead poisoning should also be considered in children with unexplained neurologic symptoms, recurrent abdominal pain, hearing loss, anemia, developmental delay, autism, or other behavior disorders. (*Chapter 21, Page 201.*)

4.91 The patient is a 9-year-old child with bed wetting almost every night. The parents have tried a battery-operated alarm with only modest success. You might appropriately tell this family that

(A) nocturnal enuresis usually resolves spontaneously
(B) a 9-year-old child cannot reasonably be expected to participate in the treatment of the condition
(C) awakening the child frequently at night is generally helpful
(D) practicing stream interruption during voiding may help the child gain greater urinary control at night

Answer: (A-True, B-False, C-False, D-True). Nocturnal enuresis usually resolves spontaneously, so reassurance and education of the child and parents are important. Most parents in the United States view bed wetting as a significant problem, and some deal with it by punishment. The child must not be blamed but should be encouraged to participate in the treatment of his or her condition. Placing stars on a calendar for dry nights followed by a small reward for consecutive dry nights provides positive reinforcement. The child should void before going to bed, but frequent awakening at night to prevent wetting is seldom helpful. A child who has a small bladder capacity may benefit by increasing the time between daytime voiding and practicing stream interruption during voiding. (*Chapter 21, Page 204.*)

5
Care of the Adolescent

The questions in this chapter constitute a review of the following chapters in *Family Medicine: Principles and Practice, Fifth Edition:*

Health Care of the Adolescent (Chapter 22)
Sexual Concerns of Adolescents (Chapter 23)

DIRECTIONS (Items 5.1 through 5.7): Each of the questions or incomplete statements in this section is followed by five suggested answers or completions. Select the ONE that is BEST in each case.

5.1 The most frequent reason older adolescents visit physicians is

(A) injuries
(B) infectious mononucleosis
(C) prenatal care
(D) human immunodeficiency virus infection and acquired immunodeficiency syndrome (AIDS)
(E) preventive health examinations

Answer: (C). Routine prenatal care examination was the most frequent reason for older adolescents visiting physicians. Although 15% of physician office visits by adolescents could be considered for health supervision, few visits include preventive services or anticipatory guidance. (*Chapter 22, Page 207.*)

5.2 In boys at puberty, there is an increase in testicular size and development of the testicular Leydig cells, which produce testosterone, which, in turn, leads to the development of secondary sex characteristics. The hormone that most directly leads to these changes is

(A) luteinizing hormone (LH)
(B) gonadotropin-releasing hormone (GnRH)

(C) follicle-stimulating hormone (FSH)
(D) thyroid-stimulating hormone
(E) progesterone

Answer: (A). In boys, LH leads to an increase in testicular size and development of the testicular Leydig cells, which produce testosterone, which, in turn, leads to the development of secondary sex characteristics. FSH stimulates development of the seminiferous tubules of the testes, leading to spermatogenesis and fertility during mid- to late adolescence. (*Chapter 22, Page 208.*)

5.3 The patient is a 13.5-year old girl. She has early development of breast buds but is concerned that her periods have not begun. You should tell her that

(A) she has delayed puberty and should be referred to an endocrinologist
(B) menarche is likely to occur within 2 to 5 years
(C) she should begin cyclic estrogen and progesterone therapy
(D) she might have a thyroid deficiency and appropriate blood tests should be obtained
(E) she can expect her menses within the next 6 months

Answer: (B). Common complaints in girls include problems with delay of onset of menarche. If the girl is age 13 to 14 and has signs of pubertal development such as breast buds (Tanner stage 2), she can be reassured that menarche will occur within 2 to 5 years. (*Chapter 22, Page 209.*)

5.4 In the adolescent girl without symptoms, the first pelvic examination should be done

(A) after the onset of sexual activity
(B) with the parent present in the room
(C) at the first prenatal vist
(D) at age 13
(E) at age 16

Answer: (A). For girls the first pelvic examination should be done after the onset of sexual activity or as symptoms dictate to obtain a Papanicolaou (Pap) smear and cultures as appropriate. In the absence of symptoms, a pelvic examination is not needed prior to sexual activity. (*Chapter 22, Page 211.*)

5.5 Which of the following diets would be most appropriate for an adolescent?

(A) 30% carbohydrates, 40% fat, 30% protein
(B) 60% carbohydrates, 20% fat, 20% protein
(C) 70% carbohydrates, 15% fat, 15% protein
(D) 50% carbohydrates, 35% fat, 15% protein
(E) 50% carbohydrates, 10% fat, 40% protein

Answer: (B). A daily diet comprised of 50 to 60% carbohydrates, 15 to 25% fat, and 15 to 20% protein meets the needs of any active teenager. Nutritional supplements are usually unnecessary if the adolescent follows a balanced diet. (*Chapter 22, Page 211.*)

5.6 Which of the following is the strongest predictor of adolescent depression?

(A) poor school performance
(B) depression in one or both parents
(C) failure to make a sports team
(D) short stature
(E) low socioeconomic status

Answer: (B). The relative contribution of genetics and environment to depression are not fully known, but one of the strongest predictive factors is depression in one or both parents. A child has a one in four chance of becoming depressed if one parent is depressed but a three in four chance if both are depressed. Low parental support predicts adolescent depression. Another strong predictor is loss of a parent through death or separation. (*Chapter 22, Page 214.*)

5.7 Which of the following kills the greatest number of Americans each year?

(A) alcohol
(B) cocaine
(C) homicide
(D) car accidents
(E) tobacco

Answer: (E). It is estimated that tobacco use kills more Americans each year than alcohol, cocaine, crack, heroin, homicide, suicide, car accidents, firearms, and AIDS combined. Despite laws that prohibit minors from purchasing tobacco, 85% of current smokers began smoking before age 21. (*Chapter 22, Page 215.*)

DIRECTIONS (Items 5.8 through 5.19): Each of the items in this section is a multiple true–false problem that consists of a stem and four lettered options. Indicate whether each of the four options is TRUE or FALSE.

5.8 With the beginning of puberty, there is an increase in certain hormones. These include

(A) GnRH
(B) FSH
(C) LH
(D) sex hormones

Answer: (A-True, B-True, C-True, D-True). At the onset of puberty, there is an increase in GnRH, FSH, LH, and the sex hormones. (*Chapter 22, Page 208.*)

5.9 The patient is a 13-year-old boy who has breast bud development and tenderness. This condition

(A) is uncommon in boys
(B) can persist for about 18 months
(C) is more often unilateral than bilateral
(D) should be biopsied to rule out malignant change

Answer: (A-False, B-True, C-False, D-False). Temporary breast tenderness and thelarche (breast bud development) is a common and temporary condition that occurs in 40% of boys and can persist approximately 1.5 years. Thelarche is most likely caused by estrogen stimulation, but there is no evidence of hormonal difference between those with and without this condition. Thelarche is more often bilateral than unilateral and occurs in thin as well as obese boys. All boys should be offered reassurance about this benign self-limited problem. (*Chapter 22, Page 208.*)

5.10 Pubertal delay

(A) in girls is defined as no breast development by age 13 or more than 5 years between thelarche and menarche
(B) in boys is defined as the absence of testicular enlargement by age 13.5 years or more than 5 years from the beginning to completion of pubertal development

(C) for both genders, the definition includes short stature, greater than 2 standard deviations below the mean

(D) may be related to disease in the hypothalamic-pituitary-gonadal axis

Answer: (A-True, B-True, C-False, D-True). Pubertal delay in girls is defined as no breast development by age 13 or if more than 5 years has elapsed between the beginning of breast development and menarche; in boys, pubertal delay is defined as the absence of testicular enlargement by age 13.5 or if more than 5 years has elapsed from the beginning to completion of pubertal developments. For both genders, organic diseases of the hypothalamic-pituitary-gonadal axis and other major systemic illnesses must be ruled out as a specific cause of delay in growth or sexual maturation. (*Chapter 22, Page 209.*)

5.11 Important immunizations and testing for adolescents include

(A) tuberculin testing for all children between the ages of 11 and 15

(B) diphtheria-pertussis-tetanus (DPT) booster before entering college or military service

(C) measles/mumps/rubella (MMR) repeat immunization if no booster since infancy

(D) hepatitis A immunization

Answer: (A-False, B-False, C-True, D-False). As many as 20% of adolescents are inadequately immunized. Important immunizations in this age group include a tetanus and diphtheria booster between ages 11 and 12. Rubella screening by the history, prior immunizations, or antibody levels should be documented in all girls. MMR immunization should be repeated if the patient has not had a booster since infancy. Hepatitis B immunization is recommended for all adolescents not previously immunized. Tuberculin skin testing (PPD) and immunizations such as influenza should be provided to adolescents in high-risk categories. (*Chapter 22, Page 211.*)

5.12 The patient is a 15-year-old girl, very thin, without breast bud development. Despite being thin, she is concerned about weight control. This patient

(A) may have anorexia nervosa

(B) is unlikely to suffer irreversible effects on her growth

(C) may have a disease that has proved fatal in some patients

(D) should be managed by serial weight determinations at 4-month intervals

Answer: (A-True, B-False, C-True, D-False). Consider an eating disorder in any teenager who fails to attain or maintain a healthy weight, height, body composition, or stage of sexual maturation for gender and age. Eating disorders may lead to irreversible effects on the physical and emotional growth and development of adolescents. In some cases, these disorders are fatal. Therefore, the threshold for intervention in adolescents should be lower than that in adults. (*Chapter 22, Page 214.*)

5.13 An adolescent with an eating disorder should be hospitalized

(A) rarely, because the best therapy for an eating disorder is in the family setting

(B) if there is significant malnutrition or dehydration

(C) if there is acute food refusal

(D) if there is family dysfunction that prevents effective treatment

Answer: (A-False, B-True, C-True, D-True). Hospitalization of an adolescent with an eating disorder is required in the presence of significant malnutrition; physiologic or physical evidence of medical compromise (e.g., vital sign instability, dehydration, or electrolyte disturbances) even in the absence of significant weight loss; arrested growth and development; failure of outpatient treatment; acute food refusal; uncontrollable binging, vomiting, or purging; family dysfunction that prevents effective treatment; and acute medical or psychiatric emergencies. (*Chapter 22, Page 214.*)

5.14 Depression in adolescents

(A) is often bipolar

(B) occurs equally among female and male adolescents

(C) can have significant morbidity and mortality

(D) currently is significantly overdiagnosed

Answer: (A-False, B-False, C-True, D-False). Depression is increasingly being recognized as a problem that affects adolescents. Most studies of unipolar depression have focused on psychiatric clients, not on general adolescent populations. One general population study found that 27% of high school students were moderately depressed and 5% severely depressed. From currently available studies, bipolar affective disorders are not major health problems among adolescents. Depression is more common in female adolescents. Adolescent depression, despite its association with high morbidity and mortality, remains significantly underdiagnosed. (*Chapter 22, Page 214.*)

5.15 Which of the following is/are true regarding suicide in adolescents?

(A) Suicide predominantly affects individuals with low economic status.
(B) The number of adolescent suicides has remained level for the past decade.
(C) Many "accidental" deaths are actually suicides.
(D) Suicide attempts by boys are more likely to have fatal outcomes than those by girls.

Answer: (A-False, B-False, C-True, D-True). Suicide affects young people from all races and socioeconomic groups. The number of adolescent suicides is increasing dramatically. For youths 15 to 19 years of age, suicide rates have tripled from between 1960 and 1980. Suicide is the third leading cause of death among adolescents and the second leading cause among young adults. Only accidental deaths and homicide are more frequent. Many experts believe that numerous "accidental" deaths are actually suicides. Boys tend to have more fatal outcomes than girls when attempting suicide because of their use of more lethal weapons, namely, firearms and hanging. Adolescent girls most often attempt suicide by ingesting pills. (*Chapter 22, Page 214.*)

5.16 You receive a call from a 17-year-old boy, who reports that his high school football team plans to use urine testing for drugs. He has a number of questions about the implications of this testing. Which of the following is/are true?

(A) Urine testing alone can establish the presence of drug dependence.
(B) Adolescents should be tested without their knowledge because prior knowledge of testing can lead to false-negative results.
(C) False-positive tests are rare.
(D) An adolescent who is prescribed a cough medicine may test positive for codeine.

Answer: (A-False, B-False, C-False, D-True). Urine testing alone should not be used to establish drug dependence, and adolescents should never be tested without their knowledge and consent. False-positives as well as false-negatives can occur. An adolescent who is prescribed cough medicine may test positive for codeine. Different drugs remain in the system for different lengths of time. An adolescent who last smoked marijuana several weeks before the examina-

tion may test positive at the time of urine testing. (*Chapter 22, Page 215.*)

5.17 The patient is a 16-year-old girl who has been in your practice since birth. She is here to discuss her concerns about beginning a sexual relationship with a boy in her high school class. Which of the following statements regarding adolescent sexual behavior is/are true?

(A) Today's mass media sends a clear message that sexual intercourse is rite of passage to adulthood.
(B) Teenage sexual experimentation may actually be the "pursuit of normalcy."
(C) Sexual activity may be equated by the adolescent with a sense of social belonging.
(D) Discussions with the family physician regarding boundaries and resistance to peer pressure are unlikely to be helpful.

Answer: (A-True, B-True, C-True, D-False). An adolescent trying to develop his or her "modus operandi" for feeling and appearing more sophisticated may experiment with behaviors and roles that have potentially adverse effects on health. In terms of sexual behavior, when one of the clear messages in the mass media is that intercourse is a rite of passage to adulthood and when many youths believe their peers to be sexually active, it is not a surprise that the "pursuit of normalcy" results in sexual experimentation. Girls, in particular, are vulnerable to equating a sense of social belonging with providing sexual favors to adolescent boys and men, regardless of whether the experience is healthy or pleasurable for them. It is in the context of this developmental task that discussions about boundaries, about the ability to resist peer pressure, can be protective of health. (*Chapter 23, Pages 220–221.*)

5.18 In your office are middle-aged parents who have just discovered that their 17-year-old son is gay. They are concerned about the impact on his health and his life. Which of the following statements is/are true regarding gay and lesbian youths?

(A) Self-identification as gay or lesbian has been shown to have no effect on the health of the adolescent.
(B) Social rejection may be perceived to be a significant problem by the gay or lesbian adolescent.
(C) Suicide attempts among gay youths are no more common than among heterosexual adolescents.
(D) In some areas, a high percentage of homeless youths may identify as gay or lesbian.

Answer: (A-False, B-True, C-False, D-True). The toll on the health of adolescents who identify themselves as gay or lesbian is high, primarily because of the social rejection that occurs. Suicide attempts among gay youths are two to three times those of heterosexual youths. In New York City, 40 to 50% of homeless youths identify as lesbian or gay; and the incidence of "survival sex," particularly with older male partners, is high with both gay and lesbian youths who are living on the streets. Thus, whether to disclose sexual orientation becomes not simply a discretionary decision but often a matter of survival for adolescents who identify themselves as gay or lesbian. (*Chapter 23, Pages 221–222.*)

5.19 Which of the following is/are true about talking with adolescents about sexuality in the office setting?

- (A) Adolescents generally welcome conversations about sexuality with physicians.
- (B) Conversations with adolescents about sexuality do not help them in making good decisions about their sexual health.
- (C) Providing information and discussion about sexuality increases student interest and is perceived as giving permission for sexual experimentation.
- (D) The discussion of adolescent sexuality should be limited to visits regarding physical development and health maintenance.

Answer: (A-True, B-False, C-False, D-False). Several studies have shown that adolescents welcome conversations about sexuality with physicians and that these conversations do make a difference in helping youths to make good decisions about their sexual health. One might presume, then, that the absence of conversation *cannot help* youths make good decisions and that correct information and the opportunity to talk about sexuality with a concerned and informed health care provider *cannot harm* young people. Given the morbidity of sexually risky behaviors, the mandate is clear in terms of the importance of finding opportunities during the course of routine health care to talk about physical, emotional, and sexual development. (*Chapter 23, Page 223.*)

6
Care of the Elderly

The questions in this chapter constitute a review of the following chapters in *Family Medicine: Principles and Practice, Fifth Edition:*

Common Problems of the Elderly (Chapter 24)
Alzheimer's Disease and Related Dementias (Chapter 25)

DIRECTIONS (Items 6.1 through 6.14): Each of the questions or incomplete statements in this section is followed by five suggested answers or completions. Select the ONE that is BEST in each case.

6.1 Falls are a common problem in the elderly. In this age group, most falls occur

(A) in unfamiliar surroundings, such as public buildings
(B) in the faller's home
(C) while walking outdoors, on the sidewalk, or along the road
(D) during the course of an acute illness
(E) none of the above

Answer: (B). Most falls occur in the faller's home, and the home environment is usually a factor in these falls. Many falls occur on stairs, with injuries more likely to occur while descending rather than climbing stairs. Other hazards are electrical cords, uneven surfaces such as throw rugs or carpeting, or objects left on the floor. Poor lighting may contribute to these hazards. (*Chapter 24, Page 227.*)

6.2 Postural hypotension in the elderly is defined as a drop in systolic blood pressure of at least 20 mm Hg 1 minute after a patient changes from a supine to a standing position. Which of the following five choices is the most common cause of postural hypotension in the elderly?

(A) deconditioning
(B) hypertension
(C) excessive salt intake in the diet
(D) anxiety
(E) unipolar depression

Answer: (A). The most common causes of postural hypotension in older people are deconditioning, with loss of compensating autonomic reflexes, and medications, especially diuretics, tricyclic antidepressants, neuroleptics, antihypertensives, and dopaminergic drugs (e.g., levodopa). Treatment is the same for these patients. Deconditioned patients should be encouraged to gradually increase their activity, under the supervision of a physical therapist if necessary. (*Chapter 24, Page 228.*)

6.3 The most common cause of problematic incontinence is

(A) stress incontinence
(B) overflow incontinence
(C) factitial incontinence
(D) urge incontinence
(E) functional incontinence

Answer: (D). Urge incontinence, also referred to as detrusor instability, occurs when the involuntary bladder contractions overcome the normal resistance of the urethra. This type of incontinence is likely the most common cause of problematic incontinence, affecting up to 70% of persons with incontinence. The three basic mechanisms of action for this type of incontinence are loss of brain inhibition, involuntary detrusor contractions, and loss of the normal voiding reflexes. It is characterized by a strong desire to void followed by a loss of urine, often on the way to the bathroom. (*Chapter 24, Page 228.*)

6.4 The most common cause of incontinence in postmenopausal women is

(A) use of diuretics
(B) complications of diabetes mellitus
(C) involuntary bladder contractions
(D) urethral stricture
(E) stress incontinence

Answer: (E). Stress incontinence, also referred to as sphincter insufficiency, is most frequently encountered in postmenopausal women and is the result of reduced intraurethral pressure and an associated increase in intra-abdominal pressure. There is usually a small amount of urine loss during coughing, sneezing, laughing, or other activities that lead to an increase in intra-abdominal pressure. (*Chapter 24, Page 228.*)

6.5 The patient is an 81-year-old white man with an upper respiratory infection that he has self-medicated with an antihistamine-decongestant capsule containing a drying agent. He has become incontinent of urine. This type of incontinence is properly called

(A) urge incontinence
(B) stress incontinence
(C) overflow incontinence
(D) functional incontinence
(E) factitial incontinence

Answer: (C). Overflow incontinence is the result of the bladder not emptying properly. It can be secondary to an atonic or hypotonic detrusor or an obstruction of the bladder outlet from an enlarged prostate, urethral stricture, or stone. Detrusor hypoactivity can result from diabetes mellitus, lower spinal cord injury, or drugs. Overflow incontinence is characterized by a variety of symptoms that may be confused with symptoms more frequently associated with urge or stress incontinence. The urinary stream is often weak, and there is the sensation of incomplete emptying of the bladder. (*Chapter 24, Pages 228–229.*)

6.6 In the management of incontinence, bladder training is most effective in patients with

(A) urge incontinence
(B) stress incontinence
(C) overflow incontinence

(D) functional incontinence
(E) facticial incontinence

Answer: (A). Clinical guidelines from the Agency for Health Care Policy and Research recommend behavioral therapy in the form of bladder training, prompted voiding, or pelvic muscle exercises for most forms of urinary incontinence. Bladder training is most effective in the setting of urge incontinence but also may be helpful for other forms of urinary incontinence. (*Chapter 24, Page 230.*)

6.7 The patient is an 84-year-old white man with overflow incontinence related to an enlarged prostate. Medication that may be useful in management includes

(A) alpha-adrenergic blockers such as prazosin
(B) anticholinergic agents such as propantheline
(C) antidepressants such as amitriptyline
(D) vitamin C, 3,000 mg daily
(E) vitamin E, 800 IU daily

Answer: (A). Men with prostatic hypertrophy and overflow incontinence can likely benefit from the alpha-adrenergic blockers prazosin, terazosin, or doxazosin. (*Chapter 24, Page 230.*)

6.8 In the care of the elderly, there is evidence to support the value of which of the following interventions?

(A) immunizations for influenza and pneumococcal disease
(B) prostate-specific antigen screening
(C) mammography screening for breast cancer in women older than 69 years
(D) cholesterol screening for men older than age 65 years
(E) all of the above

Answer: (A). Among the interventions that are probably helpful in the elderly are (1) immunizations for influenza, pneumococcal disease, and tetanus-diphtheria; (2) counseling for injury prevention (car safety belts, smoke detectors); (3) counseling for smoking cessation; (4) cervical cancer screening for women who have not been previously screened; (5) guiaic stool testing or sigmoidoscopy to detect colorectal cancer; and (6) hormone replacement therapy and calcium supplementation for women at risk of osteoporosis. Currently, no evidence exists for the elderly to support the use of prostate-specific antigen screening, mammography screening for breast cancer in women older than 69 years, or cholesterol screening, although physicians may choose to screen some older individuals for these conditions. (*Chapter 24, Page 232.*)

6.9 The lifetime risk of an older person being admitted to a nursing home is about

    (A) less than 10%
    (B) 20%
    (C) 40%
    (D) 60%
    (E) 80% or greater

Answer: (C). Only about 5% of the elderly reside in nursing homes, but the lifetime chance of an older person being admitted to a nursing home is about 40%. (*Chapter 24, Page 233.*)

6.10 There are four primary mechanisms in the development of pressure sores. These include all the following EXCEPT

    (A) obesity
    (B) pressure
    (C) shearing forces
    (D) friction
    (E) moisture

Answer: (A). There are four primary mechanisms in the development of pressure sores: pressure, shearing forces, friction, and moisture. More than 90% of pressure sores occur over the bony prominences of the lower part of the body. The amount of time and pressure necessary to cause tissue damage depends on the number of risk factors present. (*Chapter 24, Page 233.*)

6.11 In most older adults with chronic cognitive impairment, the underlying cause is

    (A) hyperthyroidism
    (B) Parkinson's disease
    (C) drug reaction
    (D) irreversible change in brain structure and function
    (E) reversible

Answer: (D). In most chronic cognitively impaired older adults, the observed deterioration is not secondary to a reversible disease or to drug reactions. The underlying cause of chronic progressive deterioration of cognitive functioning is an irreversible change in the structure and function of the brain. An estimated 5% of adults 65 years of age and older suffer severe, chronic, irreversible cognitive impairment. (*Chapter 25, Page 239.*)

6.12 Chronic dementia in the elderly is most likely to begin with

    (A) loss of recent memory
    (B) loss of insight
    (C) impaired judgment
    (D) change in personality
    (E) impaired ability to control bladder or bowel function

Answer: (A). Impaired memory, especially recent memory, typically indicates initially the clinical syndrome of chronic dementia. Other changes are impaired judgment, loss of insight, flattening of affect, and eventually change in personality. As the illness progresses, these changes are commonly followed by trouble swallowing, walking, controlling bladder and bowel functions, and maintaining mobility. Alzheimer's disease (AD), the most frequent cause of dementia in this age group, probably accounts for at least 50% of the progressive dementias in the elderly. (*Chapter 25, Page 239.*)

6.13 The brains of AD patients examined at autopsy have revealed a high accumulation of

    (A) selenium
    (B) aluminum
    (C) calcium
    (D) magnesium
    (E) manganese

Answer: (B). The fact that there is an accumulation of aluminum—30 times the normal amount—in the brains of AD patients examined at autopsy initially suggested aluminum toxicity as a cause, but a causal relation has not been established; accumulation of aluminum may be a secondary phenomenon. (*Chapter 25, Page 239.*)

6.14 The most common form of child maltreatment is

    (A) neglect
    (B) fracture of the femur
    (C) cigarette burns
    (D) head injury
    (E) sexual abuse

Answer: (A). Neglect is the most common form of maltreatment, representing 49% of reported cases of child abuse. Even at this level, neglect is seriously underreported. Neglect, defined as the failure of a parent or guardian to provide for the child's basic needs, manifests as lacking adequate food, clothing, shelter, medical care, education, safety, and nurturing. Identifying neglect is understandably difficult and must take into account the socioeconomic, educational, and functional levels of the parents. (*Chapter 25, Pages 244–245.*)

DIRECTIONS (Items 6.15 through 6.25): Each of the items in this section is a multiple true–false problem that consists of a stem and four lettered options. Indicate whether each of the options is TRUE or FALSE.

6.15 Which of the following are useful in treating the elderly patient with postural hypotension?

(A) dietary salt restriction
(B) raising the head of the bed on blocks
(C) treating hypertension with a diuretic
(D) reminding the patient to change positions slowly

Answer: (A-False, B-True, C-False, D-True). Salt intake can be liberalized for most patients without heart failure. Raising the head of the bed on blocks 4 to 6 inches high also helps improve postural hypotension by stimulating autonomic reflexes and fluid retention. Offending drugs should be eliminated whenever possible. Patients with hypertension can be switched from a diuretic to a calcium channel blocker, angiotensin converting enzyme inhibitor, or a beta-blocker, as these classes of antihypertensives have a low incidence of postural hypotension when used alone. Until the postural hypotension improves, patients should be reminded to change positions slowly to give compensating mechanisms some time to work. (*Chapter 24, Page 228.*)

6.16 The patient is a 78-year-old white man with metastatic cancer of the prostate. Part of his management includes medication to control pain. Which of the following is/are true?

(A) Because of the similarities among elderly individuals, most geriatric patients respond similarly to the same analgesics.
(B) Patients who have constant pain should receive their drugs regularly in anticipation of the pain.
(C) Side effects of analgesics subside within a day or two, and attempts to manage these side effects are ill advised because they generally cause additional problems.
(D) Opioid-induced sedation may be helped by the addition of a stimulant such as caffeine.

Answer: (A-False, B-True, C-False, D-True). Several principles help the physician provide optimal relief of cancer pain. Wide variation exists in the response of

elderly patients to analgesics. Titration must be done carefully, with frequent follow-up to ensure that the drug is effective. Patients who have pain most of the day should receive their drugs regularly, not as needed. Side effects are treated aggressively. For example, sedation due to opioids can be particularly bothersome but can be treated by adding a stimulant such as caffeine or dextroamphetamine. (*Chapter 24, Page 231.*)

6.17 The patient is a 79-year-old white man with early AD, who has been living alone in a single room occupancy hotel. You have not seen him before and are concerned that he may be malnourished. Tests to help evaluate his nutrition include

(A) skinfold thickness
(B) total lymphocyte count
(C) serum albumin
(D) serum thyroxin

Answer: (A-True, B-True, C-True, D-False). Physical signs of malnutrition may be difficult to recognize in the elderly. Anthropometric measures such as weight, height, and skinfold thickness can be helpful for the initial assessment. The total lymphocyte count, hemoglobin, serum albumin, and cholesterol levels are important tests in the biochemical assessment of nutritional status. The farther the results are below normal values, the greater is the degree of malnutrition present. (*Chapter 24, Page 232.*)

6.18 Factors that may contribute to the development of pressure sores include

(A) nutritional deficiencies
(B) polycythemia
(C) sedation
(D) consumption of more than 4 cups of coffee daily

Answer: (A-True, B-False, C-True, D-False). Factors that may contribute to the likelihood of developing pressure sores include nutritional deficiencies, volume depletion, increased or decreased body weight, anemia, fecal incontinence, renal failure, diabetes, malignancy, sedation, major surgery, numerous metabolic disorders, cigarette smoking, and being bed- or chairbound. Finally, the aging skin itself, because of reduced epidermal thickness and elasticity, increases the risk for pressure changes. (*Chapter 24, Page 233.*)

6.19 The patient is a 90-year-old white woman with AD who is a resident of a nursing home. She has developed a pressure sore over the heel, and some infection is present. Therapeutic considerations include which of the following?

(A) The goal is to promote healthy granulation tissue.
(B) The ulcer should be scrubbed vigorously twice daily with hydrogen peroxide.
(C) Wound irrigation and whirlpool baths are likely to be helpful.
(D) Povidone-iodine applied twice daily helps combat infection.

Answer: (A-True, B-False, C-True, D-False). The primary goal of therapy for pressure sores is to create an environment that promotes healthy granulation tissue. Wounds are cleansed as atraumatically as possible with normal saline-soaked gauze, wound irrigation, and whirlpool baths. Most antiseptics, such as hydrogen peroxide and povidone-iodine, are cytotoxic and should be avoided. (*Chapter 24, Page 234.*)

6.20 In the elderly patient, the most common reversible causes of impaired cognitive function are

(A) hypoglycemia
(B) medication use
(C) Parkinson's disease
(D) depressive illness

Answer: (A-False, B-True, C-False, D-True). There is a long list of potentially reversible conditions that can present as chronic deterioration of cognitive function, the most common of which are the memory impairments associated with medications or depressive illness. The other reversible causes of chronic confusion are rare in patients older than age 70, probably accounting for fewer than 5% of all cases. (*Chapter 25, Page 237.*)

6.21 The patient is a 77-year-old white woman who is having difficulty with memory. Her family is concerned that she may have AD. Which of the following statements regarding AD is/are true?

(A) Gait disturbances are common early in the course of AD.
(B) The family should be warned regarding the possibility of seizures during the early course of AD.
(C) Periods of steady improvement are consistent with the diagnosis of AD.
(D) The general trend in AD is likely to be slow deterioration.

Answer: (A-False, B-False, C-False, D-True). Focal neurologic findings, seizures, and gait disturbance are features that are rare early in the course of AD. Although the clinical course of AD may consist of good and bad days, the general trend should be slow deterioration. Periods of steady improvement are not consistent with the diagnosis. (*Chapter 25, Page 237.*)

6.22 True statements regarding AD include which of the following?

(A) The incidence of AD is actually higher among the age group 65 to 69 years of age than among those persons 85 to 89 years of age, because of deaths in the latter age group.
(B) Half of all persons in long-term care facilities have cognitive impairment.
(C) Most older individuals with cognitive impairment live in long-term care facilities.
(D) The estimated prevalence of cognitive impairment in 80-year-old persons is 22%.

Answer: (A-False, B-True, C-False, D-True). Cognitive impairment is age-correlated as well; the estimated prevalence in 80-year-olds increases to 22%. The incidence of AD is approximately 14 times higher among persons older than 85 years than among those 65 to 69 years of age. Although half of persons in long-term care facilities display cognitive impairment, most impaired adults are at home and are unknown to or uninvestigated by clinicians. (*Chapter 25, Page 239.*)

6.23 The patient is an 87-year-old white man with early AD. His family has searched the Internet and found information about tacrine and donepezil. They request a prescription for one of these medications. True statements regarding tacrine and donepezil include which of the following?

(A) About one-third of patients who reach therapeutic levels obtain some benefit.
(B) Dramatic improvement occurs often with these medications.
(C) The most worrisome side effect with tacrine is renal toxicity.
(D) Routine liver function studies are required every 6 weeks during the first year in patients taking donepezil.

Answer: (A-True, B-False, C-False, D-False). Specific treatment of the memory loss associated with AD is currently limited to the use of tacrine (Cognex) and donepezil (Aricept), acetylcholine agonists. About one-third of patients who reach a therapeutic level (80 to 120 mg/day of tacrine or 5 to 10 mg/day of donepezil) obtain some benefit from these medications. Dramatic responses are rare. The most serious adverse event seen with tacrine is hepatotoxicity associated with elevations in alanine aminotransferase (ALT). ALT levels should be measured every other week for at least the first 16 weeks of tacrine therapy. Elevations above three times normal require dose reduction or withdrawal of the medication. Hepatotoxicity has not been reported with donepezil, and routine hepatic enzyme monitoring is not required. (*Chapter 25, Page 240.*)

6.24 Depression often accompanies dementia in the elderly, particularly in the early stages. Appropriate early treatment might include which of the following?

(A) nortriptyline (10 to 50 mg/day)
(B) desipramine (500 to 800 mg/day)
(C) sertraline (50 to 100 mg/day)
(D) propranolol (60 to 80 mg/day)

Answer: (A-True, B-False, C-True, D-False). It may be necessary to initiate treatment with antidepressant medications in patients with mild or moderate dementia who appear depressed. Sometimes the patient's mood elevates and cognition improves. Nortriptyline (10 to 50 mg/day), desipramine (25 to 75 mg/day), and serotonin uptake inhibitors (e.g., sertraline 50 to 100 mg/day) are good choices. (*Chapter 25, Page 240.*)

6.25 Wandering is a frequent and serious problem with AD patients. True statements concerning this problem include which of the following?

(A) The patient should be evaluated for pain.
(B) Wandering may occur when the patient is moved to a new place.
(C) Daily exercise may help promote sleep and reduce wandering.
(D) Patients who wander should be restrained to prevent injury.

Answer: (A-True, B-True, C-True, D-False). Wandering is a frequent serious problem that deserves careful consideration. Patients should be evaluated for pain or other discomfort. When confused patients are taken to new places, they may feel lost or believe that they are not where they are supposed to be. Patients with AD who are hospitalized require frequent general reassurance about where they are, which sometimes increases their comfort and ease of management. When wandering appears to be aimless, it is sometimes helpful to plan daily exercise for the patient to see if it can reduce wandering during other parts of the day. Physical restraints are a last resort and are used only in consultation with the patient's family. (*Chapter 25, Page 241.*)

7

Family Conflict and Violence

The questions in this chapter constitute a review of the following chapters in *Family Medicine: Principles and Practice, Fifth Edition:*

Child Abuse and Neglect (Chapter 26)
Domestic Violence (Chapter 27)
Elder Abuse (Chapter 28)
Sexual Assault (Chapter 29)
Family Stress and Counseling (Chapter 30)

DIRECTIONS (Items 7.1 through 7.10): Each of the questions or incomplete statements in this section is followed by five suggested answers or completions. Select the ONE that is BEST in each case.

7.1 Most deaths caused by physical abuse of children are related to

(A) burns
(B) intracranial injury
(C) infection
(D) malnutrition
(E) fractures

Answer: (B). Most deaths caused by physical abuse of children are secondary to intracranial injury. Unfortunately, infants can have a fatal head injury without external evidence of trauma, as in the shaken baby syndrome. This syndrome is most common in infants younger than 6 months of age. The baby presents with lethargy, vomiting, seizures, and coma and may have a bulging fontanel and enlarging head. These acceleration-deceleration injuries result in a high rate of mortality and an even higher rate of morbidity with lifelong disability. Accidental trauma rarely causes intracranial injuries in infants unless it occurs in a motor vehicle accident or similar major trauma. (*Chapter 26, Page 246.*)

7.2 The most common cause of subdural hematoma in children is

(A) intercranial infection
(B) hematologic disorder
(C) otitis media
(D) idiopathic thrombocytopenic purpura
(E) physical abuse

Answer: (E). The most common cause of subdural hematoma in children is abuse, and most of these children present with a tense fontanel and seizures. In children younger than 2 years of age, the subdural hematomas frequently are bilateral. (*Chapter 26, Page 246.*)

7.3 The patient is a 9-month-old infant who is brought to the emergency department by her parents. Although there is no evidence of trauma, the patient is crying and refuses to use her left leg. Her radiograph examination reveals a fracture of the left femur. This fracture is most likely to be related to

(A) child abuse
(B) osteogenesis imperfecta
(C) osteomyelitis
(D) rickets
(E) neoplasia

Answer: (A). Nontraumatic causes of fracture are uncommon to rare. They include osteogenesis imperfecta, osteomyelitis, syphilis, scurvy, rickets, and neoplasia. (*Chapter 26, Page 247.*)

7.4 In performing a routine examination on a 4-year-old girl, you note that when the child is touched lateral to the vaginal introitus, there is reflex relaxation of the pelvic muscles. You should suspect

(A) past trauma to the pelvic muscles with incomplete healing
(B) imperforate hymen
(C) childhood sexual abuse
(D) malnutrition
(E) Hirschsprung's disease

Answer: (C). When a child is touched lateral to the introitus and reflex relaxation of the pelvic muscles occurs, sexual abuse should be suspected. Children who have been chronically sodomized may have a similar reflex relaxation of the anal sphincter with lateral retraction of the buttocks. Loss of gag reflex may indicate chronic oral copulation. Genital scarring, changes in pigment, and discharge may indicate abuse. (*Chapter 26, Page 248.*)

7.5 Childhood sexual abuse should be expected in a 3-year-old girl who has

(A) perianal itching at night
(B) *Candida* dermatitis in the "diaper area"
(C) dysuria
(D) night terrors
(E) a hymenal diameter of more than 1 cm

Answer: (E). Commonly with child sexual abuse, there are no physical findings. Anatomic hymenal variations are normal, and clinical experience on the part of the examiner is essential if the diagnosis of an abnormal hymen secondary to abuse is to be made. However, child abuse is suspected if a prepubescent girl has a hymenal diameter of more that 1 cm. Hymenal lacerations most commonly occur with digital or penile penetration and are evident in the posterior hymenal segment. Straddle injuries may result in laceration of the anterior hymenal segment. (*Chapter 26, Page 248.*)

7.6 In the United States, the single greatest cause of injury to women is

(A) automobile accidents
(B) battery
(C) firearms
(D) falls
(E) athletic injuries

Answer: (B). In the United States today, violent crimes occur more frequently within families than among strangers. According to U.S. Federal Bureau of Investigation statistics, 52% of female murder victims in

1990 were killed by a current or former partner, and men kill their female partners more than twice as often as women kill their male partners. Battery is the single greatest cause of injury to women. (*Chapter 27, Page 250.*)

7.7 You are working in an emergency department and treating a battered woman brought in by the police. The assailant, her boyfriend, has not been found. In counseling this woman, you might reasonably recommend that she

(A) purchase a pistol for protection
(B) develop a safe plan
(C) enroll in a self-defense class
(D) undertake counseling to identify behaviors that provoke battering
(E) confront the batterer

Answer: (B). The battered woman needs to develop a safe plan so she can escape quickly. It may save her life. A safe plan consists not only of consideration of where to flee but includes such things as a set of clothes packed for her and her children; an extra set of keys to home and car; evidence of abuse, such as names and addresses of witnesses, pictures of injuries, and medical reports; cash, checkbook, and other valuables; legal documents such as birth certificates, social security cards, driver's license, insurance policies, protection orders, prescriptions; something meaningful for each child (blanket, toy, book); a list of important telephone numbers, and places to stay. If the children are old enough, she should talk to them about safety: how to call for help and where to go to keep themselves safe. (*Chapter 27, Page 253.*)

7.8 Half of all sexual assaults

(A) involve firearms
(B) involve a person who is not a stranger to the victim
(C) involve use of alcohol or drugs by the victim
(D) occur on commercial property
(E) occur before 6 pm

Answer: (B). Half of all sexual assaults involve a non-stranger, with more than 65% of these assaults occurring at the home of the victim, a friend, relative, or neighbor. Sexual assaults by strangers are more likely to occur on the street or commercial property. Nearly two-thirds of sexual assaults occur after 6 o'clock at night and more commonly before midnight. The economic burden of sexual assault includes health care costs, income lost from work, and legal or court-related activities. (*Chapter 29, Page 261.*)

7.9 In the examination of a woman following sexual assault, the perineal and inner thigh area may be examined for semen stains using

(A) a colposcope
(B) acetic acid
(C) gentian violet
(D) a Wood's lamp
(E) a saturated solution of potassium iodine

Answer: (D). A Wood's lamp should be used to examine the perineal and inner thigh area for semen stains. Any fluorescent areas are then swabbed with cotton swabs for collection. (*Chapter 29, Page 263.*)

7.10 Sexual assault can have significant psychological sequelae. The single most important factor in recovery is

(A) identification of the assailant and a conviction in court
(B) the prompt administration of appropriate antianxiety medication
(C) the victim's support system
(D) the absence of sexually transmitted disease
(E) an early return to work

Answer: (C). Personal characteristics of the victim, characteristics of the sexual assault, and the victim's social support system influence the post-traumatic response. More severe responses are seen in patients with a history of severe psychiatric symptoms, previous sexual violation, and concurrent life stresses. The single most important factor in recovery is the victim's social support system. (*Chapter 29, Page 263.*)

DIRECTIONS (Items 7.11 through 7.27): Each of the items in this section is a multiple true–false problem that consists of a stem and four lettered options. Indicate whether each of the options is TRUE or FALSE.

7.11 Evidence of child neglect may include

(A) malnutrition
(B) poor hygiene
(C) clothing inappropriate for the environment
(D) poor school attendance

Answer: (A-True, B-True, C-True, D-True). The physical signs of neglect include malnutrition, poor hygiene, and inadequate clothing as appropriate for the environment. Behavioral signs relate to lack of supervision, poor school attendance, and exploitation, such as when a child is asked to beg or steal. Repeated ingestion of toxic substances demonstrates a lack of supervision. A child with excessive home responsibilities, such as child care for siblings, housework, or role reversal, in which the child becomes responsible for the parent, are all examples of neglect. (*Chapter 26, Page 245.*)

7.12 True statements regarding bruising as a manifestation of child abuse include which of the following?

(A) The shape of the injury may give a clue as to the object used to inflict injury.
(B) The common objects to be suspected in child abuse include electrical cords, coat hangers, and fly swatters.
(C) Bruising injuries caused by child abuse are generally all in same stage of healing.
(D) When bruising seems to be the chief manifestation of physical abuse, a bleeding disorder should be suspected.

Answer: (A-True, B-True, C-False, D-True). The skin mirrors the objects used to inflict injury. Common objects include belts, buckles, looped cords (electric), sticks, whips, fly swatters, coat hangers, spatulas, spoons, brushes, combs, teeth, and hands. Identifying injuries in different stages of healing supports the suspicion of ongoing intentional injury. Bruising caused by bleeding disorders may be mistaken for physical abuse. When bruising is the major manifestation, hematologic evaluation is required. (*Chapter 26, Page 245.*)

7.13 The patient is a 13-month-old girl brought to the emergency department by police. She has evidence of bruises in different stages of healing and three round burns that are about 1 cm in diameter. Your evaluation of this child should include

(A) a complete skeletal survey including the entire axial and appendicular skeleton
(B) a single radiograph that includes all skeletal structures
(C) local burn care, a tetanus booster, and a return appointment in 48 hours for follow-up
(D) investigation for additional evidence of abuse and neglect

Answer: (A-True, B-False, C-False, D-True). A complete skeletal survey is indicated for all children younger than 2 years of age when physical abuse or neglect is suspected. The survey should include the entire axial and appendicular skeleton. A "baby-gram" or single radiograph is not adequate. Skeletal surveys are rarely indicated after 5 years of age. Instead, request appropriate specific imaging. (*Chapter 26, Page 247.*)

7.14 Which of the following might suggest child abuse in a 2.5-year-old girl?

(A) herpes simplex infection
(B) syphilis
(C) varicella
(D) bacterial vaginosis

Answer: (A-True, B-True, C-False, D-True). Herpes simplex may also be acquired during the birth process; syphilis and human immunodeficiency virus (HIV) can be acquired in the birth canal and go unnoticed for years. These diseases may also represent sexual abuse, however, and so require further evaluation. Children with non-neonatal cases of trichomoniasis have a high probability of sexual abuse. Bacterial vaginosis does not appear to be naturally occurring in prepubertal girls and may be considered an indicator of sexual abuse. (*Chapter 26, Page 248.*)

7.15 True statements regarding domestic violence include which of the following?

(A) As many as 35% of women who visit emergency departments are battered.
(B) There is a lifetime prevalence of 11 to 54% of battery in U.S. women.
(C) Battery is uncommon in women in mental health centers.
(D) Although battery may occur during pregnancy, the abuse seldom continues during the postpartum period as attention is focused on the infant.

Answer: (A-True, B-True, C-False, D-False). As many as 35% of women who visit emergency departments are battered, and studies in these settings reveal a lifetime prevalence of 11 to 54%, depending on the definition of abuse and the survey method used. Two surveys in family practice settings revealed current abuse in 25 to 48% of women, with a lifetime prevalence of 38.8%. One-third to one-half of women presenting to mental health centers have been battered. As many as one in five women are battered during pregnancy, and this abuse may become more frequent during the postpartum period. (*Chapter 27, Page 250.*)

7.16 The woman who is physically abused may report that

(A) pregnancy incited the initial episodes of abuse
(B) an earlier problem with abuse became less prevalent during pregnancy

(C) when pregnant, she delayed seeking prenatal care
(D) while in the same abusive relationship, she had a miscarriage or a low-birth-weight infant during a previous pregnancy

Answer: (A-True, B-False, C-True, D-True). Pregnancy may incite the initial episodes of abuse or cause ongoing abuse to increase. Abused women are twice as likely to delay seeking prenatal care, twice as likely to miscarry, and four times as likely to have a low-birth-weight infant; and these infants are 40% more likely to die during the first year of life. (*Chapter 27, Page 251.*)

7.17 True statements regarding abusing men who batter women include which of the following?

(A) Battering occurs because the man loses control.
(B) Batterers are often dependent on and jealous of their partners.
(C) Batterers tend to believe in traditional gender roles.
(D) Most men who batter have a criminal record.

Answer: (A-False, B-True, C-True, D-False). Batterers do not lose control; rather, they take control. Common characteristics among batterers include dependence on and jealousy of their partners, a belief in traditional gender roles, an extreme need for control, hostility, difficulty with trust, and refusal to accept responsibility for their violent behaviors. Ninety percent of men who batter have no criminal record. (*Chapter 27, Page 252.*)

7.18 Which of the following increase the risk of an individual being the victim of elder abuse?

(A) male gender
(B) being very old
(C) living independently
(D) suffering dementia

Answer: (A-False, B-True, C-False, D-True). Although no older person is immune to the possibility of abuse, certain characteristics appear to increase the risk:
• being female;
• being very old;
• being dependent on others for care and protection;
• suffering dementia;
• exhibiting "difficult" behaviors known to induce caregiver stress (disturbed nights, aggressive or belligerent behavior, resistive or impulsive behavior, incontinence, and wandering);
• being physically dependent for self-care activities of daily living: washing, dressing, toileting, transferring, feeding. (*Chapter 28, Pages 257–258.*)

7.19 Elder abuse might be suspected in which of the following circumstances?

(A) unexplained weight loss
(B) bruising on the flexor surfaces of the extremities
(C) delay in treatment of medical problems or injuries
(D) accidental overdose of medication

Answer: (A-True, B-True, C-True, D-True). Abuse must be added to the differential diagnosis in all cases of significant weight loss, malnutrition, or dehydration; in cases in which there is unexplained or recurrent trauma such as bruising or fracture, especially if the bruising is on the inner (flexor) surfaces of the extremities or body rather than on the extensor surfaces where bruising is much more common, and in which fractures are discovered of a type in which direct trauma is a potential etiology (e.g., midshaft of the humerus or femur, or spiral humeral fracture); situations in which there has been delay in presentation or neglect in the treatment of medical problems and conversely when multiple visits are made to emergency departments, with signs of excessively poor hygiene; or if there is misuse of medication (overdosing or noncompliance). (*Chapter 28, Page 258.*)

7.20 True statements regarding spousal sexual assault include which of the following?

(A) In some marriages, sex may be used as a bargaining tool against anger or extramarital affairs.
(B) Marital sexual assault is uncommon in marriages involving alcoholic husbands, owing to the tendency of alcoholic husbands to have sexual dysfunction.
(C) Because of the ongoing commitment of marriage, the victims of marital sexual assault generally do not suffer significant long-term effects.
(D) Victims of spousal sexual assault may develop sexual dysfunction.

Answer: (A-True, B-False, C-False, D-True). Women often feel socially pressured to have sexual relations with their husbands, regardless of their feelings about the situation or the type of sexual activity. Sex may be used as a bargaining tool against anger, extramarital affairs, or limitations of money and other resources. Marital sexual assault is more frequent in marriages characterized by other forms of violence or involving alcoholic husbands. The effects on victims of marital sexual assault may be more severe than victims of stranger sexual assault. Long-term effects include dis-

trust of men, an increased phobia of intimacy, and sexual dysfunction. (*Chapter 29, Page 262.*)

7.21 True statements regarding sexual assault include which of the following?

(A) Sexual assault is a violent act.
(B) Sexual assault is a sexual act.
(C) Sexual assault is the fastest growing crime in the United States.
(D) Rape is a legal determination.

Answer: (A-True, B-False, C-True, D-True). Sexual assault is a violent, not a sexual, act and is the fastest growing crime in the United States. Family physicians must recognize that rape, a term used interchangeably with sexual assault, is a legal determination. (*Chapter 29, Page 265.*)

7.22 True statements regarding the impact on family stress and loss include which of the following?

(A) Widowers are especially at a higher risk of dying following the death of a spouse.
(B) The increased risk of death during a period of bereavement may be associated with a decrease in cellular immunity.
(C) Single persons have a higher death rate than separated or divorced individuals.
(D) Separated and divorced individuals may have poor immune function.

Answer: (A-True, B-True, C-False, D-True). Numerous studies have shown that after the death of a spouse, widows and particularly widowers are at significantly higher risk of dying, especially during the first 6 months of bereavement. This risk is associated with a decrease in cellular immunity during bereavement. Separated and divorced individuals also have higher death rates (than single, married, or widowed persons) from many diseases; they have been shown to engage in more health risk behaviors and have significantly poorer immune function. (*Chapter 30, Page 267.*)

7.23 The family physician should be alert to the development of family stress; the first signal may be a "red flag" indicating the need for a more detailed psychosocial assessment. These "red flags" include

(A) headache
(B) unexplained physical symptoms
(C) presentation of the clinical history in a manner that does not vary from visit to visit
(D) noting that the same family member accompanies the patient to each visit

Answer: (A-True, B-True, C-False, D-False). "Red flags" that may suggest family stress include common stress-related symptoms such as headaches, unexplained or inconsistent physical symptoms, change in the patient's affect or the manner in which the clinical history is presented, and who accompanies the patient to the visit. (*Chapter 30, Page 267.*)

7.24 The patient is a 34-year-old white woman. Her height is 5'6" and her weight is 202 lb. For months, she and her husband have been arguing regarding several issues that include finances, over-time work, and a suspicion of infidelity. Recently, the patient has noted headaches, fatigue, and early morning awakening. Which of the following statements regarding this patient is/are true?

  (A) The patient has several clinical problems that are probably unrelated.

  (B) The incidence of depression in women in distressed marriages is about the same as those that are happily married.

  (C) Treatment of this patient with antidepressant medication is likely to achieve significant improvement within 3 to 4 weeks.

  (D) Management is likely to be ineffective if the partner is not involved and the marital problems not addressed.

Answer: (A-False, B-False, C-False, D-True). Research has shown that these three problems—marital distress, depression, and obesity—affect each other and are difficult to treat independently of each other. For example, epidemiologic studies have shown that women in distressed marriages are 20 times more likely to be depressed than happily married women. Other studies have demonstrated that treating depressed patients who have marital problems with antidepressant medication or individual psychotherapy is ineffective if the partner is not involved and the marital problems are not addressed. (*Chapter 30, Page 268.*)

7.25 In family therapy, the physician is often presented with situations in which a patient blames another family member ("My husband drinks too much" or "Our son won't listen to us anymore"). They are looking for the physician's support and suggestions as to how the "other" family members should change. In this setting, the physician should

  (A) empathize with the patient

  (B) validate the patient's assessment of the problem

  (C) maintain the alliance with each family member and avoid taking sides in a conflict

  (D) recognize that it is the family physician's job to make objective determinations regarding value conflicts within a family

Answer: (A-False, B-False, C-True, D-False). The physician's usual instinct is to listen to the patient's story, empathize with him or her, and support or validate his or her assessment of the problem, inadvertently taking the patient's side in the problem or conflict. Taking any side, that of the patient or of another party, is rarely helpful when there are family conflicts. In fact, it can make it more difficult for the patient to resolve the problems. By accepting and agreeing with the patient's view of an interpersonal problem, the patient may use the physician's comments against the other person ("My doctor said you are wrong"). (*Chapter 30, Page 268.*)

7.26 Some family or marital problems can be managed by primary care counseling whereas others require referral to a mental health professional. Those problems that can often be managed by a family physician have which of the following characteristics?

  (A) The problem is situational and has a recent onset.

  (B) The problem is specific rather than general.

  (C) The couple has a good relationship and is motivated to change.

  (D) One or both members of the couple have honest concerns about "communication problems."

Answer: (A-True, B-True, C-True, D-False). Marital or couples problems can be usually managed by the family physician when (1) the problem is situational and has a recent onset. These areas include difficulty related to recent changes or life-cycle transitions, such as coping with a new baby, recent illness, or death in the family. (2) The problem is specific rather than general. The more clearly a couple can define the problem, the more likely it is that brief office counseling can be effective. Vague concerns about "communication problems" or being "unhappy with the relationship" are likely to be more difficult to treat. (3) The couple has a good relationship and is motivated to change. Couples who have a long-standing history of difficulties or in which one partner seems uninterested in counseling should be referred to a marital therapist. (*Chapter 30, Pages 271–272.*)

7.27 Effective primary care couples counseling tends to have which of the following characteristics?

  (A) long term

  (B) a focus on problem solving

(C) a specific contract that describes goals and the format of counseling
(D) flexibility in the number of sessions and frequency of visits

Answer: (A-False, B-True, C-True, D-False). In general, primary care couples counseling should be short term with the focus on problem solving. A specific contract with the goals and format of counseling can be negotiated with the couple. This contract includes the number of sessions (usually four to eight), the frequency of visits (weekly to monthly), and the length of visits (30 to 45 minutes). The couple should decide together what changes they want to make during counseling, and these goals are used to determine whether progress is being made. If significant progress has not been made at the end of the agreed-on visits, the couple should be referred to a marital therapist. (*Chapter 30, Page 272.*)

8

Behavioral and Psychiatric Problems

The questions in this chapter constitute a review of the following chapters in *Family Medicine: Principles and Practice, Fifth Edition:*

Anxiety Disorders (Chapter 31)
Depression (Chapter 32)
Suicidal Patient (Chapter 33)
Somatoform Disorders and Related Syndromes (Chapter 34)
Selected Behavioral and Psychiatric Problems (Chapter 35)

DIRECTIONS (Items 8.1 through 8.27): Each of the questions or incomplete statements in this section is followed by five suggested answers or completions. Select the ONE that is BEST in each case.

8.1 Behavioral therapy of panic disorder (PD) can sometimes be very useful. Of the following which is the most appropriate?

(A) applied relaxation and cognitive therapy
(B) individual cycle therapy
(C) insight therapy
(D) avoidance therapy
(E) reward therapy

Answer: (A). Behavioral therapy can be successful. Individual psychotherapy and insight therapy are probably not helpful, but applied relaxation and cognitive therapy are appropriate in the PD patient. Also, patients with agoraphobia eventually need some form of behavioral therapy following resolution of their panic attacks. Systematic desensitization, in which agoraphobic patients are progressively exposed to their situational fears, is effective when coupled with physician and family support. Even if drug therapy is used, exposure to phobic situations should be encouraged in all patients with PD. (*Chapter 31, Page 275.*)

8.2 Which of the following medications is effective in aborting a panic attack once it has begun?

(A) imipramine (Tofranil) 100 mg
(B) paroxetine (Paxil) 20 mg
(C) alprazolam (Xanax) 5 mg
(D) clonazepam (Klonopin) 4 mg
(E) none of the above

Answer: (E). A variety of medications successfully prevents recurrent panic attacks in susceptible individuals. No medication is effective in aborting a panic attack once it has begun. (*Chapter 31, Page 275.*)

8.3 Behavioral therapy may be useful in treating generalized anxiety disorder (GAD). The best modality is likely to be

(A) progressive relaxation
(B) stress management counseling
(C) assertiveness training
(D) hypnosis
(E) cognitive therapy

Answer: (E). A variety of modalities exist to help the GAD patient cope with stress and anxiety. Progressive relaxation, stress management, and assertiveness training with or without hypnosis are frequently used, as are family and group therapy and other forms of supportive psychotherapy. Studies with cognitive behavioral therapy, during which anxious thoughts are identified and then changed, suggest that such cognitive therapy may be superior to other forms of behavioral therapy. (*Chapter 31, Page 277.*)

8.4 The patient is a 42-year-old white female factory worker with GAD and chronic depression. She is taking no medications at this time. Your first-choice drug should be chosen from which of the following families?

(A) beta-blockers
(B) tricyclic antidepressants
(C) benzodiazepines
(D) phenothiazines
(E) monoamine oxidase inhibitors

Answer: (B). There is no evidence that beta-blockers are effective for management of GAD. Tricyclic antidepressants may be of some benefit in patients with GAD. If present, depression must be treated aggressively. Hence the drug of choice for management of GAD with major depression is a tricyclic antidepressant. Buspirone is the next alternative. Because benzodiazepines may worsen depression, they should not be first-line agents in patients with GAD and depression. (*Chapter 31, Page 277.*)

8.5 The patient is a 32-year-old divorced male college teacher who describes recurrent intrusive thoughts which include fear of contamination and thoughts of harming others. You should suspect which of the following diagnoses?

(A) panic disorder (PD)
(B) depression
(C) obsessive-compulsive disorder (OCD)
(D) GAD
(E) acquired immunodeficiency syndrome (AIDS)

Answer: (C). The hallmark of OCD is the presence of recurrent obsessions or compulsions (or both) that markedly distress or significantly interfere with the patient's life. Obsessions—intrusive ideas or thoughts—occur in more than half of OCD patients. Fears of contamination are common, as are thoughts of harming others, counting, praying, and blasphemous or sexual thoughts. Compulsions—repetitive intentional behaviors designed to neutralize discomfort—also occur in more than half of these patients. (*Chapter 31, Page 278.*)

8.6 The behavioral therapy most likely to be helpful in the treatment of OCD is

(A) insight therapy
(B) exposure therapy with response prevention
(C) individual psychotherapy with psychoanalysis
(D) dynamic psychotherapy
(E) systematic desensitization

Answer: (B). Whereas flooding therapy—sudden intense exposure to objects of fear until anxiety dissipates—may be helpful for OCD patients, insight therapy, dynamic psychotherapy, and systematic desensitization are not. Exposure therapy with response prevention is the behavioral technique of choice. (*Chapter 31, Page 280.*)

8.7 Which of the following medications is most likely to be helpful in treating the OCD patient who has been unable to comply with behavioral therapy?

(A) sertraline
(B) buspirone
(C) diazepam
(D) clomipramine
(E) electroconvulsive therapy (ECT)

Answer: (D). Drug therapy is helpful in patients who are purely obsessional, have a history of substance abuse, or cannot comply with behavioral therapy. Clomipramine in doses of up to 250 mg/day is more effective than other tricyclic antidepressants in OCD patients. (*Chapter 31, Page 280.*)

8.8 Which of the following is considered *uncommon* in post-traumatic stress disorder (PTSD)?

(A) depression
(B) anxiety
(C) violent behavior
(D) criminality without prior predilection
(E) OCD

Answer: (D). Although patients with PTSD frequently develop depression, GAD, and violent behavior, criminality without a prior predilection is uncommon. In general, men are at greater risk for developing depression and drug abuse, whereas women are at greater risk of developing PD and phobias. An increased risk of alcoholism and OCD appears similarly in both genders. (*Chapter 31, Page 281.*)

8.9 The patient is a 54-year-old white woman with recurrent depression. You began therapy with amitriptyline (Elavil) 100 mg at bedtime 2 months ago. She has returned to your office and reports that she is feeling less depressed and sleeping better. At this visit, you should

(A) increase the dose of medication to 200 mg at bedtime
(B) continue the medication at the current dose
(C) taper the medication over the next 2 weeks

(D) taper the medication over the next 2 months

(E) stop the medication today

Answer: (B). When the patient has achieved remission of the depression, the medication should be continued for a minimum of 4 to 5 months. In cases of recurring or severe depression, continued medication for longer, possibly years, may be best. Once the decision to stop treatment has been made, dosage should be reduced slowly over several weeks while observing for any signs of relapse for several months. (*Chapter 32, Page 289.*)

8.10 The patient is a 32-year-old black man with recurrent depression. He also complains of chronic tiredness. You have decided to initiate treatment with a selective serotonin reuptake inhibitor (SSRI). Which of the following statements regarding SSRIs is true?

(A) An unfavorable side effect profile limits use.

(B) Initial doses should be given on a three-times-daily basis.

(C) There is a relatively low incidence of anticholinergic properties.

(D) Cardiovascular side effects are a significant concern.

(E) There is a high risk of death from overdose.

Answer: (C). Due to their side effect profile and ease of use (once-a-day dosing), they have become a frequent first choice, despite their cost. They have low sedative and anticholinergic properties. Plasma levels are unaffected by age or renal impairment, and there is minimal cardiovascular effect. There is also a very low risk of death from overdose. (*Chapter 32, Page 289.*)

8.11 In the United States, suicide rates are highest in which one of the following age groups?

(A) ages 12 to 20

(B) ages 21 to 30

(C) ages 31 to 45

(D) ages 46 to 64

(E) ages 65 and older

Answer: (E). Suicide rates are highest in the elderly (age 65 years and older) and are continuing to rise, especially for those 75 years of age and older. (*Chapter 33, Page 293.*)

8.12 The most significant risk factor for suicide is

(A) advanced age

(B) depression

(C) cancer

(D) social isolation

(E) chronic alcoholism

Answer: (B). Psychiatric disorders comprise the most significant risk factor for suicide, with estimates suggesting that more than 90% of suicide victims suffer from them. Depression is the most common diagnosis, but the lifetime risk of suicide in patients with schizophrenia or chronic alcoholism is approximately 15%. (*Chapter 33, Page 293.*)

8.13 According to the *Diagnostic and Statistical Manual of Mental Disorders,* 4th Edition (DSM-IV), somatoform disorders include all the following EXCEPT

(A) body dysmorphic disorder

(B) factitious disorders (FD)

(C) conversion disorder

(D) hypochondriasis

(E) pain disorder

Answer: (B). The DSM-IV lists the following as somatoform disorders: body dysmorphic disorder, conversion disorder, hypochondriasis, pain disorder, somatization disorder, somatoform disorder not otherwise specified, and undifferentiated somatoform disorder. (*Chapter 34, Page 297.*)

8.14 The patient is a 48-year-old white male farmer with a sixth grade education, who reports paralysis in his right upper extremity for the past 3 weeks. Although the patient seems unable to move the right hand or arm, your physical examination fails to reveal a motor or sensory defect. The remainder of the examination is unremarkable. This patient most likely has

(A) body dysmorphic disorder

(B) FD

(C) hypochondriasis

(D) conversion disorder

(E) cerebrovascular accident involving the left hemisphere of the brain

Answer: (D). A patient with conversion disorder unintentionally develops symptoms or deficits affecting voluntary motor or sensory function that suggest a neurologic or other medical condition but that cannot be explained by a medical condition, by effects of a substance, or as a culturally sanctioned behavior. Examples include paralysis of an extremity, pseudoseizure, pseudocyesis, complaints of blindness, aphonia, and sensory complaints that do not follow neurologic parameters. (*Chapter 34, Page 298.*)

8.15 The patient is a 27-year-old white female clerical worker who is a member of a health maintenance organization plan. She has come to you as her primary care health provider seeking referral to a plastic surgeon for augmentation mammoplasty. She explains, "I have always hated my small breasts." She goes on to explain that she has stopped dating and avoids social functions because of her "flat-chested" appearance. On physical examination, although her breasts are smaller than average, they are symmetrical and seem within normal size range for her body morphology. There is no mass present. This patient

(A) has an appropriate request and should be referred to a plastic surgeon
(B) has symptoms consistent with body dysmorphic disorder
(C) is apparently attempting to receive inappropriate benefits from her insurer
(D) should have a referral to a dietician for nutritional therapy to achieve weight gain
(E) has symptoms consistent with the diagnosis of hypochondriasis

Answer: (B). Patients with body dysmorphic disorder have a loathing or preoccupation with an imagined defect in their appearance or excessive concern about a slight physical anomaly. This preoccupation causes significant distress or impairment in social, occupational, or other areas of function. (*Chapter 34, Page 298.*)

8.16 Neurasthenia is a synonym for

(A) pernicious anemia
(B) Guillain-Barré syndrome
(C) diabetic neuropathy
(D) cluster headache
(E) hypochondriasis

Answer: (E). The World Health Organization–sponsored *International Classification of Diseases and Related Health Problems* (ICD-10) includes a diagnosis of neurasthenia (literally, a lack of nerve energy), which is rarely made in the United States but is often used in other countries for patients with hypochondriasis. (*Chapter 34, Page 301.*)

8.17 The most important element in the successful management of somatizing patients is

(A) prompt psychiatric examination and referral
(B) appropriate selection of psychotropic medication
(C) confronting the patient with the psychophysiologic origins of the multiple somatic complaints

(D) establishing a solid therapeutic alliance between the patient and the personal physician
(E) individual psychotherapy

Answer: (D). After the thorough medical evaluation and the assessment or diagnosis is presented to the patient, a solid therapeutic alliance is established, which is the most essential ingredient for successful management of somatizing patients. The somatizing patient is then scheduled to see the family physician at regular intervals, the length of which varies depending on how well the patient's illness is compensated. (*Chapter 34, Page 301.*)

8.18 The distinguishing feature of FD is

(A) the high prevalence in men
(B) low prevalence in health care workers
(C) intentional production of physical or psychological symptoms
(D) inconsistency of the medical history over time
(E) the ready identification of secondary gain

Answer: (C). The essential element for the diagnosis of FD is *intentional* production of physical or psychological symptoms, with the hope of having psychological needs met by assuming a sick role. Secondary gain is not apparent, which distinguishes FD from malingering. FD is more common in women, and it seems to occur more frequently among health care workers than other populations. (*Chapter 34, Page 302.*)

8.19 Patients with eating disorders tend to have all the following characteristics EXCEPT

(A) a reluctance to reveal symptoms
(B) a tendency to come for treatment of conditions other than their eating disorders
(C) often come to the physician's office under pressure from family members
(D) typically have an isolated problem unrelated to other family dynamics
(E) often have a distorted body image

Answer: (D). Patients with eating disorders are often reluctant to reveal symptoms; they come for treatment of other conditions or under pressure from family members. Typically, practitioners do not routinely assess patients for these problems. Family systems problems predominate, especially in adolescent patients, and distorted body image is prominent as well. (*Chapter 35, Page 304.*)

8.20 The personality style of the patient with anorexia nervosa is often

(A) overcontrolled and rigid
(B) social and extroverted
(C) depressed and withdrawn
(D) open and sharing
(E) thoughtful and intuitive

Answer: (A). The personality style of the anorexia nervosa patient is often overcontrolled and rigid, with an unexpressive temperament. (*Chapter 35, Page 305.*)

8.21 The patient is a 24-year-old waitress in the office because of an upper respiratory infection. You note incidentally a loss of dental enamel from the lingual surfaces of the front teeth. This might be a sign of

(A) domestic violence
(B) bulimia
(C) pernicious anemia
(D) anorexia nervosa
(E) type 1 diabetes mellitus

Answer: (B). Common physical findings in bulimia include loss of dental enamel especially from lingual surfaces of the front teeth. The teeth may become chipped and appear ragged and "moth-eaten." (*Chapter 35, Page 306.*)

8.22 The patient is a 28-year-old white male maintenance worker in your office for the first time. He is here for the treatment of low back pain. You note that he seems humorless and perhaps irritable and hostile. He seems unable to relax and seems to scan the room while you are talking with him. He expresses a suspicion and mistrust of physicians in general and of his employers at work. He is also jealous of co-workers, who seem to get the "easy assignments." You suspect that this patient may have

(A) schizoid personality disorder (SPD)
(B) antisocial personality disorder
(C) histrionic personality disorder
(D) paranoid personality disorder (PPD)
(E) borderline personality disorder (BPD)

Answer: (D). PPD patients are suspicious and mistrustful. They refuse responsibility for their own feelings and are often hostile, irritable, and angry. Muscular tension, inability to relax, and the need to scan the environment for clues may be evident on examination. Affect is often humorless and serious. Pathologic jealousy is often present. (*Chapter 35, Page 307.*)

8.23 SPD is characterized by

(A) active involvement in community activities
(B) social withdrawal
(C) overinvolvement with family
(D) a tendency to dominate conversation during the office visit
(E) personal warmth

Answer: (B). SPD is characterized by a lifelong pattern of social withdrawal. These individuals are often seen by others as eccentric, isolated, or lonely. Prevalence may be as high as 7.5% in the general population. Patients tend to select solitary jobs. It is difficult for them to tolerate eye contact during office visits, and spontaneous conversation is avoided. (*Chapter 35, Page 307.*)

8.24 The diagnosis of BPD relies heavily on

(A) patient reports of anhedonia and sleep disturbance
(B) serial measurements of weight
(C) overwhelming anxiety, palpitations, and avoidance of selected social situations
(D) social withdrawal
(E) observing the patient's style of interacting with providers and family

Answer: (E). In contrast to such disorders as depression, which can be diagnosed from a review of relatively easily reported symptoms, the diagnosis of BPD relies heavily on observing the patient's style of interaction with providers and family. (*Chapter 35, Page 308.*)

8.25 The chief treatment for schizophrenia is

(A) drug therapy
(B) ECT
(C) family therapy
(D) individual cognitive psychotherapy
(E) commitment to an institution

Answer: (A). Drug therapy is the mainstay of treatment for schizophrenia. Treatment varies by the phase of the disease. Medication is not usually initiated during the prodromal phase of the illness, as the diagnosis cannot be made definitively. With acute exacerbation of the positive symptoms that characterize the active phase, relatively high doses of medication are often used to obtain initial control of symptoms. During the residual phase, negative symptoms tend to predominate, and lower doses of medications are used.

Some have tried "drug holidays" in an attempt to lessen short- and long-term side effects of medications, but the rate of relapse is high with low-dose maintenance and even higher with intermittent therapy. (*Chapter 35, Pages 309–310.*)

8.26 The short-term side effects of neuroleptic medications used for the treatment of schizophrenia include all of the following EXCEPT

(A) sedation
(B) transient hypertension
(C) dry mouth
(D) blurred vision
(E) urinary retention

Answer: (B). General short-term side effects of neuroleptics include sedation, orthostatic hypotension, anticholinergic symptoms such as dry mouth, blurred vision, and urinary retention. Galactorrhea and amenorrhea may occur. (*Chapter 35, Page 311.*)

8.27 The most common acute extrapyramidal side effect of neuroleptic antipsychotic medication is

(A) headache
(B) seizures
(C) intention tremor
(D) bradykinesia
(E) dystonia

Answer: (E). The most common acute extrapyramidal side effect of neuroleptics is dystonia, characterized by intermittent or sustained muscle spasms of a variety of facial or truncal muscle groups. An example is oculogyric crisis. Dystonia is reversible with administration of anticholinergics. (*Chapter 35, Pages 311–312.*)

DIRECTIONS (Items 8.28 through 8.48): Each of the items in this section is a multiple true–false problem that consists of a stem and four lettered options. Indicate whether each of the options is TRUE or FALSE.

8.28 The patient is a 24-year-old white female accountant who has a recent diagnosis of PD. She is fearful of crowds and avoids shopping whenever possible. Her work is suffering because of her fear of speaking in meetings. She asks about the long-term course of PD. Which of the following is/are true?

(A) PD is self-limited, and recovery can be expected within 12 to 18 months with or without therapy.
(B) PD patients may report previous suicide attempts, irrespective of the presence of depression.

(C) The response to anxiotic medication is generally very good.
(D) Depression rarely occurs in patients with PD.

Answer: (A-False, B-True, C-False, D-False). The longitudinal course of PD is one of persistent or recurring disability, with quality of life frequently being impaired. As many as 90% of PD patients have a history of major depression, and 20% of PD patients report previous suicide attempts, irrespective of the presence of depression. Up to 20% of PD patients abuse alcohol. When patients associate their panic attacks with the situations in which they occurred, fear and avoidance of those situations may develop as the patient attempts to prevent another panic attack. When this phobic avoidance becomes severe enough to restrict the patient's life, agoraphobia has developed. Up to two-thirds of PD patients have some degree of phobic avoidance. (*Chapter 31, Page 274.*)

8.29 True statements regarding PD include which of the following?

(A) There may be a strong family pattern.
(B) Children of PD patients frequently have behavioral problems.
(C) PD has been linked to domestic violence.
(D) Families with one or both parents with panic disorder have a decreased prevalence of childhood sexual abuse.

Answer: (A-True, B-True, C-True, D-False). Studies have shown a strong familial pattern for both PD and agoraphobia. Children of PD patients frequently have behavioral problems associated with avoidance behavior in the parents. PD has been linked to domestic violence; the prevalence of childhood sexual abuse is increased in those with PD, as is the frequency of current violence. (*Chapter 31, Page 276.*)

8.30 The patient is a 32-year-old white man with GAD. You have decided to treat him with a benzodiazepine. Factors that help predict a favorable response include

(A) absence of a precipitating stress
(B) absence of significant depression
(C) the patient is aware of the psychological nature of the symptoms
(D) a prior response to benzodiazepines

Answer: (A-False, B-True, C-True, D-True). At least 70% of GAD patients respond to benzodiazepines. Such response is more likely if a precipitating stress exists, significant depression is lacking, patients are aware of the psychological nature of their symptoms, there has been a prior response to benzodiazepines, and the patient expects recovery. Most patients who respond to benzodiazepines note improvement within the first week of therapy. (*Chapter 31, Page 277.*)

8.31 True statements regarding PTSD include which of the following?

(A) The severity of the trauma is highly correlated with the development of PTSD.
(B) The duration and intensity are highly correlated with the development of PTSD.
(C) Stress during a vulnerable time in the patient's life increases the risk of PTSD.
(D) In rape victims, PTSD is more likely to develop if rape is done by an acquaintance than done by a stranger.

Answer: (A-False, B-True, C-True, D-False). Although the severity of the trauma itself does not predict development of PTSD, its duration and intensity does. If the stress occurs during a vulnerable time in the patient's life or bears a similarity to an earlier traumatic event, PTSD is more likely. In rape victims, PTSD is more likely to develop if the rape is done by a stranger, involves physical force or injury, includes the display of weapons, or is associated with a sense of helplessness by the victim. (*Chapter 31, Page 281.*)

8.32 True statements regarding PTSD include which of the following?

(A) Symptoms generally begin 1 to 2 months following the stressor.
(B) Once established, PTSD may persist for years.
(C) Loss of interest and emotional detachment are uncommon.
(D) The patient often exhibits avoidance behavior of situations associated with the stressor.

Answer: (A-False, B-True, C-False, D-True). Although symptoms usually begin immediately after the stressor, there may be a delayed onset. Once established, PTSD frequently persists for years. Left untreated, half of those with PTSD after a motor vehicle accident no longer meet criteria 6 months later. Symptomatically, 90% of patients note sleep disturbance, loss of interest, emotional detachment, avoidance behavior of situations associated with the stressor, and reexperiencing the event. (*Chapter 31, Page 281.*)

8.33 True statements regarding ECT of depression include which of the following?

(A) Because of the success of newer antidepressant medications, ECT is no longer considered useful treatment for depression.
(B) ECT is contraindicated in patients with a recent myocardial infarction.
(C) Following ECT therapy, patients frequently exhibit long-term memory loss.
(D) Following ECT, antidepressant medication should not be resumed for 3 months.

Answer: (A-False, B-True, C-False, D-False). ECT remains a useful effective procedure for treatment of severe depression and mania. Studies have shown it to be as effective or superior to other antidepressant treatments. It is contraindicated in patients with recent stroke, space-occupying intracranial lesions, or recent myocardial infarction. There are no scientifically valid studies showing longer-term memory loss or disturbances in the ability to learn new information. Maintenance antidepressant treatment should follow to prevent relapse. (*Chapter 32, Page 291.*)

8.34 True statements regarding the use of lithium in treating bipolar disorder include which of the following?

(A) Lithium is metabolized in the liver and excreted through the gastrointestinal tract.
(B) Changes in fluid balance and dietary salt intake can affect the lithium level.
(C) Patients may experience a fine hand tremor as a side effect of lithium therapy.
(D) Up to 20% of patients taking lithium develop hypothyroidism.

Answer: (A-False, B-True, C-True, D-True). Lithium is excreted renally, so changes in fluid balance or dietary salt intake can dramatically affect the lithium level and produce toxicity. Dose-dependent side effects include gastrointestinal disturbances such as diarrhea and a fine hand tremor. Hypothyroidism occurs in up to 20% of patients. Thyroid levels must be checked before and every 6 months during treatment. Nephrogenic diabetes insipidus is infrequent, although up to 60% of patients on lithium complain of increased urination. (*Chapter 32, Page 291.*)

8.35 Important risk factors for suicide in young persons include

(A) substance abuse
(B) family dysfunction and conflict
(C) a history of physical or sexual abuse
(D) recent personal or media exposure to the suicide of others

Answer: (A-True, B-True, C-True, D-True). Important suicide risk factors in young persons include substance abuse, family dysfunction and conflict, a history of physical or sexual abuse, relationship problems (particularly with parents and boyfriends/girlfriends), and school-related problems. Feelings of extreme hopelessness and helplessness, rejection, and humiliation, coupled with a high degree of impulsivity, are common. The young are also at greater risk for "copycat" or "cluster" suicides triggered by recent personal or media exposure to the suicide of others. (*Chapter 33, Page 293.*)

8.36 True statements regarding suicide include which of the following?

(A) Men attempt suicide more often than women.
(B) Women complete suicide more often than men.
(C) About 40% of suicide attempters have made a previous attempt.
(D) Those who survive a suicide attempt rarely attempt or complete suicide in the future.

Answer: (A-False, B-False, C-True, D-False). Although the major risk factors for attempted suicide and completed suicide are the same, there are some differences between the two groups. Demographically, men complete suicide more often, but women attempt it three to seven times more often. Approximately 40% of suicide attempters have made a previous attempt; about 1% of attempters complete suicide within the following year; and somewhere between 2 to 10% complete it sometime in the future. (*Chapter 33, Page 294.*)

8.37 Your patient is a 28-year-old white male graduate student who has had a history of recurrent depression and is a survivor of a suicide attempt 4 years ago. Recently, his depression has been worse, and he is taking a tricyclic antidepressant. Although the patient denies current suicidal ideation, you are concerned about suicide risk. Worrisome clues would include which of the following?

(A) Change in appearance and self-care
(B) Change in behavior
(C) Change in cognitive function
(D) Change in emotional function

Answer: (A-True, B-True, C-True, D-True). A continuous physician–patient relationship that enables the physician to notice changes in appearance and self-care and changes in behavioral, cognitive, and emotional functioning may be the most accurate tool in assessing suicide risk. (*Chapter 33, Page 294.*)

8.38 Physicians are not immune from suicide. True statements regarding physician suicide include which of the following?

(A) Physicians commit suicide much less often than the general population.
(B) Physicians who commit suicide often have chronic mental or physical health problems.
(C) Because physicians rarely use lethal weapons (firearms) in suicide attempts, they are seldom successful on their first suicide attempt.
(D) A malpractice suit or a financial loss can be a risk factor for physician suicide.

Answer: (A-False, B-True, C-False, D-True). Physicians commit suicide at least as often as the general population; in fact, female physicians have higher suicide rates than women in general. Most physicians who commit suicide have a chronic physical or mental health disorder, and most are successful on their first attempt. Many have a history of drug or alcohol problems; others have experienced personal humiliation from financial losses or a malpractice suit. (*Chapter 33, Page 296.*)

8.39 True statements regarding hypochondriasis include which of the following?

(A) Hypochondriasis rarely begins before age 40.
(B) Hypochondriasis occurs much more commonly in women than men.
(C) Once hypochondriasis is established, significant recovery is rare.
(D) Hypochondriasis may be the chief symptom of major depression.

Answer: (A-False, B-False, C-False, D-True). Hypochondriasis can begin at any age and is seen in both sexes equally. It may fluctuate; and it may become chronic, although an estimated one-third to one-half of all patients recover significantly. Hypochondriasis may be the primary symptom of major depression, and studies have shown that almost one-half of patients with transient hypochondriasis had an anxiety or depressive disorder; 75% had at least one axis I diagnosis (a psychiatric clinical disorder or other condition that is the focus of clinical attention). (*Chapter 34, Page 300.*)

8.40 True statements regarding FD include which of the following?

(A) The disease is acute and self-limited.
(B) FD is a benign condition with low morbidity and no reported cases of fatality.

(C) No specific treatment is considered effective.

(D) Best results are achieved by confronting the patient with his or her behavior.

Answer: (A-False, B-False, C-True, D-False). The course of FD is usually chronic, and morbidity is high. Data are lacking on mortality, but case reports document that some patients die of their behavior (e.g., fatal factitious hypoglycemia) and suicides have occurred. No specific treatment is considered effective. Several controversial approaches to the patient have been advocated, including direct confrontation or "blacklisting" the patient (neither of which is recommended), behavior modification, prolonged psychiatric hospitalization, and individual or group psychotherapy. A gentler method, treatment without confrontation, uses inexact interpretations of the patient's behavior in which the patient's symptoms are partially explained; it stops short of actually confronting the factitious behavior. (*Chapter 34, Page 302.*)

8.41 The patient is a 45-year-old machinist who insists he is unable to work because of a back injury approximately 1 year ago. Your examination, supported by diagnostic imaging, fails to reveal a persistent disability. You suspect the patient is malingering. Appropriate management would include

(A) ruling out medical disorders that might be present

(B) screening for psychiatric disorders

(C) confronting the patient with your diagnosis of malingering

(D) indicating to the patient that the symptoms are not consistent with serious disease

Answer: (A-True, B-True, C-False, D-True). It is crucial to be certain that medical and psychiatric disorders do not coexist with malingering. Beyond this step, several authors agree that there is no treatment as such for malingering. It has been suggested that the individual be presented with a diagnosis of malingering only indirectly: The physician can subtly imply that he or she is aware of the simulation of illness and that the symptoms are not consistent with serious disease. Depriving the individual of the usual benefits of the sick role and in some settings (e.g., military) discussing the natural consequences of continued illness often result in rapid recovery. (*Chapter 34, Page 302.*)

8.42 Your patient is a 21-year-old female college student in your office for a sports physical examination. She is a member of the track team and reports that she runs daily. You are concerned because her weight is well below the average for her height, and there has been a loss of 22 lb since she visited your office 18 months ago. You are concerned about an eating disorder. True statements regarding eating disorders include which of the following?

(A) The prevalence of anorexia nervosa in the general population may be as high as 5%.

(B) Patients in weight loss programs have developed a "take charge" attitude toward weight control and therefore rarely have eating disorders.

(C) Approximately 90% of patients with eating disorders are female.

(D) Female athletes are at decreased risk of eating disorders when compared with their nonathlete peers.

Answer: (A-True, B-False, C-True, D-False). Estimates of prevalence are 5% for anorexia and 2% for bulimia in the general population. Prevalence is likely to be much higher among patients in weight loss programs. Patients are 90% female. Female athletes may be at increased risk. (*Chapter 35, Page 304.*)

8.43 Characteristics of anorexia nervosa include which of the following?

(A) loss of appetite

(B) fear of gaining weight

(C) disturbed perception of body morphology

(D) amenorrhea in pubescent girls

Answer: (A-False, B-True, C-True, D-True). Despite the syndrome's name, actual loss of appetite is rare. The patient is typically intensely afraid of gaining weight and exhibits a significant disturbance in the perception of the shape or size of his or her body. Amenorrhea is present among pubescent girls. (*Chapter 35, Page 305.*)

8.44 In addition to cognitive behavioral therapy, medication is often prescribed for patients with anorexia nervosa. Logical choices might include

(A) methylphenidate (Ritalin)

(B) zinc supplementation

(C) phenothiazines

(D) antidepressants

Answer: (A-False, B-True, C-False, D-True). Zinc supplementation may be useful for helping the patient to gain weight. Antidepressants, particularly SSRIs, in combination with cognitive behavioral psychotherapy, are effective. (*Chapter 35, Page 305.*)

8.45 True statements regarding BPD include which of the following?

(A) There is instability of affect and behavior.
(B) A synonym for BPD is "emotionally unstable personality disorder."
(C) BPD occurs with equal prevalence in women and men.
(D) In the United States, most patients with BPD are currently under care by psychiatrists.

Answer: (A-True, B-True, C-False, D-False). The essential characteristic of BPD is instability of affect, mood, behavior, object relations, and self-image. In the ICD-10, BPD is called "emotionally unstable personality disorder." The disorder is twice as common in women as in men; in the general population, the prevalence estimate is 2%. The prevalence may be higher in a primary care population, as these patients are attracted to medical settings. There is some evidence, not clear-cut, for genetic aspects of BPD. BPD patients tend to give primary care providers the most difficulty; and ironically, family physicians are more likely to see them than any other specialist. (*Chapter 35, Page 308.*)

8.46 True statements regarding avoidant personality disorder (APD) include which of the following?

(A) The patient has a low need for companionship.
(B) The patient has extreme sensitivity to rejection.
(C) Family members may believe the patient has an "inferiority complex."
(D) A synonym for APD is "antisocial personality disorder."

Answer: (A-False, B-True, C-True, D-False). The prevalence of APD may be lower in a primary care population, as these patients may be afraid to ask questions and delay seeking medical attention. A key feature of the disorder is extreme sensitivity to rejection coupled with a strong desire for companionship. These patients are commonly referred to as having an inferiority complex. The ICD-10 classifies it as "anxious personality disorder." (*Chapter 35, Page 308.*)

8.47 True statements regarding the management of difficult or personality disordered patients include which of the following?

(A) Assume the disorder is a true symptom.

(B) Assume that patients with these disorders are unlikely to respond to therapy of any kind.
(C) Be flexible in selecting a therapeutic approach, with a willingness to make management changes from visit to visit.
(D) Develop a collaborative relationship with the patient.

Answer: (A-True, B-False, C-False, D-True). Several authors have suggested detailed management strategies for "difficult patients," many if not all of whom are likely to be personality-disordered. Principles of management include the following:

1. Assume that the disorder is a true symptom and not a deliberate attempt to infuriate you.
2. Assume that the disorder can be managed; it is chronic and sometimes unremitting (especially without long-term psychotherapy) but is amenable to structured intervention.
3. Be consistent in implementing the chosen approach.
4. Develop a collaborative relationship with the patient (e.g., ask for feedback on how they feel about their medical care). (*Chapter 35, Page 309.*)

8.48 Neuroleptic malignant syndrome (NMS) is a feared complication of antipsychotic medications. True statements regarding NMS include which of the following?

(A) It is probably related to increased dopaminergic activity resulting from increased dopamine receptor transmission.
(B) It may also occur with abrupt withdrawal of dopaminergic medications such as L-Dopa.
(C) Patients generally recover with appropriate treatment.
(D) Although the signs and symptoms are temporarily disabling, mortality is rare.

Answer: (A-False, B-True, C-True, D-False). NMS is an uncommon but dangerous complication of treatment with neuroleptic medications. It is thought to be related to reduced dopaminergic activity resulting from dopamine receptor blockade by neuroleptics. It may also occur with abrupt withdrawal of dopaminergic medications such as L-Dopa or bromocriptine. Although patients generally recover with appropriate treatment, up to 20% fatality rates have been reported. (*Chapter 35, Page 312.*)

9

Allergy

The questions in this chapter constitute a review of the following chapters in *Family Medicine: Principles and Practice, Fifth Edition:*

Allergic Rhinitis and Hay Fever (Chapter 36)
Anaphylaxis and Anaphylactoid Reactions
(Chapter 37)

DIRECTIONS (Items 9.1 and 9.2): Each of the questions or incomplete statements in this section is followed by five suggested answers or completions. Select the ONE that is BEST in each case.

9.1 The patient is a 34-year-old white female attorney with sneezing, rhinorrhea, and nasal congestion present for 3 to 4 months. Based on the history and physical examination, you believe that the patient has allergic rhinitis. The patient, always a precise and fair person, asks for confirmation of the diagnosis. The chief method of confirming the diagnosis of allergic rhinitis is

(A) radioallergosorbent test
(B) skin tests
(C) elevated total IgE levels
(D) radiographs of the paranasal sinuses
(E) nasal challenge with allergens

Answer: (B). Skin tests are the major confirmatory study for allergic rhinitis. Epicutaneous (prick, puncture, or scratch) and intradermal techniques are used, with epicutaneous testing being more specific but less sensitive than the intradermal method and the prick method having the highest correlation with allergic symptoms. Antihistamines in standard doses can suppress positive skin reactivity for up to 1 to 3 weeks and should be discontinued before skin testing. (*Chapter 36, Page 315.*)

9.2 Up to 4% of the population is allergic to the venom of one or more stinging insects and may have re-sting reactions when stung again by the same species. Which of the following population groups is LEAST likely to experience a re-sting reaction?

(A) children younger than 16 years of age
(B) pregnant women
(C) athletes
(D) persons 65 years of age and older
(E) African Americans

Answer: (A). Children younger than 16 years of age are least likely to experience re-sting reactions. (*Chapter 37, Pages 321–322.*)

DIRECTIONS (Items 9.3 through 9.10): Each of the items in this section is a multiple true–false problem that consists of a stem and four lettered options. Indicate whether each of the options is TRUE or FALSE.

9.3 The patient is a 48-year-old black man who is taking a second-generation antihistamine for allergic rhinitis. He should be cautioned to avoid

(A) ketoconazole (Nizoral)
(B) clarithromycin (Biaxin)
(C) cimetidine (Tagamet)
(D) ibuprofen (Motrin, Advil)

Answer: (A-True, B-True, C-True, D-False). Caution should be exercised when prescribing second-generation antihistamines for patients who are concurrently taking drugs that undergo significant hepatic metabolism, such as ketoconazole, itraconazole, clarithromycin, erythromycin, cimetidine, and disulfuram (Antabuse). (*Chapter 36, Page 316.*)

9.4 The patient is a 39-year-old white man who is using topical corticosteroids in the treatment of allergic rhinitis. True statements concerning such use include which of the following?

(A) With long-term use, these drugs produce worrisome systemic adverse effects.
(B) There is a low incidence of local adverse reactions such as nasal burning or epistaxis.
(C) Response to these agents usually begins within 2 to 3 days of initiating therapy.
(D) The maximum benefit is achieved within 3 to 5 days of regular use.

Answer: (A-False, B-True, C-True, D-False). Topical corticosteroids are effective, are delivered via inhalers, have potent anti-inflammatory activity, produce no systemic adverse effects, have a low adverse effect profile (i.e., nasal burning or irritation, sneezing, and epistaxis), and substantially reduce symptoms of sneezing, rhinorrhea, and congestion. Steroids used topically in the nose reduce symptoms and mediator release during the early and late phases of the allergic reaction. Patients must understand that the response to these agents and relief of symptoms usually begins within 2 to 3 days of initiating therapy, and the maximum response may require 2 to 3 weeks of regular use. (*Chapter 36, Page 316.*)

9.5 Cromolyn sodium is sometimes prescribed for the treatment of allergic rhinitis. This drug

(A) seems to act by stabilization of the membranes of sensitized mast cells
(B) has a rapid onset of action (within 2 to 4 hours)
(C) should be reserved for use following the onset of seasonal symptoms
(D) is safe for long-term use

Answer: (A-True, B-False, C-False, D-True). The proposed mode of action of cromolyn sodium is stabilization of membranes of sensitized mast cells and prevention of degranulation and mediator release in response to an allergen challenge. As a 4% nasal spray in a metered-dose inhaler (Nasalcrom), the efficacy of cromolyn varies, and the onset of action is slow (up to 4 weeks), so it is most effective when used before the onset of seasonal symptoms and as prophylaxis before exposures. Cromolyn has few minor adverse effects (e.g., nasal irritation, sneezing) and is safe for long-term use; patient compliance can be an issue, however,

because of dosing three to four times a day. (*Chapter 36, Page 316.*)

9.6 The patient is a 32-year-old white female teacher with severe allergic rhinitis who finds that antihistamine medication causes excessive drowsiness. You are considering immunotherapy. Criteria for the use of immunotherapy include which of the following?

(A) allergy to airborne pollens
(B) significant symptoms after exposure
(C) sensitivity documented by personal and family history
(D) inability to avoid allergens

Answer: (A-True, B-True, C-False, D-True). Immunotherapy should be reserved for patients who have allergy to airborne allergens, significant symptoms after exposure, a sensitivity proved by skin testing, and those who find it difficult or impossible to avoid allergens or do not respond adequately to pharmacotherapy. (*Chapter 36, Page 318.*)

9.7 True statements regarding food-induced anaphylaxis include which of the following?

(A) Patients usually lack a history of prior reaction to foods.
(B) Patients are likely to have history of asthma or eczema.
(C) Most episodes of food-induced anaphylaxis occur in the home.
(D) Common food allergens in children include peanuts, cows' milk, and eggs.

Answer: (A-False, B-True, C-False, D-True). The incidence of food-induced anaphylaxis is unknown. What is known is that individuals with food-induced anaphylaxis usually have a history of reactions to one or more foods and are likely to have a history of asthma, rhinorrhea, or eczema. Most episodes of food-induced anaphylaxis occur away from home in situations in which the food allergen is inadvertently ingested in candy, cereals, cookies, or pastry. The most common food allergens in children are peanuts, tree nuts (walnuts, cashews, hazelnuts, almonds), cows' milk, soy, and eggs. (*Chapter 37, Page 321.*)

9.8 The immediate therapy of an anaphylactic reaction due to an insect sting includes which of the following?

(A) identification of the sting location
(B) placement of a tourniquet proximal to the sting site

(C) remove the stinger with sterile forceps

(D) injection of epinephrine intradermally at the sting site

Answer: (A-True, B-True, C-False, D-True). Once it is discovered that the anaphylactic reaction is due to an insect sting, the sting location should be found, a tourniquet applied proximal to the sting site, the stinger dug out with a surgical blade (using forceps may only serve to release further venom from the venom sack), and epinephrine 1:1000 solution 0.005 ml/kg injected intradermally at the site of the sting (maximum dose, 0.15 to 0.25 ml). (*Chapter 37, Page 322.*)

9.9 Which of the following statements regarding exercise-induced anaphylaxis (EIA) is true?

(A) EIA occurs 30 to 60 minutes following the onset of exercise.

(B) EIA is unrelated to exercise-induced asthma.

(C) EIA is unrelated to consumption of food or medication.

(D) The incidence of EIA has increased over the past few decades.

Answer: (A-False, B-False, C-False, D-True). EIA occurs within 5 to 8 minutes of the onset of exercise. EIA is a worsening of exercise-induced asthma. EIA often occurs when certain foods or medications are consumed prior to exercise. The incidence is unknown, but it has been on the rise since exercise became more fashionable during the 1970s. The usual patient profile prevails with a history of atopy, positive family history, and female sex. (*Chapter 37, Page 322.*)

9.10 The patient is a 60-year-old white man with a suspected urinary calculus. You plan to refer the patient for a intravenous pyelogram when he informs you of an "allergic reaction" with a "kidney x-ray" about 20 years ago. True statements regarding the management of this patient include which of the following?

(A) Anaphylactoid reactions to radiocontrast media are generally dose-related.

(B) Anaphylactoid reactions to radiocontrast media are always immediate.

(C) Pretreatment orally with corticosteroids or antihistamines may reduce the risk of anaphylactoid reaction to radiocontrast media.

(D) The patient with a prior history of anaphylactoid reactions to radiocontrast media rarely rereacts.

Answer: (A-False, B-False, C-True, D-False). One million diagnostic procedures in the United States per year involve the use of radiocontrast material: 1 to 2% of patients have an anaphylactoid reaction, and 1:10,000 patients die. Anaphylactoid reactions are neither dose-related nor always immediate. Pretreatment orally with corticosteroids, diphenhydramine, and ephedrine decreases the allergic reaction rate to 5%. A reported 16 to 44% of patients with a history of anaphylactoid reaction to radiocontrast media rereact. (*Chapter 37, Page 323.*)

10
Infectious Diseases

The questions in this chapter constitute a review of the following chapters in *Family Medicine: Principles and Practice, Fifth Edition:*

Epstein-Barr Virus Infection and Infectious Mononucleosis (Chapter 38)

Viral Infections of the Respiratory Tract (Chapter 39)

Sinusitis and Pharyngitis (Chapter 40)

Sexually Transmitted Diseases (Chapter 41)

Human Immunodeficiency Virus Infection and Acquired Immunodeficiency Syndrome (Chapter 42)

Bacteremia and Sepsis (Chapter 43)

Selected Infectious Diseases (Chapter 44)

DIRECTIONS (Items 10.1 through 10.46): Each of the questions or incomplete statements in this section is followed by five suggested answers or completions. Select the ONE that is BEST in each case.

10.1 The Paul-Bunnell-Davidsohn test and the identification of Downey lymphocytes may be useful in the diagnosis of

(A) allergic rhinitis
(B) herpes simplex
(C) ECHO virus infection
(D) chronic lymphocytic leukemia
(E) infectious mononucleosis (IM)

Answer: (E). IM can be diagnosed with confidence when patients have a compatible illness and laboratory tests show the following: relative and absolute lymphocytosis on differential white blood cell count from a peripheral blood smear; lymphocyte atypia (Downey lymphocytes) of more than 20%; and heterophile antibody titers of at least 1:56 by the traditional Paul-Bunnell-Davidsohn test or a positive rapid slide assay. (*Chapter 38, Page 326.*)

10.2 The patient is a 17-year-old white male high school student who has a severe sore throat with other clinical criteria for IM. He is heterophile antibody-positive. You should avoid treating this patient with ampicillin and amoxicillin because of the risk of producing a rash, which is

(A) a drug-induced anaphylactoid reaction
(B) an allergy
(C) a lifelong contraindication to further use of ampicillin or amoxicillin
(D) a temporary intolerance to aminopenicillins
(E) an indication that the patient has atopic dermatitis

Answer: (D). There is no specific therapy for IM except supportive care to the extent required by individual patients. Antibiotics are prescribed only to treat bacterial complications. Ampicillin and amoxicillin should always be avoided in patients with IM or symptoms suggestive of IM because of the risk of producing a generalized, intensely pruritic, maculopapular, erythematous rash. This reaction is a temporary intolerance to aminopenicillins, not an allergy, and later use is not contraindicated. (*Chapter 38, Page 327.*)

10.3 The patient with IM should be advised to refrain from contact sports because of the risk of

(A) splenic rupture
(B) subarachnoid hemorrhage
(C) purpura
(D) transmission to other players
(E) development of chronic fatigue syndrome

Answer: (A). All patients with IM should be advised to refrain from contact sports until splenic involution is complete, although there is no harm for most patients to resume physical exercise to the degree tolerated when they feel well enough to do so. (*Chapter 38, Page 327.*)

10.4 A 2-year-old child presents with clinical findings of bronchiolitis, and the chest radiograph shows a small area of pneumonia in the right lower lobe. The most likely cause is

(A) group A beta-hemolytic *Streptococcus* (GABHS)
(B) *Haemophilus influenzae*
(C) respiratory syncytial virus (RSV)
(D) *Streptococcus pneumoniae*
(E) Coxsackie virus

Answer: (C). RSV, a single-stranded RNA paramyxovirus, is the leading cause of pneumonia and bronchiolitis in infants and children. Two antigenically distinct groups of RSV (A and B) are recognized. Community outbreaks of RSV usually appear during the winter and spring in temperate climates. (*Chapter 39, Pages 328–329.*)

10.5 The single most important infection control measure for RSV infection is

(A) hand washing
(B) prophylactic antibiotics for household contacts of infected individuals
(C) strict isolation of infected individuals
(D) culture of nasopharyngeal secretions of all contacts of infected persons
(E) use of masks by family members and health care providers

Answer: (A). Strategies for controlling spread of RSV should be aimed at interrupting hand carriage of the virus and self-inoculation of the eyes and nose. Masks commonly used for respiratory viruses have not been shown to be an effective measure for curtailing RSV outbreaks on pediatric wards. Hand washing is probably the single most important infection control measure for RSV. (*Chapter 39, Page 329.*)

10.6 During an influenza epidemic, most deaths are due to

(A) ischemic heart disease
(B) pneumonia
(C) thrombophlebitis
(D) stroke
(E) acquired immunodeficiency syndrome (AIDS)

Answer: (A). Pneumonia is usually blamed for excess mortality, but twice as many deaths during an influenza epidemic are attributable to ischemic heart disease than to pneumonia. (*Chapter 39, Page 332.*)

10.7 The most frequent cause of upper respiratory infection (URI) in adults is

(A) GABHS
(B) *Haemophilus influenzae*
(C) Coxsackie virus
(D) rhinovirus
(E) RSV

Answer: (D). Rhinovirus is the most frequent cause of upper respiratory tract infection in adults and can be a cause of coughing without bronchitis. (*Chapter 39, Page 333.*)

10.8 The patient is an 18-month-old white girl with severe cough, tachypnea, and rapid shallow respirations. There are tight respiratory sounds and some rhonchi. On physical examination, there are intercostal retractions and nasal flaring. The chest roentgenogram shows hyperinflation but no infiltrates. This child most likely has

(A) spasmodic croup
(B) laryngotracheobronchitis
(C) *Haemophilus influenzae* infection
(D) bronchiolitis
(E) rhinovirus infection

Answer: (D). Bronchiolitis is an acute viral respiratory disease generally found in children younger than 2 years old. The typical clinical presentation is a URI with cough that progresses to a more severe cough and tachypnea. Respirations become rapid and shallow with a prolonged expiratory phase. Because the infants are not able to breathe well, they are also unable to suck or drink and can become dehydrated. Physical findings include intercostal retractions and nasal flaring, which suggest pneumonia. A chest roentgenogram shows only hyperinflation with no infiltrates. Tight respiratory sounds (not entirely typical of wheezes found with asthma) are usually present, as are some rhonchi. (*Chapter 39, Pages 333–334.*)

10.9 The patient is a 44-year-old white female school teacher who has had a mild URI for 4 to 5 days. The chief manifestation has been hoarseness, which is a problem because of her need to talk while teaching. The most important aspect of managing this patient's problem will be

(A) saline gargles
(B) voice rest
(C) inhaled corticosteroids
(D) antihistamines
(E) decongestants

Answer: (B). Voice rest makes the greatest impact on recover from laryngitis. Patients who are able to gargle with warm weak saline solution find it soothing. Patients should be told that laryngitis is not a serious disease and that adequate time to recover is the only therapy in most cases. (*Chapter 39, Page 334.*)

10.10 Acute sinusitis most commonly involves the

(A) maxillary sinuses
(B) ethmoidal sinuses
(C) sphenoidal sinuses
(D) frontal sinuses
(E) mastoid sinuses

Answer: (A). Maxillary sinuses are most commonly infected, followed by ethmoidal, sphenoidal, and frontal sinuses. (*Chapter 40, Page 337.*)

10.11 The radiographic view most specific to the maxillary sinuses is the

(A) Caldwell view
(B) Waters view
(C) lateral view
(D) submentovertical view
(E) coronal view

Answer: (B). Plain sinus radiographs may show air-fluid levels, mucosal thickening, and possibly anatomic abnormalities that predispose to the condition, such as nasal polyps. Views specific to each sinus are the Caldwell (frontal), Waters (maxillary), lateral (sphenoid), and submentovertical (ethmoid). (*Chapter 40, Page 337.*)

10.12 Appropriate antibiotics for the treatment of acute sinusitis include all the following EXCEPT

(A) amoxicillin-clavulanate
(B) trimethoprim-sulfamethoxazole (TMP-SMX)
(C) ketoconazole
(D) clarithromycin
(E) a second- or third-generation cephalosporin

Answer: (C). Amoxicillin-clavulanate, TMP-SMX, clarithromycin, or a second- or third-generation cephalosporin (e.g., cefaclor, cefuroxime axetil, loracarbef) are primary antibiotics for acute bacterial sinusitis. Dura-

tion of treatment is 14 to 21 days. Ampicillin may be used if beta-lactamase organisms are locally uncommon. (*Chapter 40, Page 338.*)

10.13 The patient is a 9-year-old girl with a URI that has lasted for almost 3 weeks. Currently, she has a fever with a temperature of 39.2°C, cough, and complaints of facial pain. You should suspect that this child has

(A) an immune deficiency
(B) ECHO virus infection
(C) streptococcal sore throat
(D) acute mastoiditis
(E) acute sinusitis

Answer: (E). If a URI is severe or persists beyond 10 days in a child, suspect sinusitis. Common symptoms include fever greater than 39°C, periorbital edema, facial pain, and daytime cough. Periorbital cellulitis is seen in infants with ethmoidal disease. (*Chapter 40, Page 339.*)

10.14 The initial antibiotic therapy of an 11-year-old boy with acute sinusitis should be

(A) erythromycin
(B) cefaclor
(C) TMP-SMX
(D) amoxicillin
(E) norfloxacin

Answer: (D). Amoxicillin is the initial antibiotic of choice. TMP-SMX, erythromycin-sulfisoxazole, amoxicillin-clavulanate, cefaclor, and cefuroxime axetil are useful in penicillin-allergic individuals or if beta-lactamase–producing organisms are suspected. All antibiotics are given for 14 to 21 days. (*Chapter 40, Page 339.*)

10.15 The rash of scarlet fever typically has all the following characteristics EXCEPT

(A) a fine blanching appearance
(B) present on palms of the hands and soles of the feet
(C) sandpaper texture
(D) circumoral pallor
(E) hyperpigmentation in the skin creases

Answer: (B). Scarlet fever produces a rash characterized by a fine blanching appearance and sandpaper texture, circumoral pallor, and hyperpigmentation in the skin creases. (*Chapter 40, Page 340.*)

10.16 The "gold standard" for diagnosing GABHS pharyngitis is

(A) throat culture
(B) elevated antistreptolysin-o titer
(C) clinical response to penicillin or similar antibiotic within 36 hours
(D) presence of gram-positive cocci on Gram stain
(E) streptococcal rapid antigen test

Answer: (A). The "gold standard" for diagnosing acute GABHS pharyngitis is a properly processed and interpreted throat culture on sheep blood agar. For best throat culture results, use a Dacron swab and thoroughly swab the palatine tonsils and pharyngeal wall, avoiding the tongue. Plating even a dry swab may be delayed as long as 24 hours without affecting culture results. (*Chapter 40, Page 340.*)

10.17 The antibiotic of choice for GABHS pharyngitis is

(A) ampicillin
(B) amoxicillin-clavulanate
(C) clarithromycin
(D) penicillin
(E) a second- or third-generation cephalosporin

Answer: (D). The choice of antibiotic for GABHS pharyngitis should include cost, side effects profile, and patient compliance. Penicillin remains the drug of choice because it is effective in preventing acute rheumatic fever, inexpensive, and relatively safe. No evidence of penicillin-resistant GABHS has been identified. (*Chapter 40, Page 341.*)

10.18 The patient is a 10-year-old boy with acute pharyngitis that is very painful. You and the family agree that analgesia is needed. Which of the following analgesics should be AVOIDED in this patient?

(A) ibuprofen
(B) naproxen
(C) aspirin
(D) acetaminophen
(E) hydrocodone

Answer: (C). Aspirin should be avoided in children and teenagers because of the risk for Reye syndrome. Ibuprofen 400 mg every 6 hours is superior to acetaminophen for alleviating throat pain. Available suspension analgesics include ibuprofen 100 mg/5 ml, naproxen 125 mg/5 ml, acetaminophen with codeine elixir, and acetaminophen with hydrocodone elixir. Warm liquids are an effective adjuvant treatment in combination with analgesics. (*Chapter 40, Page 341.*)

10.19 The most commonly occurring sexually transmitted disease (STD) in the United States is

(A) *Chlamydia*
(B) gonorrhea
(C) syphilis
(D) human immunodeficiency virus (HIV) infection
(E) genital warts

Answer: (A). *Chlamydia* infection is the most common STD in the United States. Infection rates range from 3% of women and men in asymptomatic populations to 20% of those screened in STD clinics. The prevalence is highest in sexually active, adolescent girls. Up to two-thirds of infected women and one-fourth of infected men remain asymptomatic. Continued sexual activity by untreated asymptomatic individuals contributes to continued transmission of *Chlamydia* infections. (*Chapter 40, Page 345.*)

10.20 The gold standard for the diagnosis of *Chlamydia trachomatis* infection is

(A) a prompt response to broad-spectrum antibiotic therapy
(B) culture
(C) direct fluorescent antibody (DFA) test
(D) the enzyme immunoassay (EIA) test
(E) the nucleic acid hybridization (DNA probe) test

Answer: (B). Culture is the gold standard for the diagnosis of *Chlamydia trachomatis* infection, with a specificity approaching 100%. However, cultures are technically difficult and require 3 to 7 days to obtain results. Cultures are recommended for specimens from the urethra in women and asymptomatic men, the nasopharynx in infants, the rectum at all ages, and the vagina in prepubertal girls. Culture is also indicated in low-risk populations in which documentation of a true positive is necessary and in medicolegal cases. For populations at high risk, a sensitive, more rapid diagnosis can be made with nonculture tests, including the DFA test, the EIA test, and the nucleic acid hybridization (DNA probe) test. These tests are about as specific (90 to 99%) as culture but are less sensitive (70 to 90%). (*Chapter 41, Page 345.*)

10.21 The most commonly *reported* STD in the United States is

(A) syphilis
(B) gonorrhea
(C) HIV infection
(D) *Chlamydia*
(E) herpes virus infection

Answer: (B). Gonorrhea is the most commonly reported STD in the United States. Although the rate of reported gonorrhea decreased 65% in the United States from 1975 to 1993, gonorrhea rates in the United States remain highest among developed countries. Sexually active men and women 20 to 24 years of age have the highest attack rate of the disease. (*Chapter 41, Page 346.*)

10.22 The most common symptom of women with pelvic inflammatory disease (PID) is

(A) menstrual irregularity
(B) vaginal discharge
(C) dyspareunia
(D) dull, constant lower abdominal pain
(E) right upper quadrant abdominal pain with peritoneal signs

Answer: (D). A clinical diagnosis of PID is difficult owing to the wide range in symptomatology. Women may be asymptomatic, have mild or nonspecific symptoms such as abnormal bleeding, dyspareunia, or vaginal discharge, or have severe symptoms with peritoneal signs. The most common symptom is dull constant lower abdominal pain for less than 2 weeks. (*Chapter 41, Page 347.*)

10.23 The patient is a 26-year-old white man informed yesterday by the County Health Department that a sexual partner has been diagnosed with early latent syphilis. Your patient should be

(A) treated even if seronegative
(B) treated only if seropositive
(C) not treated if seronegative
(D) not treated if seropositive
(E) observed and treated if lesions of primary or secondary syphilis are detected

Answer: (A). Individuals sexually exposed to a person with primary, secondary, or early latent syphilis within the preceding 90 days should be presumptively treated even if seronegative. If the exposure was more than 90 days, treat presumptively if serologic testing is not immediately available or if follow-up is uncertain. (*Chapter 41, Page 350.*)

10.24 The patient is a 32-year-old black female sales clerk with a history of human papilloma virus (HPV) infection. A Papanicolaou (Pap) smear shows inflammation with reactive cellular changes. Appropriate treatment for this patient would be which of the following?

(A) Refer the patient for cervical conization.
(B) Treat nightly with vaginal cleocin cream for 7 days.

(C) Treat with ampicillin and metronidazole therapy for 10 days.
(D) Treat any underlying infection and repeat the Pap smear in 3 months.
(E) Self-treat the uterine cervix with podophyllin 10% weekly for 6 weeks.

Answer: (D). Pap smears should be examined yearly not only for all women with a history of HPV infection but also for all women with a history of any STD. If a Pap smear shows inflammation with reactive cellular changes, any underlying infection should be treated and the Pap smear repeated in 3 months. (*Chapter 41, Page 351.*)

10.25 The patient is a 28-year-old single white woman who is sexually active with her boyfriend. They have been in a monogamous relationship for 6 months. Her complaint today is an ulcer of the left labia that has been present for 2 weeks and is painful, especially on urination. Physical examination confirms the presence of a superficial ulceration of the left labia with a few nearby vesicles. This patient's most likely diagnosis is

(A) primary syphilis
(B) herpes simplex virus (HSV) infection
(C) domestic violence causing vaginal trauma
(D) diabetes mellitus
(E) Bartholin cyst infection

Answer: (B). Primary infection with HSV is often severe. Patients experience a prodrome consisting of malaise, fever, headache, myalgias, and genital paresthesias followed by outbreaks of multiple painful vesicles that erode and ulcerate. (*Chapter 41, Page 352.*)

10.26 *Haemophilus ducreyi* is the organism responsible for

(A) lymphogranuloma venereum (LGV)
(B) yaws
(C) Lyme disease
(D) chancroid
(E) Kaposi's sarcoma (KS)

Answer: (D). Chancroid is caused by *Haemophilus ducreyi*, which is endemic in parts of the United States and is a cofactor for HIV transmission. LGV is caused by specific serovars of *C. trachomatis*. (*Chapter 41, Page 353.*)

10.27 The average time from HIV infection to AIDS-defining illnesses appears to be about

(A) 6 to 9 months
(B) 2 to 3 years
(C) 5 to 7 years

(D) 8 to 11 years
(E) 15 to 20 years

Answer: (D). The average time from infection to AIDS-defining illnesses appears to be about 8 to 11 years. (*Chapter 42, Page 357.*)

10.28 Patients who have acquired HIV have a "window period" between the time of infection and seroconversion. For most patients, the length of this "window period" is

(A) 2 to 3 weeks
(B) 6 weeks to 3 months
(C) 4 to 8 months
(D) 12 to 18 months
(E) 2 to 3 years

Answer: (B). A "window period" of 6 weeks to 3 months exists between the time of infection and seroconversion. During this time, patients can be infected but do not have a sufficient antibody response to result in positive serologic testing. For seronegative patients with recent at-risk activities, retesting at 3 to 6 months is advised. In a few patients, serologic evidence of HIV infection may not occur for 6 months to 1 year or longer and, rarely, not at all. (*Chapter 42, Page 358.*)

10.29 The patient is a 36-year-old white man with advanced HIV disease and a CD4+ lymphocyte count of fewer than 200 cells/mm³. You have decided to initiate prophylaxis against *Pneumocystis carinii* pneumonia (PCP). The drug of choice for this purpose is

(A) zidovudine
(B) didanosine
(C) TMP-SMX
(D) ampicillin-clavulanate
(E) ganciclovir

Answer: (C). Preventing PCP and other opportunistic infections decreases morbidity and mortality. When CD4+ lymphocyte counts fall to fewer than 200 cells/mm³ or when patients develop symptoms of advanced HIV disease, prophylaxis against PCP should be initiated. Prophylaxis has been shown to delay or prevent the development of PCP and improve the survival and health of HIV-infected persons. TMP-SMX, one double-strength tablet daily, is the drug of choice. (*Chapter 42, Page 359.*)

10.30 The most frequent first manifestation of HIV disease is

(A) cough
(B) weight loss
(C) fever
(D) diarrhea
(E) skin and oral cavity lesions

Answer: (E). Skin and oral cavity lesions are the most frequent first manifestations of HIV disease. A form of seborrheic dermatitis is the most common skin condition found in HIV-infected persons. This condition is readily treated with a combination of low-strength hydrocortisone cream plus ketoconazole cream. (*Chapter 42, Page 362.*)

10.31 The most common cause of morbidity and death in HIV-infected persons is

(A) intracranial bleeding
(B) coronary artery disease
(C) diarrhea
(D) pulmonary disease
(E) encephalopathy

Answer: (D). Pulmonary disease is the most common cause of morbidity and mortality in HIV-infected persons. Pulmonary symptoms and signs can vary from only minimal shortness of breath or nonproductive cough to severe respiratory distress. (*Chapter 42, Page 363.*)

10.32 In the human immunodeficiency virus (HIV) infected patient, the most common renal problem is

(A) drug toxicity
(B) thrombosis of one or both renal arteries
(C) urolithiasis
(D) cytomegalovirus infection
(E) nephrotic syndrome

Answer: (A). The most common renal problem is drug toxicity. Special attention is required when patients are taking TMP-SMX, nonsteroidal anti-inflammatory drugs (NSAID), or other drugs known to cause nephrotoxicity. (*Chapter 42, Page 364.*)

10.33 Establishing the diagnosis of HIV infection in infants is important but problematic. Testing for antibodies in infants can reflect maternal antibodies until approximately what age?

(A) 2 weeks
(B) 2 months
(C) 9 months
(D) 15 months
(E) 3 years

Answer: (D). Establishing the diagnosis of HIV infection in infants can be problematic, because testing for antibodies measures maternal antibodies until approximately 15 months of age. Special testing with the DNA polymerase chain reaction can identify infected infants by 1 month of age. The diagnosis in infants is confirmed by viral culture or clinical syndromes. (*Chapter 42, Page 364.*)

10.34 Your patient is a 58-year-old white man with fever, tachycardia, oliguria, and hypotension indicating septic shock. You should begin intravenous fluids to maintain a urine output of at least

(A) 0.5 ml/kg/hour
(B) 2 ml/kg/hour
(C) 5 ml/kg/hour
(D) a quantity equal to twice the infused volume of fluid plus 600 ml for insensible loss
(E) 2 L over 24 hours

Answer: (A). Volume infusion to restore blood pressure, capillary refill, mental function, and urine output to a minimum of 0.5 ml/kg/hour is mandatory. (*Chapter 43, Page 367.*)

10.35 Most children with septic shock have infections with

(A) group B *Streptococcus pneumoniae*
(B) *Escherichia coli*
(C) gram-negative enteric bacteria
(D) gram-positive rods
(E) *Staphylococcus aureus*

Answer: (C). Most children with septic shock have infections with gram-negative bacteria such as *Pseudomonas aeruginosa, H. influenzae* B, and *N. meningitidis.* (*Chapter 43, Page 368.*)

10.36 There is an increased risk of bacterial sepsis and meningitis during the first 5 years of life in infants and children who have

(A) patent foramen ovale
(B) pyloric stenosis
(C) failure to thrive
(D) fracture of the femur of unknown cause
(E) sickle cell disease

Answer: (E). Infants and children with sickle cell disease are at great risk for developing bacterial sepsis and meningitis within the first 5 years of life. The attack rate from *S. pneumoniae* and *H. influenzae* B ranges from 15 to 30%. When sepsis occurs, mortality is 30 to 50%. (*Chapter 43, Page 370.*)

10.37 The characteristic ocular lesion of toxoplasmosis is

(A) macular degeneration
(B) hyphema
(C) closed-angle glaucoma
(D) chorioretinitis
(E) nuclear cataracts

Answer: (D). Chorioretinitis usually accompanies the congenital form of toxoplasmosis and frequently is seen in the chronic form. (*Chapter 44, Page 372.*)

10.38 The most common source of toxoplasmosis infection is

(A) cat's saliva
(B) undercooked meat
(C) droplet infection
(D) body fluids
(E) breast milk

Answer: (B). *Toxoplasma gondii* is contracted most commonly by ingestion of tissue cysts in meat that is undercooked or raw (mainly lamb or pork, rarely cattle). Oocysts may also be transferred to the mouth after handling cats or cat feces while changing cat litter boxes. (*Chapter 44, Page 372b.*)

10.39 The most common finding in acute acquired toxoplasmosis is

(A) lymphadenopathy
(B) headache
(C) visual impairment
(D) rash
(E) jaundice

Answer: (A). Lymphadenopathy is the most frequently occurring symptom and may be generalized or localized, usually including the cervical lymph nodes, especially the posterior nodes. Lymphadenopathy can persist for months as the only symptom. (*Chapter 44, Page 373.*)

10.40 The patient is a 28-year-old white woman at 30 weeks' gestation. She has been diagnosed with acutely acquired toxoplasmosis. The drug appropriate for fetal therapy is

(A) norfloxacin
(B) penicillin

(C) fluconazole
(D) TMP-SMX
(E) spiramycin

Answer: (E). The current recommendation for fetal therapy of toxoplasmosis is initiation of spiramycin (3 g/day in three divided doses) for acutely acquired toxoplasmosis during pregnancy, to be continued until delivery. Once the fetal infection is confirmed, repeated courses of combination pyrimethamine (25 mg b.i.d.), sulfadiazine (500 mg/week), and folinic acid (50 mg/week) are alternated with courses of spiramycin. (*Chapter 44, Page 374.*)

10.41 The hallmark symptom of trichinellosis is

(A) headache
(B) fever
(C) upper gastrointestinal bleeding
(D) myalgia
(E) motor weakness

Answer: (D). The hallmark symptom of trichinellosis is myalgia, although abdominal pain and diarrhea are common. (*Chapter 44, Page 375.*)

10.42 The clinical presentation of psittacosis is most likely to be

(A) vomiting
(B) abdominal pain
(C) arthralgia
(D) pneumonia
(E) erythema marginatum

Answer: (D). The incubation period for psittacosis is 7 to 21 days. It most commonly presents as a pneumonia, although gastrointestinal and central nervous system involvement can occur. (*Chapter 44, Page 377.*)

10.43 Most giardiasis outbreaks can be traced to

(A) undercooked pork
(B) contaminated water supplies
(C) salads
(D) parrots
(E) cat feces

Answer: (B). Contaminated water supplies have been the source of most giardiasis outbreaks. (*Chapter 44, Page 379.*)

10.44 The most commonly reported vector-borne infectious disease in the United States is

(A) Rocky Mountain spotted fever (RMSF)
(B) anthrax
(C) toxoplasmosis
(D) Lyme disease
(E) HIV

Answer: (D). Lyme disease, a multisystem disease, is the most commonly reported vector-borne infectious disease in the United States. (*Chapter 44, Page 379.*)

10.45 The patient is an 18-year-old white man with erythema chronicum migrans (ECM) with a diameter of 11 cm. He also has fever, chills, headache, muscle pains, malar rash, and enlarged lymph glands. This patient should be treated with

(A) norfloxacin
(B) clarithromycin
(C) lincomycin
(D) doxycycline
(E) cephalexin

Answer: (D). Treatment of stage I Lyme disease should be initiated as early as possible with an oral agent such as doxycycline (100 mg orally (PO) b.i.d.), amoxicillin (500 mg PO t.i.d.), or erythromycin (250 mg PO t.i.d.) for 3 to 4 weeks. Some believe that all stages should be treated for 30 days. Of the three drugs, doxycycline is the drug of choice in nonpregnant persons older than 8 years of age. (*Chapter 44, Page 381.*)

10.46 The only timely diagnostic method useful during the acute phase of RMSF is

(A) the Weil-Felix test
(B) the complement fixation test
(C) complete blood count
(D) skin biopsy
(E) latex agglutination

Answer: (D). A 3-mm punch skin biopsy with direct immunofluorescence testing is useful for early confirmation of RMSF. It is the only timely diagnostic method useful during the acute phase of the illness. Rickettsiae show up in skin lesions as early as 3 days after onset of the illness. The rickettsiae are located in the center of the lesion, which is often marked by petechiae. Failure to biopsy the lesion to its center may yield false-negative results. (*Chapter 44, Page 384.*)

DIRECTIONS (Items 10.47 through 10.72): Each of the items in this section is a multiple true–false problem that consists of a stem and four lettered options. Indicate whether each of the options is TRUE or FALSE.

10.47 IM is the self-limiting clinical expression of symptomatic primary Epstein-Barr virus (EBV) infection. True statements regarding IM and EBV include which of the following?

(A) The virus can be spread through sexual transmission or by blood transfusion.
(B) The incubation period is 7 to 15 days.
(C) IM is particularly contagious because most contacts are young persons who lack immunity.
(D) Virus shedding may persist several months after infection.

Answer: (A-True, B-False, C-False, D-True). EBV is spread mainly by saliva, although sexual transmission and transmission by blood transfusion and shared use of needles and syringes are also possible. The incubation period is 30 to 50 days. IM is not particularly contagious because most contacts of known cases are already immune, and epidemics are therefore rare. EBV can be found in oropharyngeal washings from approximately 15% of healthy seropositive individuals at any time, and virus shedding may persist many months after infection. (*Chapter 38, Page 325.*)

10.48 RSV infection in infants and children

(A) represents a specific identifiable syndrome of acute pulmonary infection
(B) may progress rapidly from mild to severe illness
(C) can be spread through self-inoculation via contaminated fomites
(D) in the acute setting, is usually diagnosed by viral culture of nasopharyngeal secretions

Answer: (A-False, B-True, C-True, D-True). The spectrum of illness associated with RSV is broad, ranging from mild nasal congestion to high fever and respiratory distress. What seems to begin as a simple cold may suddenly become a life-threatening illness. RSV tends to peak during January most years. Evidence suggests that in infants group A viruses are associated with more severe infections than group B viruses. Modes of spread are primarily via large droplet inoculation (requiring close contact) and self-inoculation via contaminated fomites or skin. RSV is recoverable from countertops for up to 6 hours from the time of contamination, from rubber gloves for up to 90 minutes, and from skin for up to 20 minutes. Viral shedding of RSV is a prolonged process averaging 7 days.

The diagnosis of RSV in the acute setting is usually obtained by viral culture of nasopharyngeal secretions. A rapid diagnostic test (Abbott test pack RSV: Directigen RSV by Becton Dickinson) using antigen detection in nasal secretions is 95% sensitive and 99% specific. Results are available in 1 hour. (*Chapter 39, Pages 328–329.*)

10.49 Influenza virus infection

(A) tends to affect a large number of school-age children during the early stages of an epidemic
(B) tends to affect adults later in an epidemic
(C) affects children in urban areas in higher percentages than in rural areas
(D) later in an epidemic, may be caused by an antigenically distinct virus that "heralds" the epidemic virus for the following year

Answer: (A-True, B-True, C-False, D-True). During the early stage of an epidemic, a disproportionate number of cases involve school-age children, 10 to 19 years old. Later in the epidemic, more cases are diagnosed in younger children and adults. The age shift suggests that the early spread of influenza viruses in a community is concentrated among schoolchildren.

Another characteristic of influenza virus is the decreased rate of infection in children living in urban areas compared with that of children in rural areas. In 1974, the rate of influenza B was four times greater for children living in rural areas of Michigan than in the urban areas.

In addition to the predominant influenza virus that invades an area each season, many types, subtypes, or variants are identified during each epidemic period. These antigenically distinct viruses produce "herald waves." For several successive years, a relatively small wave of infections with an antigenically distinct virus can occur during the second half of an epidemic and herald the epidemic virus for the following year. These "herald waves" are useful to epidemiologists for predicting the viral antigens that should be included in each season's vaccine. (*Chapter 39, Page 329.*)

10.50 An otherwise healthy 45-year-old man complains of runny nose, hoarseness, slight sore throat, and mild cough that have been present for 3 days. He has no fever, earache, or headache. Physical examination is consistent with his symptoms. Management considerations include which of the following?

(A) Antihistamines are highly effective for relieving rhinorrhea.
(B) Aspirin or acetaminophen use may actually increase the rate of viral shedding.
(C) Inhaling heated vapor may provide some symptomatic improvement.
(D) Vitamin C, taken in doses of 3 g daily, is likely to shorten the course of disease.

Answers: (A-False, B-True, C-True, D-False). There are as many ways to manage the common cold as there are physicians and mothers. Antibiotics have no effect on the causative viruses. Antihistamines have been shown to be of little use because the kinin system rather than histamine is responsible for rhinorrhea and congestion. Antihistamines cause a generalized drying of the respiratory tract that may be unpleasant. More than 800 cold preparations are available over the counter in the United States. The decongestant component in some remedies may be helpful but is dangerous for hypertensive patients. Aspirin, acetaminophen, and NSAIDs are associated with a mild reduction in symptoms but have been shown to suppress the serum neutralizing antibody response and cause a highly significant increase in the rate of viral shedding. They should not be used routinely but, rather, targeted for reducing myalgias and malaise. Even fever reduction is not a sacred reason for use of acetaminophen and anti-inflammatory agents. Elevated body temperature has been shown to protect puppies from fatal viral infection. Numerous studies have shown symptomatic improvements after raising the temperature of the nasal mucosa by inhaling heated vapor. Folk remedies such as hot chicken soup and vitamin C in large doses have large followings but no support in research literature. (*Chapter 39, Page 331.*)

10.51 True statements regarding spasmodic croup include which of the following?

(A) The disease tends to begin suddenly and unexpectedly.
(B) The patient is usually age 4 to 7.
(C) In addition to cough, there may be dyspnea and stridor.
(D) Spasmodic croup is usually preceded by a febrile illness.

Answer: (A-True, B-False, C-True, D-False). Spasmodic croup bursts into a family's life with a scary suddenness when their younger-than-3-year-old child exhibits a croupy cough and stridor and appears dyspneic. This child has not been ill and has no fever. After a few frantic hours, the croup clears, and the child is well until the next episode. (*Chapter 39, Page 333.*)

10.52 The patient is a 16-year-old white boy treated with penicillin for a GABHS pharyngitis. The patient's mother asks about a post-treatment throat culture. Following appropriate treatment of GABHS pharyngitis, post-treatment throat cultures are indicated

(A) for all patients
(B) for patients age 16 and younger

(C) for patients who are symptomatic after completion of antibiotics
(D) for patients who have had rheumatic fever and are at specially high risk for recurrence

Answer: (A-False, B-False, C-True, D-True). Post-treatment throat cultures are indicated only in those who remain symptomatic after completion of antibiotics, who develop recurrent symptoms within 6 weeks, or who have had rheumatic fever and are at unusually high risk for recurrence. (*Chapter 40, Page 342.*)

10.53 The patient is a 22-year-old white male college student with a complaint of urethral discharge. Gram stain of the urethral exudate shows leukocytes with intracellular and extracellular gram-negative diplococci. True statements regarding this patient include which of the following?

(A) The patient should also be tested for the presence of syphilis.
(B) Following recommended therapy, the patient should have a test of cure culture.
(C) If symptoms persist following treatment, antimicrobial resistance should be considered.
(D) Persistent urethritis following therapy is normal for 3 to 6 months.

Answer: (A-True, B-False, C-True, D-False). Patients treated for gonorrhea should also be tested by serologic means for syphilis. A test-of-cure culture is not necessary following the Centers for Disease Control–recommended regimens. Patients with persistent symptoms following treatment for gonorrhea should be cultured and any gonococci isolated evaluated for antimicrobial sensitivity. *C. trachomatis* infection should be considered in patients treated for gonorrhea who experience continued symptoms of urethritis, cervicitis, or proctitis after treatment. (*Chapter 41, Page 347.*)

10.54 The patient is a 28-year-old white woman who has had three sexual partners over the past year. She now has lower abdominal tenderness, left adnexal tenderness, and cervical motion tenderness. The true statements regarding this patient include which of the following?

(A) If no other cause is evident, the patient has met the minimum criteria for the diagnosis of PID.
(B) Empiric therapy should be initiated.
(C) Treatment should await the results of culture and sensitivity from material obtained from the endocervix.
(D) Clinical findings supporting the diagnosis of PID would include an elevated erythrocyte

sedimentation rate and elevated C-reactive protein level.

Answer: (A-True, B-True, C-False, D-True). The minimum criteria for diagnosis of PID includes lower abdominal tenderness, adnexal tenderness, and cervical motion tenderness. If all three criteria are present and no other cause is established, empiric treatment for PID should be initiated. Women with more severe clinical signs require further diagnostic evaluation. Additional criteria that increase the specificity of the diagnosis of PID include an oral temperature more than 38.3°C (102.6°F), abnormal cervical or vaginal discharge, elevated erythrocyte sedimentation rate, elevated C-reactive protein, and laboratory documentation of cervical infection with *N. gonorrhoeae* or *C. trachomatis*. (*Chapter 41, Page 348.*)

10.55 The patient with secondary syphilis may have

(A) fever, malaise, and generalized lymphadenopathy
(B) a macular rash
(C) mucous patches
(D) condylomata

Answer: (A-True, B-True, C-True, D-True). About 6 to 8 weeks after the chancre heals, symptoms of secondary syphilis appear. This stage is characterized by a variety of symptoms, although some patients are asymptomatic. Symptoms include fever, malaise, and generalized lymphadenopathy. A macular, papular, annular, or follicular rash is classically present on the palms of the hands and soles of the feet. Mucous patches are shallow painless ulcerations found on mucous membranes. Broad, flat, grayish plaques known as condylomata late appear on moist body areas such as the genitalia, cervix, scrotum, anus, or inner thighs. (*Chapter 41, Page 349.*)

10.56 The patient is a 72-year-old recent immigrant whose family believes he might have been treated for a STD about 20 years ago. There is some generalized weakness, and there has been a chronic progressive dementia with sensory ataxia. True statements regarding this patient's problem include which of the following?

(A) A negative Venereal Disease Research Laboratory (VDRL) test rules out the presence of syphilitic infection.
(B) Even with adequate treatment, a fluorescent treponemal antibody absorption (FTA-ABS) test is likely to be positive.

(C) Neurosyphilis is diagnosed based on computer tomography of the brain.
(D) The VDRL is negative in up to 25% of the patients with late neurosyphilis.

Answer: (A-False, B-True, C-False, D-True). In about one-fourth of untreated patients, the VDRL eventually becomes nonreactive. Treponemal tests include FTA-ABS and microhemagglutination *T. pallidum* tests. These tests are used to confirm a positive screening test and, once positive, usually remain so for life. Neurosyphilis is diagnosed based on clinical and laboratory findings. The VDRL is negative in up to 25% of patients with late neurosyphilis, but the treponemal tests remain positive. (*Chapter 41, Page 349.*)

10.57 True statements regarding the diagnosis of HSV infection include which of the following?

(A) The gold standard for the diagnosis of HSV infection is the Tzanck smear.
(B) Twenty to thirty percent of HSV cultures are negative even when infection is present.
(C) HSV cultures are ideally obtained within 7 days of the outbreak for primary HSV infection.
(D) The best yield is provided by cultures taken from a crusted herpes lesion.

Answer: (A-False, B-True, C-True, D-False). The diagnosis of HSV infection is based on the history, physical findings, and laboratory evaluation. Culture remains the gold standard for the diagnosis of HSV, although 20 to 30% of cultures are negative when infection is present. Cultures are ideally obtained within 7 days of the outbreak for primary HSV and within 2 days for recurrent infections. A specimen from an intact vesicle is desirable. Dry crusted lesions provide low yield. The Tzanck or Pap smear is useful as an adjunct to clinical diagnosis. (*Chapter 41, Page 352.*)

10.58 HIV is typically transmitted from person to person by

(A) semen
(B) vaginal secretions
(C) sweat
(D) saliva

Answer: (A-True, B-True, C-False, D-False). HIV is usually transmitted from person to person by the passage of blood or body fluids such as semen and vaginal secretions. Urine, sweat, and saliva are not generally considered to be infectious. Persons engaging in unsafe sexual activity and intravenous drug use with needle sharing account for most cases of HIV infection. (*Chapter 42, Page 357.*)

10.59 Which of the following vaccines are appropriate for the HIV-infected patient?

(A) influenza vaccine
(B) pneumococcal vaccine
(C) hepatitis B vaccine, if ongoing risk of exposure
(D) Sabin oral polio vaccine

Answer: (A-True, B-True, C-True, D-False). Influenza vaccination and one-time pneumococcal vaccination should be administered. Hepatitis B vaccine is recommended if there is an ongoing risk of exposure to hepatitis B. Polio vaccination for HIV-infected persons and their family members should be with the inactivated (intramuscular) preparation. (*Chapter 42, Page 358.*)

10.60 True statements regarding tuberculosis in HIV-infected persons include which of the following?

(A) In such patients tuberculin skin testing is considered positive at 5 mm of induration.
(B) A negative tuberculin skin test eliminates the possibility of coinfection with tuberculosis.
(C) High-risk patients may be given prophylactic isoniazid (INH) regardless of their tuberculin skin test status.
(D) A positive tuberculin skin test in the presence of HIV infection is sufficient to make the diagnosis of active tuberculosis.

Answer: (A-True, B-False, C-True, D-False). Tuberculin skin testing should be performed with the recognition that in HIV-infected persons a 5-mm (rather than the usual 10-mm) reaction to an intermediate-strength purified protein derivative (PPD) is considered indicative of tuberculous infection. For HIV-infected persons known to be at high risk for tuberculosis (injection drug users, homeless persons, and persons from countries with a high incidence of tuberculosis), even a negative tuberculin skin test cannot eliminate the possibility of coinfection with tuberculosis. High-risk patients should probably be given prophylactic INH therapy for 1 year regardless of their PPD status. Patients with positive tuberculin skin tests and those with a high risk of tuberculosis require a chest roentgenogram to exclude active tuberculosis. (*Chapter 42, Page 359.*)

10.61 In the treatment of HIV infection and AIDS, protease inhibitor drugs

(A) have proved only marginally effective
(B) require strict adherence to the prescribed regimen
(C) are reserved for selected patients with advanced disease
(D) may be associated with permanent drug resistance

Answer: (A-False, B-True, C-False, D-True). When patients can adhere to and tolerate protease inhibitor drugs, they should be offered these very effective drugs. The protease inhibitors can be difficult to take, requiring strict adherence to medication regimens. Departures from the regimen for periods as short as 1 week can render patients resistant to this class of drugs permanently. (*Chapter 42, Page 359.*)

10.62 True statements regarding KS include which of the following?

(A) KS is an AIDS-defining condition.
(B) Lesions are found on the upper and lower extremities, and the torso generally is spared.
(C) The diagnosis is made on observation in consultation with a dermatologist experienced in managing KS.
(D) KS requires aggressive treatment with flurourocil.

Answer: (A-True, B-False, C-False, D-False). KS is an AIDS-defining condition. The violaceous-to-brown lesions can occur anywhere on the body. A biopsy is required to establish the diagnosis of AIDS (when KS is the initial manifestation) and when bacillary angiomatosis (a bacterial condition that can produce lesions similar to those of KS) or other conditions are possible. KS does not require treatment unless the lesions are cosmetically bothersome, bulky, or painful or the patient wishes the lesions to be treated. (*Chapter 42, Page 362.*)

10.63 True statements regarding HIV disease in newborns include which of the following?

(A) Infection can occur transplacentally.
(B) HIV infection does not occur during breast-feeding.
(C) Without peripartum antiretroviral treatment, approximately 25% of children borne to mothers with HIV infection are infected.
(D) Cesarean section is routinely recommended with mothers with HIV infection.

Answer: (A-True, B-False, C-True, D-False). Infection with HIV can occur transplacentally, at the time of delivery, and at breast-feeding. Without peripartum antiretroviral treatment, 25% of children born to mothers with HIV infection are infected. When mothers are treated with zidovudine during pregnancy and during delivery and the baby is treated for the first 6 weeks of life, transmission can be reduced to 8.3%. Cesarean section is not recommended on a routine basis. (*Chapter 42, Page 364.*)

10.64 The systemic signs of severe sepsis are likely to include

   (A) tachycardia
   (B) bradypnea
   (C) polyuria
   (D) altered mental status

Answer: (A-True, B-False, C-False, D-True). The systemic signs of sepsis include fever, hypotension, tachycardia, or tachypnea. Oliguria or altered mental status indicate progression to severe sepsis, and persistent hypotension indicates septic shock. Although these signs may occur abruptly, they may also present with subtlety, particularly in the elderly. (*Chapter 43, Page 367.*)

10.65 The patient is a 21-day-old white male infant who is the product of a normal pregnancy and delivery. He has been sick for 24 hours and now has a temperature of 103°F. He does not appear toxic. True statements regarding this patient include which of the following?

   (A) He should be hospitalized and closely evaluated.
   (B) He should be hospitalized if he begins to appear toxic.
   (C) He should be evaluated in the emergency department and discharged to home if laboratory tests including a lumbar puncture are unremarkable.
   (D) Empiric parenteral antibiotic therapy should be initiated.

Answer: (A-True, B-False, C-False, D-True). Clinical guidelines put forth by an expert panel state that all febrile infants younger than 28 days, regardless of whether toxic-appearing, should be hospitalized and closely evaluated. Empiric parenteral antibiotics particularly effective against the common pathogens in this age group include intravenous gentamicin/ampicillin or ceftriaxone/ampicillin. A minimum of 48 to 72 hours of antibiotic coverage is recommended, even when all cultures return negative, the infant is non-toxic, and the white blood cell count and urinalysis are within normal limits. (*Chapter 43, Page 369.*)

10.66 Which of the following would support the diagnosis of trichinellosis?

   (A) eosinophilia
   (B) leukopenia
   (C) elevated muscle enzyme levels
   (D) decreased immunoglobulin levels

Answer: (A-True, B-False, C-True, D-False). Eosinophilia, leukocytosis, muscle enzyme elevations, and increased immunoglobulins, especially total IgE, are the most characteristic findings of trichinellosis. (*Chapter 43, Page 376.*)

10.67 True statements regarding the prevention of trichinellosis include which of the following?

   (A) The increased use of home freezers preserving trichina organisms in meat has increased the incidence of trichinellosis in the United States.
   (B) To prevent trichinellosis, meat should be cooked to a temperature of 130°F.
   (C) The thermal death point of trichinae is exceeded at a temperature of 170°F.
   (D) The radiation of pork can help control trichinellosis.

Answer: (A-False. B-False, C-True, D-True). The number of trichinellosis cases has been declining since 1975, most likely because of laws prohibiting feeding offal to hogs, the increased use of home freezers, and the practice of thoroughly cooking pork. To ensure that *Trichinella* is destroyed, meat should be cooked to a temperature of 170°F (77°C) to exceed the thermal death point of the trichinae. It can be accomplished by cooking the pork until the color changes from pink or red to gray. Irradiation of pork for the control of trichinellosis has now been approved by the U.S. Department of Agriculture and the U.S. Food and Drug Administration. (*Chapter 44, Page 376.*)

10.68 True statements regarding giardiasis include which of the following?

   (A) Giardiasis is the most common protozoal infection of the intestinal tract.
   (B) Severe gastrointestinal symptoms can occur.
   (C) The cause is a rickettsial organism.
   (D) Giardiasis is a common cause of chronic diarrhea.

Answer: (A-True, B-True, C-False, D-True). Giardiasis, the most common protozoal infection of the intestinal tract, can lead to severe disabling gastrointestinal symptoms. It is caused by the flagellated protozoan parasite *Giardia lamblia* and accounts for up to 7% of cases of acute diarrhea and up to 45% of cases with chronic diarrhea. (*Chapter 44, Page 378.*)

10.69 Appropriate treatment for giardiasis includes which of the following?

(A) quinacrine hydrochloride
(B) norfloxacin
(C) metronidazole
(D) doxycyline

Answer: (A-True, B-False, C-True, D-False). Approximately 90 to 95% of patients with giardiasis are cured with a 7- to 10-day course of quinacrine hydrochloride (100 mg t.i.d.) or metronidazole (250 mg t.i.d.). If symptoms are persistent after both agents have been tried, these agents can be given together for an additional 2 weeks. Furazolidine (100 mg t.i.d.) and mebendazole (200 mg t.i.d.) have been used as alternative drugs. (*Chapter 44, Page 378.*)

10.70 The most characteristic manifestation of Lyme disease is ECM. Characteristics of ECM include

(A) papular lesions, warm to the touch, occasionally with slight itching
(B) redness expanding outward from the center to a plaque 3 to 70 cm in diameter
(C) central clearing, giving the lesion a "target" appearance
(D) spontaneous resolution within 2 weeks if untreated

Answer: (A-True, B-True, C-True, D-False). The ECM lesion initially appears as a papule, warm to touch, occasionally with slight itching or burning; in some instances, it develops a raised border, a vesiculated or necrotic center, or both. During the first few days, redness expands outwardly from the center to a plaque 3 to 70 cm in diameter (mean, 15 cm). Central clearing usually occurs, giving the lesion a "target" appearance.

If untreated, lesions last 4 to 6 weeks (maximum, 14 months). Lesions disappear in several days with successful antibiotic treatment. ECM occurs in about 70% of adults and up to 90% of children with Lyme disease. (*Chapter 44, Page 380.*)

10.71 True statements regarding RMSF include which of the following?

(A) RMSF is an uncomfortable febrile disease, but mortality is rare.
(B) Prompt treatment with antibiotics can change the course of RMSF.
(C) Specific laboratory tests for *Rickettsia rickettsii* allow prompt early diagnosis if the clinician suspects the disease.
(D) Deaths from RMSF have been reported only among the immunocompromised and the elderly.

Answer: (A-False, B-True, C-False, D-False). RMSF is the most virulent form of a group of tick- and mite-borne zoonotic infections known as spotted fevers caused by various rickettsiae. RMSF has a case fatality rate of 20% unless treated promptly with appropriate antibiotics. Early diagnosis is difficult. Young, otherwise healthy individuals occasionally die from RMSF. (*Chapter 44, Page 382.*)

10.72 True statements regarding the rash of RMSF include which of the following?

(A) A rash is present in 90% of the cases.
(B) The rash appears simultaneously with the onset of fever.
(C) The rash starts on the trunk and spreads to the extremities.
(D) The rash tends to spare the face.

Answer: (A-True, B-False, C-False, D-True). RMSF gets its name from the hallmark rash that is present in 90% of the cases. It appears 3 to 5 days after onset of fever; it is initially maculopapular and evolves into a more defined petechial rash. The rash starts on the extremities (wrists and ankles) and spreads to the trunk, with facial sparing. (*Chapter 44, Page 383.*)

11

Environmental and Occupational Health Problems

The questions in this chapter constitute a review of the following chapters in *Family Medicine: Principles and Practice, Fifth Edition:*

Occupational Health Care (Chapter 45)
Problems Related to Physical Agents (Chapter 46)

DIRECTIONS (Items 11.1 through 11.7): Each of the questions or incomplete statements in this section is followed by five suggested answers or completions. Select the ONE that is BEST in each case.

11.1 The first symptom of carpal tunnel syndrome is likely to be

(A) hand pain at the end of the work day
(B) weakness leading to dropping of tools or eating utensils
(C) pain in the neck and shoulders
(D) numbness or paresthesias in the hand
(E) pallor of the involved wrist or hand

Answer: (D). Carpal tunnel syndrome usually begins with complaints of nocturnal numbness or paresthesias in the distribution of the median nerve; it often starts as a sensory neuropathy best detected with two-point discrimination or vibration. (*Chapter 45, Page 389.*)

11.2 Byssinosis is a disease caused by hypersensitivity to

(A) coal dust
(B) cotton dust
(C) silage
(D) heated plastic polymers
(E) metal oxides

Answer: (B). Byssinosis, or cotton dust hypersensitivity, was originally called brown lung disease to differentiate it from the more deadly "black lung" disease of coal workers. (*Chapter 45, Page 391.*)

11.3 The risk of heat exhaustion increases as the ambient temperature rises above 95°F. At this air temperature, the dissipation of body heat is chiefly through

(A) radiation
(B) conduction
(C) convection
(D) evaporation of sweat
(E) none of the above

Answer: (D). Dissipation of heat occurs through radiation, conduction, convection, and evaporation of sweat. At temperatures above 35°C (95°F), most body heat is lost through sweating, a mechanism that becomes inefficient when the humidity rises above 75%. (*Chapter 46, Page 397.*)

11.4 The patient is a 22-year-old college football player brought to the emergency department on a hot sunny day with confusion, a pulse of 110/min, and a respiratory rate of 38/min. His temperature is 40.5°C (105°F). The most likely diagnosis is

(A) heat exhaustion
(B) heat stroke
(C) head trauma
(D) sepsis
(E) acute myocardial infarction

Answer: (B). In heat stroke, there is usually a history of acute changes of mental status after exertion in hot weather. Examination of the patient demonstrates tachycardia, hypotension or normotension, and tachypnea. The core temperature is usually at least 40.5 °C (105.0°F) but may be lower with cooling during examination. Neurologic signs include irritability, confusion, ataxia, seizures, decorticate posturing, and coma. (*Chapter 46, Page 397.*)

11.5 The average person living at sea level receives a small amount of radiation each year. This amount is closest to which of the following?

(A) 100 rad
(B) 1,000 rad
(C) 80 mrem
(D) 1 rem
(E) 400 rem

Answer: (C). The rad is the standard unit of absorbed dose (1 rad = 100 ergs/kg tissue). One rem is that dose of any radiation that produces a biologic effect equivalent to 1 rad of x- or y-rays. Collectively, a person living at sea level receives about 80 mrem/year. Persons living at high altitudes or near deposits of radioactive ores may receive more. (*Chapter 46, Page 399.*)

11.6 Inhalation of products liberated by anaerobic microbial fermentation in silos can cause alveolar injury. These products are chiefly

(A) carbon monoxide
(B) hydrogen cyanide
(C) polyvinyl chloride
(D) ozone
(E) oxides of nitrogen

Answer: (E). Oxides of nitrogen liberated by anaerobic microbial fermentation in silos cause alveolar injury with pulmonary edema and hyaline membrane dysfunction. (*Chapter 46, Page 402.*)

11.7 Acoustic trauma accounts for one-fifth of all hearing loss and much exposure occurs in industry. The decibel (dB) level at any given time at which a person is considered in danger is

(A) 50 dB
(B) 70 dB
(C) 95 dB
(D) 125 dB
(E) 150 dB

Answer: (C). Noise exposure is measured by the dose concept (i.e., intensity multiplied by time). In industry,

two measurements of dose are used to evaluate the danger: the time-weighted average, which is a measure of exposure over the work day (85 dB), and the permissible exposure limit, which is the maximum decibels to which a person can be exposed at any given time (95 dB). (*Chapter 46, Page 402.*)

DIRECTIONS (Items 11.8 through 11.20): Each of the items in this section is a multiple true–false problem that consists of a stem and four lettered options. Indicate whether each of the options is TRUE or FALSE.

11.8 Cumulative trauma is a common occupational health problem. True statements regarding cumulative trauma include which of the following?

(A) Cumulative trauma most often affects the upper extremity.
(B) Cumulative trauma is chiefly a disease of blue-collar workers, such as factory workers.
(C) The disorder is common in jobs that require frequent, awkward, or forceful movements.
(D) The presence of a cool or cold environment can reduce the risk of cumulative trauma disorders.

Answer: (A-True, B-False, C-True, D-False). Cumulative trauma most commonly affects the upper extremity. Originally a disease of blue-collar workers such as butchers and factory workers, with the advent of the computer, cumulative trauma made the jump to the white-collar population. Traditionally, the disorder is found in positions that require frequent movements (more than 2,000 hand movements per hour) or the hands are engaged in awkward or forceful movements. Cold and vibration are additional risk factors. (*Chapter 44, Page 388.*)

11.9 Risk factors for the development of carpal tunnel syndrome include

(A) wrist tendinitis
(B) thyroid disease
(C) weight loss
(D) pregnancy

Answer: (A-True, B-True, C-False, D-True). Approximately one-third of cases of wrist tendinitis progress to carpal tunnel problems. Additional medical risk factors for carpal tunnel syndrome include thyroid disease, obesity, pregnancy, and amyloidosis. (*Chapter 44, Page 389.*)

11.10 The patient is a 32-year-old white female file clerk with an acute low back strain of moderate severity sustained 3 days ago while bending on the job.

There is no evidence of nerve root compression. Your treatment should include

(A) bed rest for 7 to 10 days
(B) traction
(C) narcotic analgesics
(D) early activity and return to work

Answer: (A-False, B-False, C-False, D-True). Past wisdom has dictated prolonged bed rest, traction, muscle relaxers, and narcotics. Outcomes-based research has modified many of these recommendations. New clinical practice guidelines from the Agency for Health Care Policy and Research, *Acute Low Back Problems in Adults*, recommend minimum bed rest (no more than a day or two) for all but the most extreme cases. In most cases, early activity and return to work are recommended. (*Chapter 45, Page 390.*)

11.11 Physicians providing occupational health care may become involved in the determination of disability. True statements regarding disability include which of the following?

(A) Disability is a specific failure in function of a body part.
(B) Disability describes failure of an organ system.
(C) Disability is an impediment that keeps the individual from interacting with his or her environment.
(D) A disability limits a person's ability to perform activities of daily living (ADL), which may include employment.

Answer: (A-False, B-False, C-True, D-True). *Impairment* is a specific failure in function of a body part or organ system. The impairment rating is a medical evaluation. *Disability*, by contrast, is an impediment that keeps individuals from interacting with their environment. A disability limits individuals' ability to perform their ADLs, which may include employment. Thus, a man missing the distal part of his fifth finger may be essentially unimpaired but is considered totally disabled if he makes his living as a violinist. (*Chapter 45, Page 395.*)

11.12 True statements regarding heat injury include which of the following?

(A) Because of intense physical conditioning, military personnel rarely suffer heat injuries.
(B) Athletes are particularly susceptible to heat injuries.
(C) Amphetamines and cocaine help protect patients against heat injury.

(D) Anticholinergics decrease sweating and increase the risk of heat injury.

Answer: (A-False, B-True, C-False, D-True). Military personnel, youth groups, athletes, the elderly, persons with heart disease, and those with outdoor occupations are particularly susceptible to heat injuries. Moreover, drugs such as amphetamines, cocaine, and anticholinergics decrease sweating and place individuals at increased risk. (*Chapter 46, Page 397.*)

11.13 In the field, the immediate treatment of heat stroke might include which of the following?

(A) blankets to reduce shivering
(B) removing unnecessary clothing
(C) applications of lukewarm water to the exposed areas
(D) fluid restriction to prevent renal overload

Answer: (A-False, B-True, C-True, D-False). In the field, it is critical to decrease the core temperature by removing unnecessary clothing, spraying the face with lukewarm water, augmenting airflow, and providing oral fluids if the person is conscious. (*Chapter 46, Page 398.*)

11.14 True statements regarding cold injuries include which of the following?

(A) Patients with diabetes mellitus are at increased risk of cold injury.
(B) Cardiac drugs reduce vasodilation and help protect against cold injury.
(C) Antipsychotic drugs reduce cold tolerance.
(D) Alcoholic drinks help protect against cold injuries.

Answer: (A-True, B-False, C-True, D-False). Occupations with exposure to cold, winter athletic activities, outdoor youth outings, and winter military operations present a greater risk for cold injuries. Alcoholics, the elderly, disabled persons, soldiers in combat, and individuals with diabetes and heart disease are more susceptible. Medications, especially cardiac and antipsychotic drugs, reduce cold tolerance. Alcoholic drinks increase heat loss from the body due to vasodilation. (*Chapter 46, Page 398.*)

11.15 Treating the patient with hypothermia may include

(A) gradual rewarming
(B) rehydration and correction of acid–base and electrolyte imbalances

(C) inhaled warm carbon dioxide
(D) peritoneal dialysis may be needed in severe cases

Answer: (A-True, B-True, C-False, D-True). In the emergency department, the patient should be rewarmed slowly over a period of 2 to 3 hours to avoid rewarming shock. Rehydration and correction of acid–base and electrolyte imbalances must be carried out concomitant with rewarming. Inhaled warm oxygen, if available, may be helpful. Peritoneal dialysis with lactated Ringer's solution at 43°C exchanged at a rate of 10 to 12 L/hour may be needed in severe cases. Warm baths, if used, should be maintained at 40° to 42°C. (*Chapter 46, Page 398.*)

11.16 Early mild cases of frostbite may be recognized by the presence of

(A) numbness
(B) stiffness
(C) itching
(D) pale white edematous skin

Answer: (A-True, B-False, C-True, D-False). In mild cases, numbness, prickling, and itching of the skin may be present. In severe cases, there may be paresthesia, stiffness, and pale white edematous skin. (*Chapter 46, Page 398.*)

11.17 Based on long-term studies of survivors of the 1945 bombing of Hiroshima, Japan, true statements include which of the following?

(A) There was an increase in malignant tumors, especially leukemias, in survivors.
(B) Late effects included cataracts and chromosomal aberrations.
(C) There was an increase in leukemia in children born to survivors more than 9 months after the attack.
(D) There was an increase in sterility and congenital abnormalities in children born to survivors more than 9 months after the attack.

Answer: (A-True, B-True, C-False, D-False). Late effects measured over a period of 50 years included increases in malignant tumors (especially leukemias of all types), cataracts, chromosomal aberrations, somatic cell mutations, mental retardation, growth retardation, and functional abnormalities to organs, especially glands. There was no increase in leukemia, sterility, or congenital abnormalities in children born

to survivors more than 9 months after the attack. (*Chapter 46, Page 400.*)

11.18 Cancer can be a late effect of radiation exposure. These cancers are

(A) often more aggressive than cancers occurring naturally
(B) have been found to arise from different cell lines than those cancers occurring naturally
(C) are treated by using special protocols designed for radiation-induced cancers
(D) are treated by using standard protocols

Answer: (A-False, B-False, C-False, D-True). Cancers induced by radiation are indistinguishable from those occurring naturally and are treated by using standard protocols. (*Chapter 46, Page 400.*)

11.19 Welder's flash, also called photokeratoconjunctivitis, is an occupational hazard of welders, particularly seen when working without adequate eye protection. True statements regarding welder's flash include which of the following?

(A) Symptoms include severe pain and photophobia.
(B) Symptoms typically begin a few minutes after exposure.
(C) Symptoms require prolonged, often cumulative exposure, usually more than 30 to 60 minutes or more.
(D) Although the conjunctiva are involved, the eyelids are spared.

Answer: (A-True, B-False, C-False, D-False). Photokeratoconjunctivitis (welder's flash) manifests with symptoms of severe pain, photophobia, tearing, and the sensation of sand in the eyes 6 to 12 hours after exposure. A single short exposure may provoke symptoms, but increases in duration and intensity shorten the latency period and increase the symptoms. The eyelids may be erythemic and swollen, and examination of the eye may be normal or reveal punctuate staining of the cornea. (*Chapter 46, Page 400.*)

11.20 True statements regarding electrical injury include which of the following?

(A) The vascular system is at greatest risk.
(B) There may be thermal burns at the entrance and exit sites.

(C) Nerve tissue is at low risk from electrical injury and is generally not affected.

(D) Myoglobinuria may occur.

Answer: (A-True, B-True, C-False, D-True). Electric current follows the course of least resistance, usually through water-laden tissues. Therefore the vascular system is most at risk, and bone is least at risk. Circular or elliptical thermal burns may occur at entrance and exit sites, and tissue necrosis and thrombosis may occur in muscles and vessels. Muscle destruction may result in necrosis and myoglobinuria. Depolarization of nerve tissue and the brain may produce tetany and seizures. Renal and liver damage may occur as a consequence of electrocution; and there may be blunt trauma resulting from falls or being thrown. (*Chapter 46, Page 401.*)

12

Injuries and Poisoning

The questions in this chapter constitute a review of the following chapters in *Family Medicine: Principles and Practice, Fifth Edition:*

Bites and Stings (Chapter 47)
Poisoning (Chapter 48)
Care of Acute Lacerations (Chapter 49)
Selected Injuries (Chapter 50)

DIRECTIONS (Items 12.1 through 12.16): Each of the questions or incomplete statements in this section is followed by five suggested answers or completions. Select the ONE that is BEST in each case.

12.1 The brown recluse spider (*Loxosceles reclusa*)

(A) is found chiefly in the western United States
(B) is a large brown spider generally approximately 3 to 4 cm in diameter
(C) has a violin-shaped pattern on the back
(D) produces a venom containing alpha-latrotoxin
(E) has a venom containing a neurotoxin

Answer: (C). The brown recluse spider (*Loxosceles reclusa*) is found primarily in the south-central regions of the United States but may be transported anywhere. It is a small (1 to 2 cm) tan to dark brown spider with a violin-shaped pattern on the back. It produces a venom containing sphingomyelinase D, which causes endothelial swelling, platelet aggregation, and thrombosis. (*Chapter 47, Page 405.*)

12.2 Of the following, which may be the management option of choice for significant envenomation due to a black widow spider?

(A) pilocarpine
(B) specific antivenin
(C) diazepam
(D) sodium bicarbonate
(E) corticosteroids prescribed as prednisone in a decreasing dose over 1 week

Answer: (B). If available, specific antivenin (Antivenin; Merck, West Point, PA) may be the management option of choice for all significant envenomations due to black widow spiders. Parenteral narcotics, intravenous (IV) diazepam, or methocarbamol are useful for muscle cramps, as are prolonged hot baths. Calcium gluconate 10% solution, 0.1 to 0.2 ml/kg IV, with cardiac monitoring may provide transient relief of symptoms. (*Chapter 47, Page 406.*)

12.3 The shared manifestation of stings by bees, wasps, hornets, and ants is the production of localized

(A) tissue necrosis
(B) erythema chronicum migrans
(C) anaphylactoid reaction
(D) bullus formation
(E) dermal wheal-and-flare reactions

Answer: (E). Stings by bees, wasps, hornets, and ants are common in most climates. Their shared manifestation is the production of localized dermal wheal-and-flare reactions. (*Chapter 47, Page 406.*)

12.4 The most common presentation of a tick bite is

(A) bullus formation
(B) erythema chronicum migrans

(C) infection with local redness, pain, and heat
(D) discovery of an attached tick
(E) lymphangitis

Answer: (D). The most common presentation of a tick bite is discovery of an attached tick. (*Chapter 47, Page 407.*)

12.5 The chief problem in acetaminophen overdose is

(A) renal toxicity
(B) hemolysis
(C) hepatotoxicity
(D) neurotoxicity
(E) seizures

Answer: (C). Acetaminophen is metabolized in the liver (96%), with only 2 to 4% excreted unchanged in the urine. Metabolism of therapeutic doses results in the formation of benign metabolites (90%) and *N*-acetyl-*p*-benzoquinonimine (10%), the compound thought to cause hepatotoxicity in overdoses. (*Chapter 48, Page 409.*)

12.6 The patient is a 34-year-old white woman whom you are seeing in the emergency department with acute benzodiazepine poisoning. She has been stabilized and now has severe central nervous system (CNS) depression. A logical treatment option would be

(A) flumazenil (Romazicon)
(B) naloxone (Norcan)
(C) phenytoin (Dilantin)
(D) dexamethasone (Decadron)
(E) methylphenidate (Ritalin)

Answer: (A). Once stabilized, selected patients with benzodiazepine overdose (documented by drug screen or reliable history) who are comatose or have severe CNS depression may be treated with flumazenil (Romazicon). Flumazenil should be avoided in patients suspected of coingesting cyclic antidepressants (CA), those with a history of benzodiazepine dependence, or those with a history of seizure disorders treated with benzodiazepines. (*Chapter 48, Page 417.*)

12.7 Midazolam (Versed) is sometimes used for sedation during office procedures. This drug

(A) is a benzodiazepine
(B) is a phencyclidine derivative
(C) is a synthetic opioid
(D) has a long elimination half-life
(E) is only given parenterally

Answer: (A). Midazolam is a benzodiazepine with typical class effects of hypnosis, amnesia, and anxiety reduction. It is readily absorbed and has a short elimination half-life. It may be given as single dose via the nasal, oral, or parenteral route. (*Chapter 49, Page 424.*)

12.8 Fentanyl is a powerful synthetic opioid that produces rapid short-lasting sedation and analgesia. About half of all patients taking this drug will develop

(A) dizziness
(B) diarrhea
(C) hypoventilation
(D) respiratory depression
(E) pruritus

Answer: (E). About half of patients develop transient pruritus, 15% notice dizziness, and at least one-third develop vomiting. The most dangerous effect is hypoventilation, which can be fatal. Oversedation or respiratory depression responds to naloxone. (*Chapter 49, Page 425.*)

12.9 The patient is a 16-year-old girl with a 2-cm laceration of her left forearm. The wound has excessively everted margins. This is best managed by

(A) parallel debridement of wound margins
(B) undermining the subdermal layer
(C) use of a vertical mattress suture
(D) use of an intracuticular running stitch
(E) use of a stitch that is wider at the top than at the base

Answer: (E). Occasionally, a wound exhibits excessively everted margins. By reversing the usual approach and taking a stitch that is wider at the top than at the base, the wound can be inverted, improving the cosmetic appearance. This is shown in the figure below. (*Chapter 49, Page 427.*)

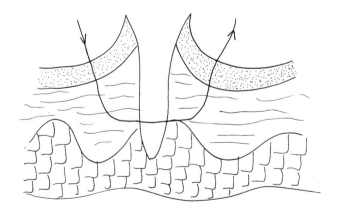

Fig. 12.1. Question 12.9. Suture placement in a wound with everted edges.

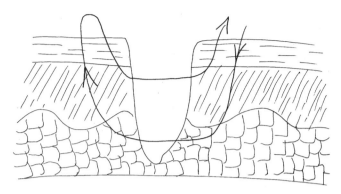

Fig. 12.2. Question 12.10.

12.10 The figure above illustrates which type of suture?

(A) surgeon's knot
(B) simple interrupted suture
(C) closure of an asymmetric wound
(D) vertical mattress suture
(E) intracuticular running suture

Answer: (D). The vertical mattress suture promotes eversion and is useful where thick layers are encountered or tension exists. Two techniques may be used. The classic method first places the deep stitch and closes with the superficial stitch. The short-hand method is performed by placing the shallow stitch first, pulling up on the suture (tenting the skin), and then placing the deeper stitch. (*Chapter 49, Page 428.*)

12.11 In care of an acute laceration or surgical wound, the intracuticular running suture

(A) uses an absorbable suture material such as chromic catgut
(B) is best used where there is significant skin tension
(C) is secured by surgeon's knots at both ends
(D) results in minimal scarring without suture marks
(E) is used when controlled tissue apposition is needed

Answer: (D). The intracuticular running suture, using a nonabsorbable suture, can be used where there is minimal skin tension. It results in minimal scarring without suture marks. Controlled tissue apposition is difficult with this method, but it is a popular technique because of the cosmetic result. The suture ends do not need to be tied but can be taped in place under slight tension. (*Chapter 49, Page 428.*)

12.12 Most near-drownings and drownings occur in which of the following settings?

(A) inadequately supervised young children in swimming pools or similar sources of water
(B) boating accidents
(C) persons older than age 65
(D) following acute convulsive seizures
(E) following alcohol use

Answer: (A). Most near-drownings and drownings occur among inadequately supervised children younger than 4 years of age in swimming pools, ocean surf, bathtubs, or hot tubs. Young men between the ages of 15 and 24 and the elderly older than age 75, especially if unable to swim, are also at risk because of alcohol or drug use while swimming, infirmity, or associated trauma or seizures. (*Chapter 50, Page 435.*)

12.13 Barotrauma—injury caused by barometric pressure changes—usually results from diving underwater, ascending into the atmosphere, or mechanical respiratory support. When descending in water, the pressure exerted on the body doubles every

(A) 2 m
(B) 10 m
(C) 40 m
(D) 80 m
(E) 120 m

Answer: (B). As one ascends into the atmosphere, the atmospheric pressure decreases gradually; and at 5,500 meters (18,000 ft), it reaches a pressure of about one-half that at sea level. By contrast, when one descends into water, the pressure of the water increases more rapidly, with a doubling of pressure every 10 m (33 ft) below the surface. (*Chapter 50, Page 436.*)

12.14 The patient is a 16-year-old white boy who had been SCUBA diving in a mountain lake. He estimates that he descended to about 30 ft of depth, perhaps deeper. He has pain in his left ear. Examination revealed petechiae and hemorrhagic blebs on the tympanic membrane (TM). The TM is intact. This patient appears to have

(A) external barotitis
(B) barotitis media
(C) inner ear barotrauma
(D) factitial external otitis
(E) decompression sickness

Answer: (A). External barotitis (ear canal squeeze) occurs when divers descend with ear canals plugged with cerumen or plugs. The diver experiences pain and bloody drainage as the pressure in the middle ear exceeds that within the canal. On examination of the TM, petechiae, hemorrhagic blebs, and rupture may be seen. (*Chapter 50, Page 437.*)

12.15 A useful agent for the topical therapy of second-degree burns is

(A) Neosporin powder
(B) neomycin ointment
(C) diphenhydramine cream
(D) hydrocortisone cream
(E) silver sulfadiazine cream

Answer: (E). Topical chemoprophylaxis is used for all but first-degree burns to prevent infection. Silver sulfadiazine cream, by far the most commonly used topical agent, is applied to the burn in a thickness of about 2 mm and is then covered with a dressing such as Telfa and soft gauze. (*Chapter 50, Page 440.*)

12.16 The patient is a 3-year-old child with two small circular burn sites on the left shoulder and an additional healing burn of the right heel that appears older than the other burns. You should

(A) instruct the family to reduce the temperature setting on the hot water tank
(B) advise the parents to observe the child when interacting with siblings and playmates
(C) suspect child abuse
(D) suspect attention deficit/hyperactivity disorder
(E) screen the child for coordination of major muscle groups

Answer: (C). As many as one in five burns of young children are the result of abusive acts, so abuse must be considered when a child has more than two burn sites, burns at various stages of healing, and burns that follow a particular pattern (e.g., "stocking-glove" distribution). (*Chapter 50, Page 441.*)

DIRECTIONS (Items 12.17 through 12.37): Each of the items in this section is a multiple true–false problem that consists of a stem and four lettered options. Indicate whether each of the options is TRUE or FALSE.

12.17 True statements regarding bite injuries include which of the following?

(A) Dog bites often tend to be lacerations with torn tissue.
(B) Although dog bites in children cause soft tissue lacerations, bone is rarely involved.
(C) Cat bites are usually puncture wounds.

(D) Human bite wounds often arise during contact sports.

Answer: (A-True, B-False, C-True, D-True). Significant dog bites tend to be lacerations, often with crushing or tearing of tissue. Bites are most often sustained on the extremities, head, and neck. In children, dog bites may penetrate the skull. Because of their needlelike teeth, cat and rodent bites are usually puncture wounds, often involving tendons or joint spaces. A multitude of organisms reside in the mouths of all higher primates. For this reason, these bites are notoriously predisposed to infection. Human bite wounds most commonly result from conflict or contact sports. (*Chapter 47, Page 404.*)

12.18 True statements regarding disease transmission during human bites include which of the following?

(A) Human bites may transmit hepatitis B.
(B) Following a human bite, prophylaxis against hepatitis B may be achieved by administering immunoglobulin and hepatitis B vaccine.
(C) Hepatitis B has not been found to be transmitted by human bites.
(D) There is significant incidence of human immunodeficiency virus (HIV) transmission by human bites.

Answer: (A-True, B-True, C-False, D-False). Human bites may transmit hepatitis B and C as well as herpes simplex virus. Prophylaxis against hepatitis B may be achieved by administering hepatitis B immunoglobulin 0.06 ml/kg and hepatitis B vaccine. The potential for HIV transmission by this route is thought to be low. The need for tetanus and rabies vaccination should be assessed. (*Chapter 47, Page 405.*)

12.19 Bats and other wild animals are currently the major source of rabies in the United States. Which of the following injuries constitute rabies exposure?

(A) a break in the skin from teeth or claws of an infected animal
(B) contact with saliva of an infected animal on mucous membranes or broken skin
(C) a bite from a raccoon feeding on the back porch who disappears into the woods
(D) a scratch sustained from a bat while exploring a cave

Answer: (A-True, B-True, C-True, D-True). Assessment of risk involves a thorough history and physical examination. A break in the skin from teeth or claws of an infected animal or contact with saliva on mucous membranes or broken skin constitutes exposure. The decision to apply prophylaxis is then guided by the specific situation and animal species. In general, bats, skunks, raccoons, foxes, and other wild carnivores should be regarded as rabid and immunoprophylaxis administered. (*Chapter 47, Page 405.*)

12.20 The treatment for most spider bites should include

- (A) local wound care
- (B) review of tetanus immunization status
- (C) infection prophylaxis with amoxicillin-clavulanate as the first-choice medication
- (D) pain control using ice and analgesics

Answer: (A-True, B-True, C-False, D-True). For most spider bites wound care, ensuring current tetanus immunization status, and monitoring for infection are the only interventions required. Local symptoms are controlled through the use of ice, analgesics, and antihistamines. (*Chapter 47, Page 406.*)

12.21 One of the two families of poisonous snakes in the United States is the crotalidae or the pit vipers. True statements regarding the crotalidae include which of the following?

- (A) This family includes rattlesnakes and copperheads.
- (B) This family includes coral snakes, chiefly found in the southern United States.
- (C) These snakes are distinguished by the "pit," which is a heat-sensing organ between the eye and the nostril.
- (D) These snakes produce a venom that blocks the transmission of nerve impulses to muscle.

Answer: (A-True, B-False, C-True, D-False). Crotalidae, or pit vipers, which include rattlesnakes, cottonmouths, and copperheads, are distinguished by heat-sensing organs, or "pits," in the area between the eye and the nostril. Crotalid toxin primarily causes hemolysis, hemorrhage, and local soft tissue damage. (*Chapter 47, Page 407.*)

12.22 The patient is a 26-year-old forest service worker in Florida bitten approximately 45 minutes ago by a coral snake. He has been brought to the emergency department by his co-workers. True statements regarding management of this patient include which of the following?

- (A) He should receive administration of specific antivenin.
- (B) He should be observed for symptoms of reaction to envenomation, with administration of antivenin if such evidence occurs.
- (C) If antivenin is used, the possibility of anaphylaxis should be anticipated.
- (D) There is no specific antivenin manufactured for coral snake bites.

Answer: (A-True, B-False, C-True, D-False). Specific antivenin should be administered to anyone sustaining a bite from a coral snake, regardless of initial presentation, as symptoms may progress rapidly once they appear. Antivenin administration is associated with anaphylaxis and serum sickness in a significant percentage of patients. (*Chapter 47, Page 407.*)

12.23 You are hiking with friends in a forest located in an area with a high incidence of Lyme disease. A member of your party has been bitten by a tick, which has been removed carefully and completely. Your further recommendations might include which of the following?

- (A) prophylactic ketoconazole therapy
- (B) penicillin therapy
- (C) prophylactic tetracycline therapy
- (D) local wound care

Answer: (A-False, B-False, C-False, D-True). Administration of prophylactic antibiotics after a tick bite, even in areas with a high incidence of Lyme disease or ehrlichiosis, is not recommended. (*Chapter 47, Page 407.*)

12.24 The treatment of acetaminophen poisoning includes

- (A) minimizing absorption from the gastrointestinal (GI) tract
- (B) appropriate use of glutathione inhibitors
- (C) appropriate use of *N*-acetylcysteine (NAC)
- (D) supportive care

Answer: (A-True, B-False, C-True, D-True). Treatment of acetaminophen poisoning embodies three principles: preventing absorption of ingested acetaminophen from the GI tract, appropriate use of the antidote NAC, and supportive care. Acetylcysteine (Mucomyst), the current treatment of choice for toxic acetaminophen ingestions, is believed to exert its protective effect by replacing the depleted glutathione stores. (*Chapter 48, Pages 409–410.*)

12.25 In poisoning due to CA, cardiac abnormalities are common. True statements regarding this problem include which of the following?

(A) Sinus bradycardia is often present.
(B) Sinus tachycardia is often present with serious overdoses.
(C) Prolongation of the QRS interval on the electrocardiogram (ECG) is characteristic of CA overdoses.
(D) Shortening of the QRS interval on the ECG is a sign of potentially serious toxicity.

Answer: (A-False, B-True, C-True, D-False). Sinus tachycardia is frequently present with serious CA overdoses but is a nonspecific finding. A limb-lead ECG QRS interval of more than 0.10 sec is more specific and is considered a sign of potentially serious toxicity. (*Chapter 48, Page 412.*)

12.26 Arrhythmias induced by CA may be treated by

(A) alkalinization of the plasma
(B) lidocaine
(C) procainamide
(D) flecainide

Answer: (A-True, B-True, C-False, D-False). Arrhythmias induced by CAs are treated by alkalinization of the plasma to pH 7.50 to 7.55, the use of antiarrhythmics, and cardioversion when necessary. If serious ventricular arrhythmias persist following alkalinization and other supportive measures, lidocaine is the initial drug of choice. The use of class IA (quinidine, procainamide, disopyramide) and IC (flecainide, encainide, propafenone) antiarrhythmic agents should be avoided whenever possible because they potentiate the cardiac effects of CAs. Beta-blockers may be used cautiously, but careful monitoring for hypotension and cardiac arrest is mandatory. (*Chapter 48, Page 413.*)

12.27 Following poison by ingestion of oral salicylate-containing medications, signs and symptoms often noted within the first 8 to 10 hours include

(A) vomiting
(B) respiratory acidosis
(C) hyperpnea
(D) low body temperature

Answer: (A-True, B-False, C-True, D-False). Signs and symptoms, which usually begin within 3 to 8 hours of ingestion, include nausea and vomiting, hyperpnea, and respiratory alkalosis. The respiratory alkalosis typically persists but is accompanied by progressive metabolic acidosis as the severity and duration of the poisoning increases. Additional findings may include tinnitus, disorientation, and hyperpyrexia. (*Chapter 48, Page 414.*)

12.28 The clinical presentation of patients with *chronic* salicylate intoxication may differ from that of patients with *acute* intoxication. True statements regarding the patient with *chronic* salicylism include which of the following?

(A) There is likely to be a more gradual onset of symptoms.
(B) Neurologic symptoms are especially prominent in young and middle-aged persons.
(C) Bizarre behavior and paranoia may occur.
(D) Chronic salicylism may be confused with alcoholism, sepsis, or dementia.

Answer: (A-True, B-False, C-True, D-True). Potential differences include a more gradual onset of symptoms, an advanced stage of intoxication at initial presentation, and a predominance of neurologic symptoms particularly in the elderly. Neurologic findings may include confusion, agitation, stupor, paranoia, and bizarre behavior. Chronic salicylism has been misdiagnosed as sepsis, alcohol withdrawal, myocardial infarction, organic psychosis, and dementia. (*Chapter 48, Page 415.*)

12.29 True statements regarding poisoning with benzodiazepines include which of the following?

(A) These drugs have a low margin of safety.
(B) Severe overdose can cause hypotension and hypothermia.
(C) Severe complications such as coma or respiratory distress are common in benzodiazepine-only ingestions.
(D) Coingestions with other drugs, notably alcohol, increase the risk of benzodiazepine complications.

Answer: (A-False, B-True, C-False, D-True). Benzodiazepines have a high margin of safety, and overdoses usually produce only mild-to-moderate signs of toxicity, including ataxia, dysarthria, drowsiness, and lethargy. However, severe overdoses can cause coma, hypotension, hypothermia, and respiratory distress requiring endotracheal intubation and assisted ventilation. Such complications are rare in benzodiazepine-only ingestions but occur much more frequently with coingestions of other drugs that cause CNS depression (especially alcohol). (*Chapter 48, Page 416.*)

12.30 Ipecac syrup is used for early management in specific cases of acute oral poisoning However, ipecac should *not* be used in patients who have ingested

(A) hydrocarbons such as kerosene or gasoline
(B) hydrocarbons containing pesticides
(C) acids or alkalis
(D) hydrocarbons containing heavy metals

Answer: (A-True, B-False, C-True, D-False). Ipecac should not be used in patients who have ingested hydrocarbons (kerosene, gasoline, paint thinner), strychnine, or acids or alkalis because of the potential of aspiration. However, emesis is indicated for ingested aromatic or halogenated hydrocarbons and hydrocarbons containing pesticides, camphor, or heavy metals. (*Chapter 48, Page 417.*)

12.31 The patient is a 4-year-old child who has ingested an unknown number of phenobarbital tablets. You are considering the use of activated charcoal and/or syrup of ipecac. True statements include which of the following?

(A) Ipecac and activated charcoal should be given simultaneously.
(B) If a patient is to receive ipecac, activated charcoal should be given 20 minutes after administering the syrup of ipecac.
(C) If a patient is to receive ipecac, activated charcoal should be withheld until ipecac-induced vomiting has stopped.
(D) Activated charcoal should be given first, followed 1 hour later by syrup of ipecac.

Answer: (A-False, B-False, C-True, D-False). If a patient is to receive ipecac, activated charcoal should be withheld until ipecac-induced vomiting has stopped (usually 1 to 2 hours after the last ipecac dose). Activated charcoal should never be given before ipecac therapy. Otherwise, there are no absolute contraindications to the use of activated charcoal. (*Chapter 48, Page 418.*)

12.32 A well-closed surgical wound has the following characteristics:

(A) The margins are approximated with tension to prevent hematoma formation.
(B) The tissue layers are accurately aligned.
(C) Dead space is eliminated.
(D) Deep sutures are placed by using a surface knot.

Answer: (A-False, B-True, C-True, D-False). A well-closed wound has three characteristics: the margins are approximated without tension; the tissue layers are accurately aligned; and dead space is eliminated. Deep stitches are placed in layers that hold the suture, such as the fat–fascial junction or the dermal–fat junction. A buried knot technique is the preferred method for placing deep sutures. Deep sutures provide most of the strength of the repair; skin sutures approximate the skin margins and improve the cosmetic result. (*Chapter 49, Page 427.*)

12.33 In acute lacerations, especially those wounds that are contaminated with sewage or feces, tetanus immunoglobulin (TIg) may be required as passive immunity. True statements regarding TIg include which of the following?

(A) The preferred vaccine is equine TIg.
(B) The usual dose of TIg is 500 units intramuscularly (IM).
(C) Tetanus toxoid and TIg should not be given simultaneously.
(D) Tetanus toxoid and TIg should be given at separate sites.

Answer: (A-False, B-True, C-False, D-True). Whenever passive immunity is required, human TIg is preferred. The usual dose of TIg is 500 units IM. Tetanus toxoid and TIg should be given through separate needles at separate sites. (*Chapter 49, Page 433.*)

12.34 True statements regarding decompression sickness (the bends) include which of the following?

(A) The disease most often occurs after divers descend to 10 m (33 ft) or deeper.
(B) The pathophysiology is related to the carbon dioxide dissolved in the blood and tissues.
(C) Decompression illness may begin as long as 12 hours after the dive.
(D) The disease is named for Dr. Joseph Bends, who first described the syndrome.

Answer: (A-True, B-False, C-True, D-False). Decompression sickness, "the bends," most often occurs after divers descend to 10 m (33 ft) or deeper. As divers increase underwater depth and time, nitrogen gradually dissolves in the blood and tissues. If ascent is too rapid, this nitrogen can become insoluble, forming bubbles in the bloodstream and the tissues. Decompression sickness usually manifests immediately or shortly after the dive but may occur as long as 12 hours later. Most commonly, the victim experiences steady or throbbing pain in the shoulders and elbows, with some relief on "bending" the affected joint. (*Chapter 50, Page 437.*)

12.35 Scarring usually occurs with

(A) first-degree burns
(B) second-degree burns
(C) third-degree burns
(D) all burns

Answer: (A-False, B-True, C-True, D-False). Scarring usually occurs with second- and third-degree burns, and excision and skin grafting may give better results than reepithelialization. (*Chapter 50, Page 440.*)

12.36 The patient is a 92-year-old white man, a denture wearer, who complains that since dinner last night it feels like a piece of food is caught "half way down." The patient can breathe and speak normally but attempts to swallow water lead to regurgitation. This patient may be treated with which of the following?

(A) proteolytic enzymes
(B) IV glucagon
(C) nifedipine administered sublingually
(D) endoscopic removal

Answer: (A-False, B-True, C-True, D-True). Endoscopic removal is preferred. The use of proteolytic enzymes, such as aqueous solution of papain (i.e., Adolph's meat tenderizer), is not recommended owing to the risk of perforation. When endoscopy is not available, IV glucagon (1.0 mg) has been suggested to relax the esophageal smooth muscle. If the food bolus has not passed in 20 minutes, an additional 2.0 mg IV is given. When not contraindicated, nifedipine (10 mg sublingually) can be given to lower esophageal pressure and the amplitude of gastroesophageal sphincter contractions. (*Chapter 50, Page 441.*)

12.37 The patient is a 3-year-old who has swallowed a button battery from a travel alarm clock. True statements regarding this clinical problem include which of the following?

(A) A button battery lodged in the esophagus is treated as an emergency.
(B) Button batteries contain calcium carbonate, which protects esophageal and gastric mucosa against damage.
(C) A button battery in the esophagus should be removed endoscopically.
(D) If a button battery has reached the stomach, it may be observed for as long as 5 days without intervention.

Answer: (A-True, B-False, C-True, D-False). Most batteries pass uneventfully through the GI tract within 46 to 72 hours. However, a button battery lodged in the esophagus is an emergency. These batteries contain 45% potassium hydroxide, which is erosive to the esophagus and especially hazardous. Button batteries should be removed endoscopically from the esophagus or if they remain in the stomach longer than 24 hours. (*Chapter 50, Page 441.*)

13

Care of the Athlete

The questions in this chapter constitute a review of the following chapters in *Family Medicine: Principles and Practice, Fifth Edition*:

Medical Problems of the Athlete (Chapter 51)
Athletic Injuries (Chapter 52)

DIRECTIONS: (Items 13.1 through 13.20): Each of the questions or incomplete statements in this section is followed by five suggested answers or completions. Select the ONE that is BEST in each case.

13.1 Asthmatic exacerbations during exercise generally occur

(A) at the initiation of exercise
(B) 2 to 5 minutes following the start of exercise
(C) at the ventilatory threshold
(D) with the development of lactic acidosis
(E) during anaerobic exercise

Answer: (C). Asthmatic exacerbations during exercise generally occur at the ventilatory threshold—that point at which the ventilatory rate abruptly increases in response to progressively increasing work or exercise. Increased physical fitness associated with a regular exercise program results in an increase in the amount of work before the ventilatory threshold is reached. (*Chapter 51, Page 446.*)

13.2 The athletic heart syndrome is

(A) associated with overexertion
(B) requires annual monitoring until the patient involved participates in athletic training
(C) necessitates antibiotic prophylaxis during dental surgery or oral surgery

(D) chiefly involves the intraventricular septum
(E) represents changes due to a normal physiologic response to training

Answer: (E). The athletic heart syndrome is a constellation of clinical variants of cardiac structure and function that is present in physically active individuals. These changes, originally thought to result from heart disease associated with "overexertion," are now thought to represent changes due to a normal physiologic response to training. (*Chapter 51, Page 446.*)

13.3 The patient is a 21-year-old college athlete with an enlarged heart with cardiac hypertrophy on electrocardiograph (ECG), bradycardia, and T-wave abnormalities. This patient also notes occasional dizziness and palpitations. He has a grade 2/6 systolic murmur that increases in volume with the Valsalva maneuver. This patient should be suspected of having

(A) the athletic heart syndrome
(B) hypertrophic cardiomyopathy
(C) mitral stenosis
(D) chronic hypertension
(E) intraventricular heart block

Answer: (B). The distinction between the athletic heart syndrome and hypertrophic cardiomyopathy is probably the most important clinical decision during cardiac evaluation of the athlete. The history, family history, and cardiac review of systems are essential for this differentiation. A good rule of thumb for the practicing family physician is that the hallmark of the athletic heart syndrome is the absence of positive cardiac symptomatology (light-headedness or dizziness, syncope, palpitations, chest pain) and a negative family history of sudden death or hypertrophic cardiomyopathy. The presence of cardiac symptoms requires close follow-up or referral. The asymptomatic individual who has abnormalities on the physical examination and ECG associated with physical activity can be followed by testing or with temporization. The finding of a systolic murmur that increases in volume with the Valsalva maneuver or an upright posture is suggestive of hypertrophic cardiomyopathy. An echocardiogram is useful for diagnosing such a cardiomyopathy when clinical judgment finds it warranted. (*Chapter 51, Page 447.*)

13.4 The patient is a 36-year-old black male postal worker whose blood pressure is 158/102. He is not currently taking antihypertension medication. At this time, this individual should avoid

- (A) all exercise
- (B) low-intensity exercise
- (C) moderate-intensity exercise
- (D) static exercise such as heavy weight training
- (E) no restrictions are appropriate

Answer: (D). Avoidance of static exercise, such as heavy weight training, is prudent for the hypertensive individual. (*Chapter 51, Page 447.*)

13.5 The most common cause of true anemia among athletes is

- (A) expansion of plasma volume associated with regular aerobic exercise
- (B) hemolytic anemia
- (C) sickle cell anemia
- (D) iron deficiency
- (E) spherocytosis

Answer: (D). The most common cause of true anemia among athletes is iron deficiency. Some endurance athletes lose iron through small amounts of gastrointestinal bleeding, menses, or the urine. (*Chapter 51, Page 448.*)

13.6 Heat syncope is an abrupt loss of consciousness observed in dehydrated individuals going from a supine or sitting position to an upright posture. It is thought to be

- (A) related to insulin resistance
- (B) caused by transient hypoglycemia
- (C) caused by a transient low serum calcium level
- (D) a vasovagal phenomenon resulting from venous pooling of blood
- (E) a manifestation of cardiac syncope

Answer: (D). It is thought to be a vasovagal phenomenon resulting from venous pooling of blood in vasodilated peripheral veins. Preload is reduced, cardiac output is diminished, and impaired cerebral perfusion can lead to syncope. (*Chapter 51, Page 449.*)

13.7 The most common sign of heat stroke is

- (A) coma
- (B) tachycardia
- (C) abdominal cramps
- (D) lassitude
- (E) headache

Answer: (B). Tachycardia is the most common sign of heat stroke. (*Chapter 51, Page 450.*)

13.8 Most sports injuries are related to

- (A) low calcium content of bone
- (B) poor conditioning
- (C) direct trauma
- (D) overuse
- (E) lax ligaments

Answer: (D). Overuse injuries comprise the most common form of sports injuries seen by the family physician. These injuries are induced by repetitive motion leading to microscopic disruption of a bone–tendon or bone–synovium interface. (*Chapter 52, Page 453.*)

13.9 The patient is a 17-year-old white female high school distance runner. She has suffered an inversion sprain of the ankle. The structures most likely to be injured are

- (A) anterior and posterior talofibular ligaments and the calcaneofibular ligament
- (B) the deltoid ligament
- (C) the tibial fibular aponeurosis
- (D) anterior and posterior talotibial ligaments and the calcaneotibial ligament
- (E) the calcaneotalor ligament

Answer: (A). The most common structures injured with inversion are the three lateral ligaments that support the ankle joint: the anterior and posterior talofibular ligaments and the calcaneofibular ligament. (*Chapter 52, Page 455.*)

13.10 The patient is a 17-year-old white male football player. He is the star half-back of the team, and while changing direction during open field running, he felt the knee "give out." There was no direct blow to the knee. This young athlete is most likely to have

(A) a medial meniscal tear
(B) a lateral meniscal tear
(C) a medial collateral ligament injury
(D) a lateral collateral ligament injury
(E) an anterior cruciate ligament (ACL) injury

Answer: (E). ACL injury is the most frequent, most severe ligamentous injury to the knee. The injury usually occurs without a direct blow to the knee; rather, it results from torsional stress coupled with a deceleration injury. These injuries are seen when an athlete changes direction while running and the knee suddenly "gives out." (*Chapter 52, Page 457.*)

13.11 The patient is an 18-year-old white male basketball player who struck his head in a fall to the floor during a game 1 hour ago. Following the injury, he had impaired balance and disturbed vision and was unable to concentrate for a few minutes. This patient

(A) probably has an epidural hematoma
(B) is best defined as "dazed"
(C) has a postconcussion syndrome
(D) has a concussion
(E) has a scalp contusion

Answer: (D). A definition of concussion is "a clinical syndrome characterized by immediate and transient posttraumatic impairment of neural function, such as the alteration of consciousness, disturbance of vision, equilibrium, etc., due to brainstem involvement."

Postconcussion syndrome consists of headache (especially with exertion), labrynthine disturbance, fatigue, irritability, and impaired memory and concentration. These symptoms can persist for weeks or even months. (*Chapter 52, Page 458.*)

13.12 The only shoulder injury that requires prompt manipulation is

(A) posterior dislocation
(B) anterior dislocation
(C) fracture of the surgical neck of the humerus
(D) acromioclavicular (AC) separation
(E) rotator cuff tear

Answer: (B). Anterior dislocation is the only shoulder injury that requires prompt manipulation. (*Chapter 52, Page 459.*)

13.13 The initial management of an AC separation involves

(A) surgery
(B) injection of corticosteroid into the joint space
(C) ultrasound therapy
(D) casting
(E) immobilization in a sling

Answer: (E). Initial management of AC separations requires the shoulder to be immobilized in a sling. (*Chapter 52, Page 460.*)

13.14 The flexion "boutonniere" deformity at the proximal interphalangeal joint occurs with which of the following types of injuries?

(A) forced abduction
(B) laceration of the flexor surface of the hand
(C) crush injury of the distal phalangeal joint
(D) avulsion of the flexor tendon of the distal phalanx
(E) avulsion of the central slip of the distal phalanx

Answer: (E). Proximal phalangeal joint injuries occur when there is avulsion of the central slip of the distal phalanx resulting in a flexion "boutonniere" deformity. (*Chapter 52, Page 461.*)

13.15 The patient is a 22-year-old white male college baseball player. He is the team's star pitcher and has a 2-month history of pain in his right (throwing) shoulder. The pain radiates deep from the subacromial space to the deltoid region. It is vague and not well localized. There is pain with abduction of the arm and especially with attempts to raise the arm above the level of the shoulder. Palpation of the subacromial bursa under the coracoacromial ligament elicits pain deep to the acromion as does internal rotation of the arm when abducted at 90° with the elbow also flexed at 90°. This patient appears to have

(A) a brachial plexus injury
(B) recurrent subluxation of the shoulder
(C) shoulder impingement syndrome
(D) bicipital tendinitis
(E) subdeltoid bursitis

Answer: (C). Patients with shoulder impingement complain of pain with abduction to varying degrees and especially with attempts to raise the arm above the level of the shoulder. The pain radiates deep from the subacromial space to the deltoid region and may be vague and not well localized. Palpation of the subacromial bursa under the coracoacromial ligament often elicits pain deep to the acromion as does internal rotation of the arm when abducted at 90 degrees with the elbow also flexed at 90 degrees. (*Chapter 52, Page 460.*)

13.16 Lateral epicondylitis is characterized by point tenderness of the lateral epicondyle at the area of attachment of the

- (A) brachioradialis muscle
- (B) extensor carpi radialis brevis
- (C) flexor carpi radialis brevis
- (D) extensor carpi ulnaris
- (E) common origin of the long flexors of the fingers and thumb

Answer: (B). Lateral epicondylitis is characterized by point tenderness of the lateral epicondyle at the attachment of the extensor carpi radialis brevis. (*Chapter 52, Page 461.*)

13.17 Which among the following athletes is at *greatest* risk of spondylolysis?

- (A) weight lifters
- (B) runners
- (C) divers
- (D) football players
- (E) preadolescent gymnasts

Answer: (E). Preadolescent gymnasts are at highest risk for developing spondylolysis, but it is also seen in weight lifters, runners, swimmers who perform the butterfly stroke, divers, and football players. (*Chapter 52, Page 461.*)

13.18 Your patient is a 32-year-old male stockbroker who runs regularly, totaling about 20 miles a week. He has some pain in the area of the patella, particularly occurring after exercise. The pain is worse when walking downhill and sometimes pain occurs spontaneously if the knee remains flexed for several minutes. Even before performing a physical examination, you might suspect that this patient has

- (A) a tear of the medial cartilage
- (B) an ACL syndrome
- (C) plantaris syndrome
- (D) retropatellar pain syndrome (RPPS)
- (E) Osgood-Schlatter's disease

Answer: (D). Patients with RPPS present with vague retropatellar or peripatellar pain, which is usually most significant several hours after exercise. Walking downhill or downstairs, bending at the knees, and kneeling can exacerbate the pain. With more ad-

vanced cases, the pain can be constant, occurring during and after exercise. Oddly, patients often experience pain if the knee is not moved enough; that is, if the knee remains flexed for several minutes, pain develops. (*Chapter 52, Page 462.*)

13.19 The patient is a 35-year-old runner who has pain in the lower extremity after recently increasing the duration of running. Your clinical diagnosis is tibial periostitis (shin splints). This patient probably also has what other orthopedic problem?

- (A) pes planus
- (B) RPPS
- (C) Osgood-Schlatter's disease
- (D) meralgia paresthetica
- (E) chondromalacia patellae

Answer: (A). Most patients with this syndrome have pes planus, which results in tibialis posterior tendonitis initially. Their pain is localized to the lower third of the medial aspect of the tibia. (*Chapter 52, Page 462.*)

13.20 The patient is a 31-year-old white male runner who has recently increased his weekly distance. For the past month, he has noted moderately severe pain near the base of the left fifth metatarsal. There is no history of direct trauma. You suspect that this patient may have

- (A) plantar fasciitis
- (B) a fracture of the proximal fifth metatarsal (Jones' fracture)
- (C) a stress fracture of the cuboid
- (D) a hairline fracture of the talus
- (E) a chronic strain of the supporting ligaments of the lateral foot

Answer: (B). Jones' fractures are primarily seen in distance runners, especially those with a recent increase in activity. There is usually a history of antecedent pain for several weeks where the peroneus brevis tendon attaches to the proximal fifth metatarsal. (*Chapter 52, Page 463.*)

DIRECTIONS: (Items 13.21 through 13.25): Each of the items in this section is a multiple true–false problem that consists of a stem and four lettered options. Indicate whether each of the four options is TRUE or FALSE.

13.21 True statements regarding asthma and exercise include which of the following?

(A) Less than 10% of patients with asthma are prone to exacerbation during exercise.
(B) Exercise-induced asthma may be the only manifestation of asthma.
(C) Many persons limit their physical activity to prevent asthma exacerbations.
(D) Asthmatic children should be encouraged to limit exercise and avoid competitive sports.

Answer: (A-False, B-True, C-True, D-False). Approximately 80% of patients with asthma are prone to exacerbation of asthmatic symptoms during exercise. In some patients (particularly those with allergic rhinitis), exercise-induced asthma may be the only manifestation of the disease. Although many adults and children with asthma have limited their physical activity to prevent asthma exacerbations, most patients with this condition should be able to participate in athletics with physician monitoring. (*Chapter 51, Page 445.*)

13.22 The patient is a 42-year-old white woman with type 2 diabetes. You recommend a moderate level of physical activity for this patient. Moderate physical activity is likely to result in

(A) increased insulin resistance
(B) decreased insulin sensitivity
(C) improved glycemic control
(D) increased serum levels of insulin

Answer: (A-False, B-False, C-True, D-False). Moderate levels of physical activity can result in decreased insulin resistance, increased insulin sensitivity, improved glycemic control, and decreased serum levels of insulin in the type 2 diabetic patient. (*Chapter 51, Page 448.*)

13.23 Contraindications to exercise during pregnancy include

(A) pregnancy-induced hypertension
(B) incompetent cervix
(C) weight gain of greater than 18 lb
(D) persistent second- or third-trimester bleeding

Answer: (A-True, B-True, C-False, D-True). Contraindications to exercise during pregnancy include pregnancy-induced hypertension, preterm rupture of membranes, preterm labor during a previous or current pregnancy, incompetent cervix, persistent second- or third-trimester bleeding, or intrauterine growth retardation. (*Chapter 51, Page 451.*)

13.24 Stress fractures

(A) generally cannot be visualized on plain films
(B) are inflammatory in nature
(C) have a lower rate of delayed union or nonunion than traumatic fractures
(D) may result in permanent degenerative changes or deformity

Answer: (A-False, B-True, C-False, D-True). True stress fractures can be visualized on plain films, whereas stress reactions (periostitis) are best seen on bone scans. Because stress fractures are inflammatory in nature, the complication rates due to delayed union or nonunion are higher than those with traumatic fractures. The results of improper treatment of these injuries can be severe, resulting in permanent degenerative changes or deformity. (*Chapter 52, Page 454.*)

13.25 The patient is a 16-year-old white male football player, who injured his left knee in a game this afternoon. With the patient lying supine, you have flexed the patient's knee to about 90° and rotated the lower leg. The patient has pain during external rotation. True statements include which of the following?

(A) The patient appears to have a medial meniscal injury.
(B) The patient appears to have a lateral meniscal injury.
(C) The patient appears to have an injury to the ACL.
(D) You have performed McMurray's test.

Answer: (A-True, B-False, C-False, D-True). When the lower leg is rotated with the knee flexed about 90 degrees, pain during external rotation indicates a medial meniscus injury (McMurray's test). (*Chapter 52, Page 456.*)

14

Common Clinical Problems

The questions in this chapter constitute a review of the following chapters in *Family Medicine: Principles and Practice, Fifth Edition:*

Care of the Obese Patient (Chapter 53)
Care of the Patient with Dysequilibrium (Chapter 54)
Care of the Patient with Fatigue (Chapter 55)
Care of the Patient with a Sleep Disorder (Chapter 56)
Medical Care of the Surgical Patient (Chapter 57)
Counseling Patients with Sexual Concerns (Chapter 58)
Care of the Alcoholic Patient (Chapter 59)
Care of the Patient Who Misuses Drugs (Chapter 60)
Care of the Patient with Chronic Pain (Chapter 61)
Care of the Dying Patient (Chapter 62)

DIRECTIONS (Items 14.1 through 14.33): Each of the questions or incomplete statements in this section is followed by five suggested answers or completions. Select the ONE that is BEST in each case.

14.1 The patient is a 45-year-old white woman who is overweight and undertaking a caloric restriction program. She asks how many calories must be eliminated from her diet to lose 1 lb of weight if all other factors remain the same. The answer to her question is

(A) 500 kcal
(B) 2,000 kcal
(C) 3,500 kcal
(D) 5,000 kcal
(E) 10,000 kcal

Answer: (C). To lose 1 pound of weight, approximately 3,500 kcal must be expended. To do so requires the patient either to ingest fewer calories or increase the expenditure of calories. (*Chapter 53, Page 467.*)

14.2 Appetite suppressants may cause which of the following significant side effects?

(A) classic migraine headache
(B) peptic ulcer disease
(C) carcinoma of the colon
(D) primary pulmonary hypertension
(E) anorexia nervosa

Answer: (D). Appetite suppressants have been associated with the rare but significant side effect of primary pulmonary hypertension. The reported incidence of primary pulmonary hypertension (some irreversible) is 25 to 30 per million users. The incidence in the general population is one to two per million. (*Chapter 53, Page 468.*)

14.3 Vertigo is a specific term used to describe a feeling of

(A) weakness
(B) light-headedness
(C) being off balance
(D) motion
(E) giddiness

Answer: (D). Vertigo is a specific term used to describe a feeling of motion or rotation of one's self (subjective) or of surroundings (objective). Patients may complain that the room is spinning or that their head is spinning. (*Chapter 54, Page 471.*)

14.4 The Dix-Hallpike maneuver can be useful in the diagnosis of

(A) benign paroxysmal positional vertigo
(B) acoustic neuroma
(C) cholesteatoma
(D) Meniere's disease
(E) subclavian steal syndrome

Answer: (A). Evocative testing in the office for evaluation of dizziness and vertigo includes the Dix-Hallpike maneuvers to rule out benign paroxysmal positional vertigo. This maneuver and the abnormal nystagmic response were first described in 1952 by Dix and Hallpike. With benign paroxysmal positional vertigo, the nystagmus begins after a 10-second delay and subsides within 1 minute. (*Chapter 54, Page 472.*)

14.5 The patient is a 36-year-old white woman with a chief complaint of dizziness who describes a "whirling sensation," which has been present on and off for 6 months. In addition, she has had some difficulty with vision in the left eye and some sense of parasthesias in the upper extremities. There has also been some double vision, clumsiness, and emotional lability. On physical examination, you note decreased perception of vibration and position sense in the lower extremities plus some hyperreflexia in all extremities. The most likely diagnosis is

(A) Meniere's disease
(B) vestibular neuronitis
(C) diabetes mellitus
(D) hyperthyroidism
(E) multiple sclerosis (MS)

Answer: (E). MS may cause vertigo, which is the initial complaint in 5% of MS patients. As the disease progresses, 50% of the patients suffer vertigo. The history and physical examination may disclose symptoms of impaired vision, nystagmus, decreased perception of vibration and position sense, paresthesias, clumsiness, diplopia, emotional lability, hyperreflexia, and bladder dysfunction. (*Chapter 54, Page 474.*)

14.6 As an individual ages, his or her required hours of sleep tend to

(A) become greater
(B) stay about the same
(C) become less
(D) average about 7 hours/24-hour day
(E) average about 12 hours/24-hour day

Answer: (A). Transition into older adulthood produces a gradual increase in total daily sleep time. By age 90, the average is nearly 9 hours/day. In addition, older adults often take longer to fall asleep, take daytime naps, experience more frequent awakenings, and spend less time in the deep states of sleep. (*Chapter 56, Page 483.*)

14.7 Narcolepsy typically begins during

(A) infancy
(B) childhood or adolescence
(C) middle age
(D) after age 65
(E) at any time of life

Answer: (B). Narcolepsy is a relatively uncommon sleep disorder that typically develops during childhood or adolescence. (*Chapter 56, Page 485.*)

14.8 The patient is a 39-year-old white man whom you referred to the sleep laboratory and a diagnosis of sleep apnea has been confirmed. Your first step in managing this patient should be

(A) referral for consideration of palatal surgery
(B) a prescription for fluoxetine or similar selective serotonin reuptake inhibitor
(C) counseling to avoid factors that may increase severity of upper airway obstruction (i.e., alcohol, sedatives, and obesity)
(D) continuous positive airway pressure delivered through a mask or nasal prongs
(E) careful fitting of an oral appliance

Answer: (C). Patients with sleep apnea first must be counseled to avoid factors that increase the severity of upper airway obstruction (i.e., sleep deprivation, alcohol, sedatives, and obesity). (*Chapter 56, Pages 485–486.*)

14.9 Medications shown to benefit patients with restless leg syndrome (RLS) include all the following except

(A) propranolol
(B) levodopa/carbidopa
(C) clonazepam
(D) carbamazepine
(E) quinidine hydrochloride

Answer: (A). Discontinuation of several medications sometimes associated with RLS, such as neuroleptics, lithium, beta-blockers, tricyclics, antidepressants, anticonvulsants, and histamine blockers is sometimes helpful. At times, a hot bath before bedtime is useful. Levodopa/carbidopa, oxycodone hydrochloride, clonazepam, carbamazepine, and quinidine hydrochloride have been shown to benefit patients with RLS in randomized controlled trials. (*Chapter 56, Page 486.*)

14.10 Valvular heart disease in the surgical patient increases the risk of perioperative mortality. The greatest risk is in patients with

(A) symptomatic aortic regurgitation
(B) mitral stenosis
(C) mitral valve prolapse
(D) mitral regurgitation
(E) hemodynamically significant aortic stenosis

Answer: (E). Valvular heart disease (especially hemodynamically significant aortic stenosis) is associated with an increased risk for perioperative mortality. Mitral stenosis is not associated with increased mortality, but these patients are sensitive to preload volume changes. Patients with aortic regurgitation and mitral regurgitation are less sensitive to volume changes but require adequate left ventricular contractility, as regurgitation takes place during both diastole and systole. (*Chapter 57, Page 492.*)

14.11 In evaluating a 75-year-old white man preoperatively for venous ligation and stripping, you note that he has decreased peripheral pulses, some atrophic changes of the skin of the feet, and cool extremities. This patient has an increased risk of concomitant

(A) renal failure
(B) coronary artery disease
(C) carcinoma of the pancreas
(D) abdominal aortic aneurism
(E) von Willebrand's disease

Answer: (B). There is a high incidence of occult coronary artery disease among patients with peripheral vascular disease. Up to 60% have severe coronary artery disease; many have no clinical symptoms and frequently have normal electrocardiographs (ECG). (*Chapter 57, Page 492.*)

14.12 The patient is a 58-year-old white man whom you have treated for severe chronic depression. After trying a number of medications, the patient has been taking a monoamine oxidase (MAO) inhibitor for the past year. His depression has been stable and well controlled. He has now been found to have a mass in the left kidney, and surgery is scheduled. You should advise this patient to

(A) continue the MAO inhibitor, stopping the day before surgery
(B) continue the MAO inhibitor, taking the last pill with a sip of water on the morning of surgery
(C) recommend that the surgeon continue the use of this medication group using parenteral administration during the early postoperative period
(D) discontinue the medication a few weeks before surgery
(E) continue the MAO inhibitor and add a beta-blocker to avoid perioperative blood pressure fluctuations

Answer: (D). MAO inhibitors interfere with autonomic function and may cause perioperative hypertension and hypotension. These agents may prolong neuromuscular blockade, inhibit hepatic enzymes, and prolong the action of narcotic drugs. If possible, the medication is discontinued a few weeks before surgery. (*Chapter 57, Page 493.*)

14.13 The most common medical disorder affecting blood clotting factor production is

(A) classical hemophilia
(B) von Willebrand's disease
(C) hypofibrinogenemia
(D) severe liver disease
(E) renal failure

Answer: (D). The most common disorder affecting clotting factor production is severe liver disease. (*Chapter 57, Page 495.*)

14.14 The patient is a 35-year-old white man who reports that when he has an erection, the erect penis looks "crooked." This patient may have

(A) erythroplasia of Queyrat
(B) diabetes mellitus
(C) a reaction to antihypertensive medication
(D) acute thrombosis of the corpora callosum
(E) Peyronie's disease

Answer: (E). When a man complains of a "crooked" erection, it may indicate Peyronie's disease; to confirm it, have him take a Polaroid photograph of the erection while at home. (*Chapter 58, Page 501.*)

14.15 The lowest level of alcohol consumption and the lowest frequency of alcohol-related problems are found in which ethnic group in the United States?

(A) Hispanic Americans
(B) Native Americans
(C) African Americans
(D) Caucasians
(E) Asian Americans

Answer: (E). Asian Americans have the lowest level of alcohol consumption and the lowest frequency of alcohol-related problems of any ethnic group in the United States. Within this group, drinking seems to be more socially controlled and restricted to the company of friends on special occasions. (*Chapter 59, Page 507.*)

14.16 One "highball" drink is the equivalent of about 10 ml of absolute alcohol. The average man can metabolize this amount of alcohol in approximately

(A) 1 hour
(B) 2 hours
(C) 3 hours
(D) 4 hours
(E) 6 hours

Answer: (A). Although individuals vary greatly in their ability to metabolize alcohol, an average man can metabolize about 10 ml of absolute alcohol (or one drink) per hour. (*Chapter 59, Page 509.*)

14.17 The Wernicke-Korsakoff syndrome characteristically includes all the following except

(A) confusion
(B) elevated alkaline phosphatase levels
(C) ocular disturbances
(D) specific vitamin deficiency
(E) ataxia

Answer: (B). Organic brain syndromes among alcohol-dependent patients can usually be categorized as Wernicke-Korsakoff syndrome or alcoholic dementia. Wernicke's disease includes a triad of signs: confusion, ocular disturbances, and ataxia, caused by thiamine deficiency. Korsakoff's psychosis may be the chronic phase of Wernicke's disease. (*Chapter 59, Page 510.*)

14.18 The characteristic presentation of acute pancreatitis is

(A) anorexia and weight loss
(B) deep epigastric pain radiating to the back following alcohol ingestion or a heavy meal
(C) jaundice, with elevations of both direct and indirect bilirubin

(D) hyperglycemia unresponsive to sulfonylurea drugs
(E) chronic diarrhea with fat globules in the feces

Answer: (B). Deep epigastric pain radiating to the back following alcohol ingestion or a heavy meal is the characteristic presentation. There may be few physical findings. (*Chapter 59, Page 510.*)

14.19 The patient is a 44-year-old white man who has been involved in two recent automobile accidents while driving. His family suspects that he abuses alcohol while away from home, although the patient denies such use. Following your examination, you plan blood testing. The most sensitive laboratory screening test for alcoholism is the

(A) aspartate transaminase level
(B) alanine transaminase (ALT) level
(C) alkaline phosphatase level
(D) gamma-glutamyl transferase (GGT) level
(E) indirect bilirubin level

Answer: (D). The half-life of GGT is approximately 26 days, and an elevated GGT level may be the most sensitive laboratory screening test that indicates alcoholism. (*Chapter 59, Page 513.*)

14.20 The most sensitive indicator of *continued drinking* in an alcoholic patient who reports that he or she has been abstinent is the

(A) aspartate transaminase level
(B) ALT level
(C) alkaline phosphatase level
(D) GGT level
(E) carbohydrate-deficient transferin (CDT) level

Answer: (E). An elevated CDT level is the most sensitive indicator of continued drinking in a purportedly abstinent patient. Unlike the other biochemical markers, a CDT elevation does not seem to reflect organ damage but, rather, recent heavy (five drinks or more per day) consumption of alcohol. (*Chapter 59, Page 513.*)

14.21 The patient is a 46-year-old white man with a long history of heavy drinking who has recently been admitted to the hospital for elective surgery and has become delirious and is hallucinating and combative. He is actively hallucinating. The drug of choice in this patient is

(A) hydroxyzine
(B) phenytoin

(C) chloral hydrate
(D) haloperidol
(E) chlordiazepoxide

Answer: (D). For delirious, hallucinating, and combative patients, haloperidol is the agent of choice, in combination with withdrawal agents such as phenobarbital. Haloperidol is safe in oral, intramuscular, and intravenous doses of 70 to 80 mg/day; higher doses are not uncommon. (*Chapter 59, Page 516.*)

14.22 The patient is a 20-year-old college student admitted to the emergency department with stupor, miosis, hypotension, and bradycardia. There are needle tracks on both arms. You strongly suspect opiate intoxication. A urine toxicology screen will detect most opiates EXCEPT

(A) heroin
(B) fentanyl
(C) morphine
(D) meperidine
(E) propoxyphene

Answer: (B). The presenting signs and symptoms of opiate overdose are stupor, miosis, hypotension, bradycardia, and decreased bowel sounds. Frequently, needle marks or tracks are present. In more severe cases, respiratory depression with apnea and pulmonary edema can occur. Seizures are seen with meperidine and propoxyphene overdoses. A urine toxicology screen detects most opiates (except fentanyl). (*Chapter 60, Page 522.*)

14.23 The preferred drug treatment for acute opiate overdose is

(A) naproxen
(B) pentazocine
(C) naloxone
(D) methylphenidate
(E) methadone

Answer: (C). Naloxone is the primary treatment for opiate overdose. An initial intravenous dose of 0.4 to 2.0 mg usually reverses the opiate effects. This dose can be repeated every 2 to 3 minutes up to 10- to 20-mg total dose. Higher doses of naloxone are needed for codeine, propoxyphene, and pentazocine overdoses. (*Chapter 60, Page 522.*)

14.24 "Crank" is a street name for

(A) freebase cocaine

(B) cocaine rocks produced by dissolving cocaine hydrochloride in sodium bicarbonate and distilling off the water
(C) pentazocine capsules
(D) phencyclidine
(E) methamphetamine

Answer: (E). "Crank" is a street name for methamphetamine that can be taken as pills, injected, or snorted. "Crack" is freebase cocaine. The effects and complications of amphetamine misuse are similar to those of cocaine, except amphetamines have a longer half-life. (*Chapter 60, Page 522.*)

14.25 The most common presenting symptom of amphetamine misuse is

(A) weakness
(B) depression
(C) agitation
(D) chest pain
(E) visual symptoms

Answer: (C). Agitation is the most common presenting symptom of amphetamine misuse. Hallucinations, suicidal ideation, delusions, and confusion may be present. Cardiac symptoms include chest pain, palpitations, and myocardial infarction (MI). (*Chapter 60, Page 522.*)

14.26 The patient is a 20-year-old white female college student brought to the emergency department with severe anxiety and a sense of panic. She has frightening visual hallucinations, which she states began when she took some medication given to her by an acquaintance. On physical examination, the patient has a pulse of 110, a low-grade fever, and pupillary dilation. She is tremulous and sweaty. This patient is most likely to be having a reaction to

(A) opiates
(B) amphetamines
(C) cocaine
(D) marijuana
(E) hallucinogens

Answer: (E). Paranoia, depression, anxiety, and panic attacks are associated with bad trips. Patients experiencing adverse reactions to hallucinogens can be confused with patients having a schizophrenic reaction. Patients toxic from hallucinogens (1) have no history of mental illness, (2) tell you they have ingested the drug, and (3) have visual instead of auditory hallucinations.

On physical examination, patients have pronounced pupillary dilation, tachycardia, sweating, and fever. (*Chapter 60, Page 523.*)

14.27 The patient is a 15-year-old high school boy brought to the emergency department by friends who reported that "he passed out while we were having a party." The friends then disappeared. The patient seems excited, light-headed, and mildly confused. You suspect that the problem may be related to

(A) marijuana
(B) amphetamines
(C) cocaine
(D) volatile substances
(E) acute schizophrenia

Answer: (D). In the emergency department, solvent misuse frequently can be mistaken for acute psychiatric problems because of the altered mental state and hallucinations. Solvent abuse should be suspected in teenagers who suddenly collapse while partying. (*Chapter 60, Page 524.*)

14.28 Physical findings that suggest cocaine misuse include all EXCEPT which of the following?

(A) dehydration
(B) malnutrition
(C) bradycardia
(D) elevated blood pressure
(E) rhinorrhea

Answer: (C). Physical findings suggestive of cocaine misuse include agitation, dehydration, malnutrition, tachycardia, elevated blood pressure, rhinorrhea, singed eyebrows (from crack or freebase smoking), coughing, wheezing, poor dentation, and a generally unkempt appearance. (*Chapter 60, Page 520.*)

14.29 Cocaine can cause myocardial ischemia and cardiac arrhythmias. The drug's effect on the heart appears to be caused by

(A) alpha blockade
(B) heart block
(C) serotonin effect
(D) blocking the reuptake of norepinephrine at the neuronal synapses
(E) a secondary effect of peripheral vasodilation

Answer: (D). Cocaine's effect on the heart appears to be caused by blocking the reuptake of norepinephrine at the neuronal synapses. The norepinephrine excess produces

an increased heart rate and increased blood pressure; simultaneous coronary vasospasm decreases the myocardial oxygen supply. (*Chapter 60, Page 520.*)

14.30 Which of the following opioids is available transdermally?

(A) fentanyl
(B) hydromorphone
(C) oxycodone
(D) morphine
(E) methadone

Answer: (A). Fentanyl (TDS-Fentanyl) is the only opioid available transdermally. It has a long duration of action. It is available in patches that deliver 25 to 100 µg/hour and are changed every 3 days. (*Chapter 61, Page 529.*)

14.31 Discontinuing opioid therapy can be achieved by gradually tapering the dose. During such tapering, which of the following drugs may help inhibit withdrawal symptoms?

(A) diazepam
(B) clonidine
(C) diphenhydramine
(D) propranolol
(E) naloxone

Answer: (B). Discontinuation of chronic opioid therapy can be achieved without precipitating withdrawal symptoms by gradually tapering the dose over 1 to 4 weeks. Clonidine (oral dose 0.25 to 0.50 mg two or three times daily; transdermal dose 0.1 to 0.2 mg/day) can be used to inhibit withdrawal symptoms during opioid tapering. (*Chapter 61, Page 529.*)

14.32 Anticonvulsants are sometimes used in pain management. Carbamazepine (Tegretol) may be especially useful in the management of the pain of

(A) metastatic cancer
(B) cluster headache
(C) intermittent claudication
(D) osteoarthritis
(E) trigeminal neuralgia

Answer: (E). Anticonvulsants play a role in the management of chronic neuropathic pain, as they are thought to have a stabilizing effect of excitable nerve membranes. Conditions such as trigeminal neuralgia are commonly treated with carbamazepine (Tegretol) at a starting dose of 100 mg qd or b.i.d. with food. (*Chapter 61, Page 530.*)

14.33 In the control of pain in a patient dying of cancer, the gold standard in the United States is

(A) meperidine
(B) morphine
(C) heroin
(D) fentanyl
(E) codeine

Answer: (B). Although many opioid analgesics exist, morphine remains the gold standard, as no other narcotic is more effective. Morphine has a simple metabolic route with no accumulation of clinically significant active metabolites. There are a wide variety of preparations, making it easy to titrate or change routes of administration. (*Chapter 62, Page 535.*)

DIRECTIONS (Items 14.34 through 14.72): Each of the items in this section is a multiple true–false problem that consists of a stem and four lettered options. Indicate whether each of the four options is TRUE or FALSE.

14.34 Very low calorie (VLC) diets used for weight loss range from 400 to 800 kcal/day. True statements regarding these diets include which of the following?

(A) They are largely liquid in nature.
(B) Through supplements, they maintain the minimum recommended daily allowances of macronutrients including potassium, magnesium, and calcium.
(C) Medical complications such as arrhythmias may occur.
(D) If effective, this diet can be sustained for a prolonged period of time.

Answer: (A-True, B-False, C-True, D-False). These dietary programs, which are liquid in nature, must be medically supervised because they are deficient in recommended daily allowances of many macronutrients, including sodium, potassium, magnesium, and calcium. These deficiencies can have potential medical complications (e.g., arrhythmia). Studies have shown VLC diets to be effective for short-term weight loss, but they are difficult to sustain. (*Chapter 53, Page 467.*)

14.35 In the control of body weight, surgery

(A) has no place in management
(B) may be more successful than other methods in patients who are morbidly obese
(C) may be recommended with a patient of a body mass index (BMI) of 30 kg/m²

(D) includes procedures such as intestinal bypass, gastric stapling, or gastric balloon

Answer: (A-False, B-True, C-False, D-True). Surgery may have a place and be more successful in the treatment of patients who are morbidly obese (more than 50% over ideal body weight) or have a BMI of more than $40\,kg/m^2$. These patients have been shown to have increased morbidity and mortality from heart disease, diabetes, insulin resistance, and cancer. Current surgical procedures for obesity include intestinal bypass, gastric stapling, and gastric balloon. (*Chapter 53, Page 468.*)

14.36 Vestibular neuronitis

(A) is a synonym for Meniere's disease
(B) is characterized by light-headedness and tinnitus
(C) usually subsides over several days
(D) is often preceded by a viral respiratory infection

Answer: (A-False, B-False, C-True, D-True). Vestibular neuronitis is marked by a sudden bout of vertigo that worsens over several hours but usually subsides over several days. Patients often report a viral respiratory infection before the onset. (*Chapter 54, Page 473.*)

14.37 Fatigue is a common symptom in family practice. Fatigued patients

(A) tend to have higher levels of physical activity than nonfatigued patients
(B) have a lower level of anxiety on standardized test instruments than nonfatigued patients
(C) have a higher level of depression on standardized test instruments
(D) have no difference in the lifetime likelihood of being diagnosed with depression when compared with nonfatigued patients

Answer: (A-False, B-False, C-True, D-False). Fatigued patients tend to score lower than nonfatigued patients on tests that measure physical activity. They also score significantly higher than control patients on standardized instruments measuring anxiety and depression and have a higher lifetime likelihood of being diagnosed with these disorders. (*Chapter 55, Page 478.*)

14.38 True statements regarding chronic fatigue syndrome (CFS) and the Epstein-Barr virus (EBV) include which of the following?

(A) The altered EBV immunity changes that have been found reflect only the generalized immune changes found in chronically fatigued patients.

(B) There is good evidence to establish a meaningful clinical association between EBV and CFS.

(C) There is research evidence of retroviral DNA sequences in patients with chronic fatigue.

(D) Immune abnormalities found in CFS patients show consistent patterns among numerous research studies.

Answer: (A-True, B-False, C-False, D-False). Because of obvious similarities to infectious mononucleosis, a number of studies have searched for an association with EBV infection. Although these investigations continue, most evidence suggests that altered EBV immunity reflects only the generalized immune changes found in chronically fatigued patients. There is insufficient evidence to establish a meaningful clinical association between EBV and CFS. There is also no evidence of retroviral DNA sequences in patients with chronic fatigue. Other research has examined the immune function of patients with CFS. Although measurable immune abnormalities have been associated with CFS, no consistent pattern has been delineated from study to study. (*Chapter 55, Page 479.*)

14.39 The patient is a 44-year-old white female social worker who is having some difficulty sleeping. She uses alcohol and caffeine in moderate amounts and smokes a few cigarettes each day. True statements regarding the effect of these substances on sleep include which of the following?

(A) Alcohol taken at bedtime helps to stabilize sleep patterns and reduce early awakening.

(B) Caffeine has a relatively short half-life of 3 to 4 hours and thus can be safely consumed during afternoon hours without interfering with sleep.

(C) Nicotine in cigarettes can produce enough arousal to interfere with sleep.

(D) Nicotine gum and patches do not interfere with sleep.

Answer: (A-False, B-False, C-True, D-False). A review of the patient's drug use is essential. Alcohol, often self-prescribed to induce sleep, can produce abnormal sleep architecture and early awakening. Caffeine has a long half-life (8 to 14 hours) and can interfere with sleep onset long after consumption. Nicotine, through smoking or administered as a drug, can produce enough arousal to interfere with sleep initiation. (*Chapter 56, Page 483.*)

14.40 Hypnotic drugs are often used in the treatment of insomnia. True statements regarding hypnotic drugs include which of the following?

(A) Such drugs should be used with great caution in patients with a known or suspected history of drug abuse.

(B) These drugs can be used safely in recovering alcoholics.

(C) Hypnotics are often useful in the management of sleep apnea.

(D) Hypnotics are often prescribed to relieve the transient insomnia of pregnancy.

Answer: (A-True, B-False, C-False, D-False). Some patients are not good candidates for hypnotic drugs. These drugs are relatively contraindicated in patients with known drug abuse potential, including those with a history of alcohol dependence. Patients taking other central nervous system depressants, such as pain relievers or antidepressants, should be dosed carefully with an awareness of possible drug potentiation. Hypnotics should be avoided if sleep apnea is suspected. Pregnancy is a contraindication owing to possible effects on the fetus. (*Chapter 56, Page 484.*)

14.41 The patient is a 25-year-old graduate student who describes excessive daytime sleepiness with a tendency to fall asleep uncontrollably, even during stimulating activity. He describes irresistible episodes of sleepiness lasting 10 to 30 minutes and sometimes occurring suddenly without warning. This patient

(A) probably has CFS

(B) probably has narcolepsy

(C) is describing cataplexy

(D) should be referred to a sleep laboratory for an evaluation

Answer: (A-False, B-True, C-False, D-True). The illness is characterized by excessive daytime sleepiness with a tendency to fall asleep uncontrollably even during stimulating activities. These irresistible sleep episodes generally last 10 to 30 minutes and sometimes occur suddenly, without warning. This sudden onset can put the patient at risk while participating in dangerous activities such as working or driving. The other major symptom of narcolepsy is an emotion-associated weakness called cataplexy. Cataplexy is considered pathognomonic for the disease. Other associated symptoms can include sleep paralysis and hypnagogic hallucinations. Evaluation of patients suspected of having narcolepsy in a sleep laboratory is essential. (*Chapter 56, Page 485.*)

14.42 Sleep apnea

(A) is characteristically associated with daytime sleepiness or altered cardiopulmonary function
(B) is a rare problem
(C) is associated with an increased risk of road traffic accidents
(D) is caused by recurrent upper airway narrowing during sleep

Answer: (A-True, B-False, C-True, D-True). Sleep apnea consists of repeated episodes of obstructive apnea and hypopnea during sleep, together with either daytime sleepiness or altered cardiopulmonary function. The disorder is common and underdiagnosed. Approximately 2 to 4% of middle-aged adults have obstructive sleep apnea. This syndrome is associated with an increased risk of road traffic accidents and mortality due to cardiovascular and cerebrovascular disease. The syndrome is caused by recurrent upper airway narrowing during sleep, resulting in recurrent arousals from sleep with consequent sleep fragmentation and recurrent transient hypertension. (*Chapter 56, Page 485.*)

14.43 In performing a preoperative medical evaluation on a cardiac patient planning to undergo cholecystectomy,

(A) the primary care physician should recommend the type and route of anesthesia
(B) general anesthesia should be recommended
(C) spinal anesthesia should be recommended
(D) the type or route of anesthesia is significant in predicting adverse outcomes

Answer: (A-False, B-False, C-False, D-False). It is tempting to make recommendations about the type and route of anesthesia. There is, however, little evidence to suggest that the type or route of anesthesia is important for predicting adverse outcomes. "General" anesthetic agents are myocardial suppressants and peripheral vasodilators. Spinal anesthesia induces a sympathectomy at the level at which it is administered and causes levels of hypotension similar to those seen with general anesthetic agents. (*Chapter 57, Page 489.*)

14.44 The patient is a 72-year-old white man with no known cardiac disease. His blood pressure is 132/78, and the cardiac examination and resting ECG are normal. True statements regarding his risk during a proposed left hemicolectomy include which of the following?

(A) His risk of postoperative MI is approximately 2 to 12%.

(B) The peak time of occurrence of postoperative MI is 3 to 6 days after surgery.
(C) Postoperative MIs are due to increased activity, pain, and shifts of third-space fluid.
(D) Most postoperative MIs cause typical substernal chest pain often radiating to the chin or shoulder.

Answer: (A-False, B-True, C-True, D-False). Patients without cardiac disease have a low incidence of postoperative MI and other cardiac complications. The peak time of occurrence of MI is 3 to 6 days after surgery; it is due to increased activity, pain, and shifts of third-space fluid. Most postoperative MIs are "silent," perhaps accounting for the high mortality (up to 50%) among patients who sustain postoperative MIs. (*Chapter 57, Page 490.*)

14.45 The patient is a 76-year-old white woman with congestive heart failure (CHF) caused by valvular heart disease. She is being medically evaluated prior to a hysterectomy for large symptomatic fibroids. True statements regarding the management of this patient include which of the following?

(A) A Swan-Ganz catheter should be inserted.
(B) A low ventricular ejection fraction (EF) increases her risk of postoperative CHF.
(C) Studies have shown that jugular venous distension is not predictive of perioperative CHF.
(D) Surgery is best performed following a period of at least 2 weeks of euvolemia.

Answer: (A-True, B-True, C-False, D-True). A Swan-Ganz catheter for invasive monitoring should be inserted in surgical patients with congestive cardiac failure. Patients with low left ventricular EF are more likely to develop postoperative CHF, whereas those with EFs of 50% or more have low complication rates, even if they have had a history of CHF. The presence of jugular venous distension, current pulmonary edema, or an S_3 gallop places a patient at risk for perioperative cardiac complications. If possible, surgery is postponed until the CHF has been treated with a goal of euvolemia for a period of 2 weeks or more prior to surgery. (*Chapter 57, Page 491.*)

14.46 During surgery, the risk of severe hypertension increases significantly during which of the following times?

(A) induction of anesthesia
(B) intubation
(C) during the surgical incision
(D) during emergence from anesthesia

Answer: (A-True, B-True, C-False, D-True). Severe hypertension may occur especially during induction of anesthesia, intubation, and emergence from anesthesia. (*Chapter 57, Page 491.*)

14.47 The patient is a 58-year old white male executive. On preoperative medical examination prior to a lumbar laminectomy, you find periodic nonsustained premature ventricular contractions (PVCs). There is no history of chest pain or prior cardiac disease. There are no heart murmurs, and the ECG is normal. An event monitor confirms the presence of nonsustained PVCs. True statements regarding the management of this patient include which of the following?

(A) The patient is at risk for ventricular tachycardia.
(B) This patient is at risk for sudden death during surgery.
(C) This patient is at risk for cardiac complications only if there is underlying cardiac ischemia.
(D) The proposed surgery is contraindicated because of the arrhythmia.

Answer: (A-False, B-False, C-True, D-False). The significance of cardiac arrhythmias identified preoperatively is somewhat controversial, as it has become clear that the presence of nonsustained PVCs is not a risk factor for ventricular tachycardia or sudden death unless associated with underlying cardiac ischemia (suggesting the presence of severe coronary artery disease). (*Chapter 57, Page 491.*)

14.48 In performing a medical evaluation of a patient prior to a major surgical procedure, you would consider placement of a pacemaker in patients who have which of the following?

(A) Long sinus pauses
(B) High-grade second-degree heart block
(C) First-degree atrioventricular (AV) block
(D) Asymptomatic bifascicular block

Answer: (A-True, B-True, C-False, D-False). It is rare that patients need to have a pacemaker inserted prior to a major surgical procedure. Placement of a pacemaker should be considered in patients who have long sinus pauses, high-grade second-degree heart block, or complete heart block. There is no indication for pacemaker placement in patients with first-degree AV block or asymptomatic bifascicular block, as these patients rarely develop complete heart block. (*Chapter 57, Page 492.*)

14.49 During office surgery to remove a large cyst from the upper back, you plan to use electrocautery for hemostasis. Your patient is a 72-year-old cardiac patient with a "demand" pacemaker. True statements regarding this procedure include which of the following?

(A) The use of electrocautery during surgery will not interfere with "demand" pacemaker function.
(B) The use of electrocautery during surgery is less likely to effect pacemaker function in the fixed rate mode than in the demand mode.
(C) Placing the earth lead away from the pacemaker magnet and using short bursts of electrocautery reduce the risk of interfering with pacemaker function.
(D) Electrocautery does not affect pacemaker function.

Answer: (A-False, B-True, C-True, D-False). The use of the electrocautery machine during surgery may interfere with "demand" pacemaker function; if the earth lead is placed away from the pacemaker magnet and the surgeon administers short bursts of electrocautery, this effect is reduced. It may, however, be necessary to convert the pacemaker function to the fixed-rate mode when "demand" pacemaker responses are suboptimal. (*Chapter 57, Page 492.*)

14.50 Warfarin sodium (Coumadin)

(A) acts by directly reducing circulating prothrombin levels
(B) inhibits factors II, VII, IX, and X
(C) has an effect that lasts about 7 days after taking the last dose
(D) when appropriate, is discontinued 3 days before surgery

Answer: (A-False, B-True, C-False, D-True). Warfarin inhibits factors II, VII, IX, and X, with the effect lasting about 72 hours. If it is reasonable to discontinue the Coumadin, it is stopped 3 days before surgery and then reinstituted after surgery. (*Chapter 57, Page 493.*)

14.51 Which of the following are the typical results of general anesthesia on the pulmonary system?

(A) a 20% increase in tidal volume
(B) an increase in respiratory rate
(C) no significant change in minute ventilation
(D) an increase in lung compliance

Answer: (A-False, B-True, C-True, D-False). General anesthesia results in a 20% decrease in tidal volume, but a compensatory increase in respiratory rate occurs, such that the minute ventilation changes minimally. Lung compliance decreases by 33%, and sighing is abolished by the effects of narcotic medications. (*Chapter 57, Page 493.*)

14.52 In patients with pulmonary disease undergoing general anesthesia and surgery, incentive spirometry

(A) is contraindicated
(B) can reduce the incidence of pulmonary complications
(C) has been linked to an increased incidence post-operative atelectasisis
(D) may reduce the length of stay in hospital

Answer: (A-False, B-True, C-False, D-True). Incentive spirometry has been shown to reduce the incidence of pulmonary complications and length of stay in hospital. (*Chapter 57, Page 494.*)

14.53 True statements regarding the risk of blood transfusion include which of the following?

(A) The risk of infection with human immuno-deficiency virus (HIV) is approximately 5%.
(B) The current risk of acquiring hepatitis C is approximately 0.3% or less.
(C) There is moderate risk of hemolytic reactions.
(D) The risk of CHF accompanying blood transfusion is low.

Answer: (A-False, B-True, C-False, D-True). The risks associated with blood transfusion are low; there is a less than 1% risk of transfusion mortality associated with the HIV and a less than 0.3% risk of acquiring hepatitis C (since testing became available during the 1990s); the risk of hemolytic reactions or congestive cardiac failure is also low. (*Chapter 57, Page 494.*)

14.54 Surgical patients at increased risk for developing deep vein thrombosis (DVT) include which of the following?

(A) elderly patients
(B) very thin patients
(C) cancer patients
(D) patients with a history of CHF

Answer: (A-True, B-False, C-True, D-True). All surgical patients are at risk for developing DVT. This risk is increased for elderly patients, the obese, cigarette smokers, cancer patients, patients who are having long procedures, those with previous venous disease, and those with a history of CHF. (*Chapter 57, Page 495.*)

14.55 The patient is a 48-year-old white woman with brittle diabetes admitted for emergency abdominal surgery. To maintain optimum diabetic control, you elect to start an insulin infusion a few hours before surgery. The usual rate of infusion

(A) is 2 units of insulin/hour
(B) is 6 to 8 units of insulin/hour
(C) can be adjusted depending on serum glucose levels
(D) may be accompanied by a dextrose infusion administered simultaneously in the other arm

Answer: (A-True, B-False, C-True, D-True). For patients with "brittle" diabetes, better control may be achieved by starting an insulin infusion a few hours before surgery. The usual rate of infusion is 2 units of insulin/hour, but this dosage can be adjusted depending on the serum glucose levels. To avoid hypoglycemia, a dextrose infusion is administered simultaneously in the other arm. (*Chapter 57, Page 496.*)

14.56 In examining a female patient, the bulbocavernosus reflex

(A) is observed as a contraction of the groin muscles
(B) is elicited by digital pressure on the anal sphincter
(C) indicates that the sacral nerves responsible for the neurologic component of the human sexual responses are intact
(D) if absent, denotes pathology

Answer: (A-False, B-False, C-True, D-False). The bulbocavernosus reflex is an anal "wink" in response to gentle squeezing of the clitoris. If present, this reflex indicates that the sacral nerves (S2 to 4) responsible for the neurologic component of the human sexual response are intact. (Only 70% of normal female patients have a bulbocavernosus reflex, so its absence does not necessarily denote pathology.) (*Chapter 58, Page 501.*)

14.57 The patient is a 19-year-old mother in the office with her first baby. She reports, with some embarrassment, that during diapering and bathing her 2-month-old baby boy develops an erection. You should inform the mother that

(A) this is a normal reaction to skin touching
(B) this is an indication of hypersexuality, which is likely to become more evident at the time of puberty

(C) the infant has a conscious appreciation of the sexual nature of this response

(D) the parent should reduce the erection by the careful application of ice chips

Answer: (A-True, B-False, C-False, D-False). Ultrasonographic studies have shown that our awareness of sexual feelings begins even before birth, as fetuses in utero can be observed repeatedly touching the genital area to produce reflex erections of the male penis. After birth, male infants develop firm erections while nursing, and clitoral erection and vaginal lubrication occurs in female infants. Babies are highly responsive to skin touching, and arousal signs may occur during diapering, bathing, or play. Parents who observe these signs of sexual arousal should be told that they are reflex responses and in no way indicate hypersexuality or any conscious appreciation of the sexual nature of their responses. As the child gets older, happy expressions can be seen on the baby's face as genital self-stimulation takes place. Parents with more sexually repressive backgrounds may express alarm, disgust, or fear that their child is a masturbator. It is appropriate to provide reassurance that it is normal infant behavior and that it will disappear if ignored. (*Chapter 58, Page 501.*)

14.58 The patient is a mother of three children who reports that her 5-year-old youngest child, a boy, is acting sexually aggressive toward other children and has attempted to have oral-genital contact with two playmates. True statements regarding this child include which of the following?

(A) This is normal sexual curiousness.

(B) This may be a red flag for prior sexual abuse of the child.

(C) The mother should be reassured that the behavior will disappear if ignored.

(D) The physician should make a notation to inquire regarding this behavior at the child's next preventative care visit in 1 year.

Answer: (A-False, B-True, C-False, D-False). A word of caution is needed about children who are sexually aggressive toward other children, especially those who act as if they are trying to have intercourse or oral-genital contact. This behavior is far beyond the natural development of sexual curiosity and usually is a "red flag" for prior sexual abuse of the child by a parent or family member. (*Chapter 58, Page 502.*)

14.59 True statements regarding discussions with sexually active teens include which of the following?

(A) The prevalence of homosexuality is 5 to 6% among teens.

(B) Homosexual teens are generally open to discussions regarding sexuality with their physicians.

(C) To avoid offending teen patients, it is best to assume that every sexually active person is heterosexual.

(D) The term *boyfriend* or *girlfriend* is preferable to demeaning terms such as *sexual partner*.

Answer: (A-True, B-False, C-False, D-False). The prevalence of homosexuality is about 5 to 6% among teens, and the topic is difficult for them to discuss. Assuming that every sexually active person is heterosexual is a common error made by health care professionals. Try to use gender-neutral language and talk about the "sexual partner" rather than the "boyfriend" or "girlfriend" so as not to destroy the rapport and respect you have worked so hard to build. (*Chapter 58, Page 502.*)

14.60 True statements regarding alcohol dependence and abuse in the United States include which of the following?

(A) Approximately 18 million Americans display evidence of alcohol dependence or abuse.

(B) Half of all alcohol is consumed by 10% of the drinking population.

(C) The heaviest drinking is in the 50 to 65 year old age group.

(D) Women and men are equally likely to be problem drinkers.

Answer: (A-True, B-True, C-False, D-False). An estimated 18 million Americans display evidence of alcohol dependence or alcohol abuse. Their medical care costs up to three times more than that of the general population. Fifty percent of all alcohol is consumed by 10% of the drinking population. More people drink heavily in the 21- to 34-year-old age group, and the fewest people drink heavily in the older than 65-year-old group. Throughout all age groups, men are two to five times more likely to be "problem drinkers" than are women. (*Chapter 59, Page 507.*)

14.61 After ingestion, alcohol may be found in

(A) brain

(B) cerebrospinal fluid (CSF)

(C) fetal circulation

(D) breast milk

Answer: (A-True, B-True, C-True, D-True). Alcohol interacts with both water and lipids, allowing it to penetrate and disorder cell membranes. There is no blood-brain barrier to alcohol. Because of the brain's vascularity, the concentration of alcohol in the brain may, in fact, exceed the level in the venous peripheral blood until the alcohol equilibrates in total body water. Until this balance is reached, the blood alcohol concentration may be less than the CSF concentration. The placenta is unable to protect the fetus from exposure to alcohol in the mother's blood. Similarly, breast milk conveys some of the alcohol in the mother's blood to the infant. (*Chapter 59, Page 509.*)

14.62 Craniofacial dysmorphic features of the fetal alcohol syndrome (FAS) include microcephaly, hypoplastic maxilla, thinned upper lip, short upturned nose, and short palpebral fissure. These facial features

(A) tend to disappear during adulthood
(B) persist throughout life
(C) become accentuated after ages 35 to 40
(D) are passed as congenital defects to offspring

Answer: (A-True, B-False, C-False, D-False). Facial features associated with FAS tend to disappear during adulthood. (*Chapter 59, Page 510.*)

14.63 True statements regarding the FAS and the fetal alcohol effect (FAE) include which of the following?

(A) In patients with FAS, the magnetic resonance imaging (MRI) scan is characteristically normal.
(B) The development of FAS is significantly related to the peak blood alcohol concentration (BAC).
(C) African American women and Asian American women are relatively immune to the teratogenic effects of alcohol.
(D) The safe level of alcohol consumption for a pregnant woman is 2 oz/week or less.

Answer: (A-False, B-True, C-False, D-False). MRI scans of children with FAS show proportionally reduced basal ganglia and smaller corpus callosum effects related to the amount of alcohol consumed during pregnancy. The peak BAC contributes more to the development of FAS than does the amount consumed. The more severe morphologic defects occur with more extreme levels of alcohol consumption. There is substantial individual variation in susceptibility to alcohol's effect on the fetus. Not all women who drink heavily deliver FAS or FAE infants, but no ethnic or racial group is immune to the teratogenic effect of alcohol. In the light of the severity of the risk of FAS and FAE, it is not yet possible to recommend that any level

of alcohol consumption is safe for a pregnant woman. (*Chapter 59, Page 511.*)

14.64 You are working in the emergency department and your patient is a 24-year-old woman being treated for a laceration of her hand. While placing sutures, you become aware that she has consumed a large quantity of alcohol and is quite intoxicated. The patient drove herself to the hospital and her car is outside in the parking lot. After completion of the wound care, appropriate actions might include which of the following?

(A) Physically restrain the patient, who would be a serious hazard as a driver.
(B) Contact the police.
(C) Persuade the patient not to drive.
(D) Call a friend or family member and ensure that they arrive to take the patient home.

Answer: (A-False, B-True, C-True, D-True). The intoxicated patient cannot be legally restrained unless he or she can be committed under state law, except by police. If a patient is thought to be impaired, it becomes the provider's duty to persuade the patient not to drive, to use a taxi, to call a friend or family member, and as a last resort to contact the police and inform them of the situation (*Chapter 59, Page 518.*)

14.65 Crack cocaine

(A) is sold and consumed as "rocks"
(B) is typically dissolved and injected intravenously
(C) is produced by chemical treatment of cocaine hydrochloride
(D) is called "crack" because the "rocks" can be broken in cleavage planes into smaller units

Answer: (A-True, B-False, C-True, D-False). "Crack" cocaine is produced by dissolving cocaine hydrochloride in sodium bicarbonate and distilling off the water. It then forms "rocks," which can be smoked. The term *crack* comes from the noise the "rocks" make as they are heated and smoked. (*Chapter 60, Page 520.*)

14.66 Newborn infants born to mothers who abuse cocaine may have which of the following?

(A) voracious appetite and excessive weight gain
(B) irritability and tremulousness
(C) intense maternal-infant bonding
(D) increased risk of developmental delay

Answer: (A-False, B-True, C-False, D-True). Newborn infants may demonstrate signs of cocaine withdrawal, including irritability, tremulousness, and poor eating. Maternal–infant bonding is poor. Although long-term effects are not clear, cocaine babies may have developmental delays and attention deficit disorders. (*Chapter 60, Page 521.*)

14.67 Common physical signs of marijuana use are

(A) tachycardia
(B) heart block
(C) conjunctival irritation
(D) paranoid delusions

Answer: (A-True, B-False, C-True, D-False). The most common physical signs of marijuana use are tachycardia and conjunctival irritation (which may be masked in experienced users by using eyedrops). (*Chapter 60, Page 523.*)

14.68 Of the following nonsteroidal anti-inflammatory drugs, those with lower rates of gastrointestinal toxicity include which of the following?

(A) piroxicam
(B) ibuprofen
(C) tolmetin
(D) naproxen

Answer: (A-False, B-True, C-False, D-True). Ibuprofen (Motrin and others) and naproxen (Naprosyn) may have lower rates of gastrointestinal toxicity, whereas piroxicam (Feldene), tolmetin (Tolectin), and meclofenamate (Meclomen) may have higher rates. (*Chapter 61, Page 528.*)

14.69 Tramadol (Ultram) is an analgesic that

(A) is a NSAID
(B) produces analgesia by binding to opioid receptors
(C) is effective only for acute pain
(D) can cause urinary retention and constipation

Answer: (A-False, B-True, C-False, D-False). Tramadol (Ultram) is not an NSAID but is another type of nonopioid analgesic that produces analgesia by binding to opioid receptors. It is effective for both acute and chronic pain. Like an opioid, it can cause nausea, vomiting, sedation, and dizziness but does not cause respiratory depression, urinary retention, constipation, or physical dependence. (*Chapter 61, Page 528.*)

14.70 Patients with chronic pain often require management with opioid analgesics. True statements regarding such management include which of the following?

(A) The risk of addiction to opioids in patients with legitimate chronic pain is high.
(B) Long-term opioid therapy often induces physical dependence.
(C) Even though the patient's level of pain remains the same, tolerance for the drug develops with long-term opioid therapy, causing the need for increasing doses to achieve the same analgesic effect.
(D) In patients with chronic pain, a pattern of compulsive behavior centered around the desire for, acquisition of, and the use of the drug is common.

Answer: (A-False, B-True, C-False, D-False). The risk of addiction to opioids in patients with legitimate chronic pain is minimal. Although long-term opioid therapy often induces physical dependence (occurrence of withdrawal symptoms after cessation), tolerance (the need for increasing doses to achieve the same analgesic effect) usually does not develop if the patient's level of pain remains the same; moreover, addiction (a pattern of compulsive behaviors centered around the desire for, acquisition of, and use of the drug) is rare. Additional caution and more extensive evaluation is warranted before using chronic opioids in patients with a history of substance abuse or drug-seeking behavior. (*Chapter 61, Page 528.*)

14.71 You have been asked to speak to a senior citizens group on the topic of "Advance Directives and Living Wills." True statements on advance directives and living wills include which of the following?

(A) Advanced directives support the ethical value of patient autonomy.
(B) Advanced directives have made significant differences in the way that patients are treated at the end of life.
(C) Advanced directives seek to address the reality of needing to conserve health costs.
(D) Advanced directives have reduced health costs significantly.

Answer: (A-True, B-False, C-True, D-False). The advance directives movement seems to fit well with an emphasis on patient autonomy and the economic reality of needing to conserve health costs. Unfortunately, studies have revealed that advance directives may make little difference in the way patients are treated at the end of life and reduce costs only modestly. (*Chapter 62, Page 534.*)

14.72 True statements regarding the distinction between somatic (nociceptive) and neuropathic pain include which of the following?

    (A) Somatic pain is often described as dull or aching.
    (B) Sciatica is an example of somatic pain.
    (C) Neuropathic pain results from injury to some element of the nervous system.
    (D) Neuropathic pain is often described as dull or aching and is well localized.

Answer: (A-True, B-False, C-True, D-False). Somatic pain is often described as dull or aching and is well localized. Bone and soft tissue metastases are examples of causes of somatic pain. Visceral pain tends to be poorly localized and is often referred to dermatomal sites distant from the source of the pain. Neuropathic pain results from injury to some element of the nervous system because of the direct effect of the tumor or as a result of cancer therapy (surgery, irradiation, chemotherapy). Examples include brachial or lumbosacral plexus invasion, spinal nerve root compression, or neuropathic complications of drugs such as vincristine. Neuropathic pain is described as sharp, shooting, shocklike, or burning and is often associated with dysesthesias. (*Chapter 62, Page 535.*)

15

The Nervous System

The questions in this chapter constitute a review of the following chapters in *Family Medicine: Principles and Practice, Fifth Edition:*

Headache (Chapter 63)
Seizure Disorders (Chapter 64)
Cerebrovascular Disease (Chapter 65)
Movement Disorders (Chapter 66)
Disorders of the Peripheral Nervous System
(Chapter 67)
Selected Disorders of the Nervous System
(Chapter 68)

DIRECTIONS (Items 15.1 through 15.30): Each of the questions or incomplete statements in this section is followed by five suggested answers or completions. Select the ONE that is BEST in each case.

15.1 The patient is a 34-year-old white woman with severe headaches of recent origin. You plan to obtain diagnostic imaging and are deciding between computed tomography (CT) and magnetic resonance imaging (MRI). MRI provides superior imaging in all the following EXCEPT

(A) resolution in the posterior fossa
(B) infection
(C) post-traumatic changes
(D) acute hemorrhage
(E) detection of gliosis

Answer: (D). CT is very sensitive to acute hemorrhage and certain enhancing solid lesions; MRI provides better resolution in the posterior fossa and superior detection of gliosis, infection, post-traumatic changes, and certain tumors. (*Chapter 63, Page 541.*)

15.2 Classic migraine headache is characterized by an aura—generally with visual phenomena—that precedes the head pain. Therefore, this type of headache is now properly called *migraine headache with aura.* What percentage of migraine patients have classic migraine headache?

(A) 20%
(B) 40%
(C) 60%
(D) 80%
(E) 100%

Answer: (A). Patients in the "classic" subgroup (approximately 20% of all migraineurs) experience a characteristic aura before the onset of migraine head pain. (*Chapter 63, Page 542.*)

15.3 The patient is a 34-year-old white male college professor who complains of severe unilateral orbital headache that develops rapidly and lasts about 90 minutes. The headache has occurred most evenings for the past month, and the patient recalls similar headaches that bothered him about 1 year ago. This patient's most likely diagnosis is

(A) classic migraine headache
(B) common migraine headache
(C) retinal migraine headache
(D) cluster headache
(E) muscle contraction headache

Answer: (D). The cluster headache, a rare but dramatic form, occurs predominantly in middle-aged men. The estimated prevalence is 69 per 100,000 adults with a 6:1 male preponderance. The headache is severe, unilateral, centered around the eye or temple, and accompanied by lacrimation, rhinorrhea, red eye, and other autonomic signs on the same side as the headache. Symptoms develop rapidly, reach a peak intensity within 10 to 15 minutes, and last up to 2 hours. (*Chapter 63, Page 543.*)

15.4 In adults, the most common type of epilepsy is

(A) idiopathic
(B) vascular
(C) neoplastic
(D) traumatic
(E) postinfectious

Answer: (A). For adults, 55% of epilepsy is idiopathic, 16% vascular, 11% neoplastic, 10% traumatic, 3% congenital, 3% degenerative, and 2% postinfectious. (*Chapter 64, Page 547.*)

15.5 The patient is a 14-year-old girl whose mother describes the following problem. Over the past year she has had myoclonic jerks while brushing her teeth or combing her hair. Yesterday, she had a major tonic-clonic seizure while watching television. This patient's most likely diagnosis is

(A) hypoglycemia
(B) petit mal epilepsy
(C) juvenile myoclonic epilepsy
(D) psychic partial seizures
(E) autonomic partial seizures

Answer: (C). Juvenile myoclonic epilepsy usually afflicts persons aged 12 to 16 years and accounts for 5% of childhood epilepsy. A genetic locus on chromosome 6p has been linked to this disorder. It presents with early morning myoclonic jerks while performing simple daily tasks such as brushing the hair. Later, it may evolve into tonic-clonic epilepsy that requires lifelong treatment. Photic stimulation tends to precipitate these seizures. (*Chapter 64, Page 549.*)

15.6 The patient is a 5-year-old boy whose mother describes as having sporadic nocturnal episodes characterized by guttural noises, difficulty swallowing, and tonic contractions of the face or upper extremity. The most likely diagnosis is

(A) grand mal epilepsy
(B) petit mal epilepsy
(C) night terrors
(D) benign partial epilepsy of childhood (BPEC)
(E) psychic partial seizures

Answer: (D). BPEC, also known as sylvian or rolandic epilepsy, is an inherited disorder that affects about 15% of children with epilepsy, with its onset usually between ages 2 and 14 years. BPEC is characterized by nocturnal simple partial seizures, consisting of guttural noises, dysphagias, paresthesias about the face, and tonic face or arm contractions that may generalize. Neurologic evaluation is normal. These seizures cease during adolescence. (*Chapter 64, Page 549.*)

15.7 The drug of choice for BPEC partial epilepsy of childhood is

(A) phenytoin
(B) carbamazepine
(C) phenobarbital
(D) primidone
(E) valproate

Answer: (B). BPEC is best treated with carbamazepine for at least 2 years of seizure-free time or until the child is 16 years old, when treatment is stopped. (*Chapter 64, Page 552.*)

15.8 The drug of choice for prolonged febrile seizures is

(A) intravenous (IV) lorazepam
(B) intramuscular phenytoin
(C) IV phenytoin
(D) intramuscular phenobarbital
(E) IV valproate acid

Answer: (A). IV lorazepam is the drug of choice for prolonged febrile seizures. (*Chapter 64, Page 555.*)

15.9 The patient is a 2-week-old infant born to a 19-year-old single mother. The mother states that the baby has been "acting funny." On careful history, it seems that the baby has had some fixed eye deviation alternating with nystagmus. There have been inappropriate chewing motions and excessive salivation, and at times there are some brief jerks of the arms or legs. You should be suspicious that this 2-week-old patient has

(A) neonatal seizures
(B) hypoglycemia
(C) hypothyroidism
(D) congenital toxoplasmosis
(E) cerebral palsy

Answer: (A). During the first month of life, tonic-clonic activity is unusual, so seizures are difficult to recognize. Focal rhythmic twitching, especially of the face or arms, and brief jerks of the body or distal muscle groups are typical. Rigid posturing, fixed eye deviation, nystagmus, apnea, chewing, excessive salivation, or skin color changes typify subtle convulsive disorders. (*Chapter 64, Page 555.*)

15.10 The patient is a 36-year-old white woman with the sudden onset of severe left-sided headache associated with stiff neck, nausea, vomiting, diplopia, and photophobia. There is no prior history of headache, no fever, and no history of head trauma. You are concerned that this patient may have the first symptoms of which of the following?

(A) classic migraine headache
(B) common migraine headache
(C) meningitis
(D) subarachnoid hemorrhage
(E) domestic violence with unreported head trauma

Answer: (D). The constant and characteristic symptom in a patient with subarachnoid hemorrhage is a severe headache of sudden onset with meningism. Other symptoms include nausea, vomiting, diplopia, photophobia, and commonly changes in consciousness. (*Chapter 65, Page 560.*)

15.11 The gold standard for the evaluation of a stroke is angiography. This procedure would be appropriate for

(A) a patient with vertebrobasilar transient ischemic attack (TIA) in whom surgery is not indicated
(B) a patient with sudden hemiplegia who is a potential candidate for surgery
(C) a patient with acute hemiplegia 4 days following an acute myocardial infarction
(D) a patient who has sudden right-sided hemiplegia accompanied by respiratory depression and coma
(E) None of the above

Answer: (B). The indications for an angiogram are anticipated surgery and uncertain diagnosis. Angiography generally should not be performed in patients with the following: a vertebrobasilar TIA unless surgery is indicated, an acute MI, coma, respiration depression, or severe systemic disease. (*Chapter 65, Page 561.*)

15.12 With an acute stroke, the chief threat to life is

(A) anoxia
(B) shock
(C) hypertension
(D) respiratory depression
(E) cerebral edema

Answer: (E). The development of cerebral edema following an acute stroke is a major threat to life. Osmotic agents such as mannitol and glycerol are not routinely recommended to reduce cerebral edema. Selected cases with displacement of brain tissue may benefit from osmotic agents. (*Chapter 65, Page 561.*)

15.13 The patient is a 68-year-old white male retired machinist who recently had a TIA from which he has fully recovered. He has some peripheral atherosclerosis but no known coronary artery disease. He has no drug allergies or insensitivities. For this patient, you should prescribe

(A) no medication
(B) aspirin
(C) papaverine
(D) dipyridamole
(E) propranolol

Answer: (B). Patients at increased risk for stroke (TIA) and completed stroke should be started on a platelet antagonist. Aspirin is considered to be the standard agent, although results from studies evaluating ticlopidine reveal this agent to be more effective than aspirin or placebo for secondary stroke prevention. Aspirin has been shown to cause a 22% reduction in nonfatal strokes, and a reduction in MIs was observed as well. (*Chapter 65, Page 562.*)

15.14 The primary pathologic injury in Parkinson's disease (PD) is a loss of neurons in the

(A) brain stem
(B) cerebellum
(C) cerebral cortex
(D) rolandic fissure
(E) substantia nigra

Answer: (E). The primary pathologic injury in PD is the loss of neurons in the substantia nigra. Other pigmented nuclei are likewise affected by mechanisms not fully understood at this time. Approximately 75% of the dopaminergic neurons in the substantia nigra must be destroyed before clinical features of PD manifest. (*Chapter 66, Page 565.*)

15.15 The patient with early PD is first likely to be aware of

(A) rigidity
(B) bradykinesia
(C) postural instability
(D) tremor
(E) mental changes

Answer: (D). Tremor is the most common symptom of PD and usually the first observed. It occurs at rest and is most frequently seen in the hands. This type of tremor has classically been called a "pill-rolling" tremor because of the movement of the thumb and fingers. The tremor is of a slow frequency, occurs at rest, and disappears with active movement. (*Chapter 66, Page 565.*)

15.16 Amantadine may be useful in treating PD. It is *most* effective in reducing

(A) depression
(B) postural instability and gait disturbance
(C) rigidity and bradykinesia
(D) tremor
(E) parkinsonian dementia

Answer: (C). Amantadine's therapeutic benefits seem to derive from its ability to increase dopamine release, block dopamine reuptake, and stimulate dopamine receptors plus its possible peripheral anticholinergic properties. It appears to clinically relieve all the cardinal features of PD but is most effective in reducing rigidity and bradykinesia. (*Chapter 66, Page 567.*)

15.17 The most effective *symptomatic* drug for the treatment of PD is

(A) selegiline
(B) benztropine
(C) amantadine
(D) pergolide
(E) levodopoa

Answer: (E). Levodopa therapy continues to be the most effective symptomatic drug therapy for PD. Levodopa therapy should be withheld until significant limitations in activities of daily living and job performance become obvious. (*Chapter 66, Page 567.*)

15.18 The patient is an 82-year-old white woman who has a bilateral tremor involving the hands, voice, and head. She has found the tremor is relieved by the ingestion of alcohol. This patient has symptoms consistent with

(A) PD
(B) essential tremor
(C) parkinsonian-plus syndrome
(D) tardive dyskinesia
(E) subclinical alcoholism

Answer: (B). Essential tremor is the most common of the movement disorders. Up to 50% of patients with this condition have a positive family history, with autosomal dominant transmission apparent. An essential tremor is characterized by a bilateral action (kinetic) and positional tremor seen most commonly in the hands but also often the head and voice. Alcohol (ethanol) markedly reduces the intensity of the tremor within 30 minutes. (*Chapter 66, Page 570.*)

15.19 The patient is a 52-year-old white woman who has been using metoclopramide (Reglan) for gastrointestinal dysmotility. She has taken the drug for approximately 8 months. For the past several weeks, she has noted involuntary, purposeless movements including chewing, tongue protrusion, and lip smacking. She has noted some periodic awkwardness of movement of the hands. You suspect that this patient has

(A) an essential tremor
(B) a delayed reaction to the synthetic heroin analog MPTE
(C) parkinsonian-plus syndrome
(D) malingering
(E) tardive dyskinesia

Answer: (E). Clinically, tardive dyskinesia is characterized by repetitive, involuntary, purposeless movements, which can include chewing, tongue protrusion, lip smacking and puckering, paroxysms of rapid eye blinking, choreoathetoid limb movements, and dyskinesias of the hands. (*Chapter 66, Page 571.*)

15.20 The patient is a 58-year-old white man who describes a 1-month history of paroxysmal attacks of severe lancinating pain in the lower right side of the face, made worse by chewing, shaving, or brushing his teeth. Reasonable therapy for this patient would be

(A) propranolol
(B) carbamazepine
(C) phenytoin
(D) valproic acid
(E) selegiline

Answer: (B). Typically, trigeminal neuralgia involves the maxillary or mandibular divisions of the fifth nerve; the ophthalmic division is only rarely involved. Pain in the ophthalmic division is more likely due to incipient herpes zoster or postherpetic neuralgia. Most patients respond readily to carbamazepine (Tegretol), 200 to 300 mg three times a day. (*Chapter 67, Page 575.*)

15.21 The patient is a 36-year-old white woman who awoke this morning with a left-sided facial droop and an inability to close the left eye. There are no objective signs of sensory loss. The weakness involves the muscles of the forehead. The greatest danger to this patient involves

(A) the risk of aspiration
(B) damage to the cornea
(C) progression of the Guillain-Barré syndrome (GBS)
(D) aspiration of ingested substances
(E) progression to completed stroke

Answer: (B). The greatest danger with Bell's palsy is to the cornea; careful eye care is of the utmost importance. The eye should be kept moist and lubricated with an ophthalmic ointment or artificial tears. It is often helpful to protect the eye with a shield or to tape the lid shut, particularly during sleep. (*Chapter 67, Page 576.*)

15.22 The patient is a 17-year-old high school baseball pitcher who complains of numbness and tingling in the fourth and fifth fingers of the right (pitching) hand and a weakness of grasp with some clumsiness of the right fingers and hand. The most likely diagnosis in this patient is

(A) carpal tunnel syndrome
(B) polyneuropathy
(C) meralgia paresthetica
(D) posterior interosseus syndrome
(E) cubital tunnel syndrome

Answer: (E). Cubital tunnel syndrome is caused by entrapment of the ulnar nerve about the cubital tunnel, just distal to the medial epicondyle. Young athletes involved in overhand activities, such as pitching, are particularly prone to this disorder. The patient experiences intermittent paresthesia in the fourth and fifth fingers, including the dorsoulnar aspect of the hand and forearm. The patient may also have a generalized weakness of grasp and clumsiness of the hand and fingers with fine manipulation. (*Chapter 67, Page 577.*)

15.23 The patient is a 52-year-old male deputy sheriff. He is diabetic and moderately overweight and is here today because of a pain in the lateral right thigh associated with some localized numbness and tingling. The most likely diagnosis is

(A) diabetic neuropathy
(B) a herniated lumbar disc at the L1-L2 level
(C) sciatic neuropathy
(D) meralgia paresthetica
(E) obstruction of the right common iliac artery

Answer: (D). Compression neuropathy of the lateral femoral cutaneous nerve of the thigh is relatively common; entrapment may occur where it passes underneath the inguinal ligament or where it pierces the fascia lata. It occurs most frequently in overweight or diabetic individuals. Patients experience increasingly severe numbness, pain, and paresthesias, as well as decreased sensation of the anterolateral thigh; there is no objective weakness. (*Chapter 67, Page 577.*)

15.24 The patient is a tall, thin, white male computer operator who spends most of his day sitting with one leg crossed over the other. He recently has noted some weakness of dorsiflexion of the right foot. This patient probably has

(A) pernicious anemia with neuropathy
(B) peroneal neuropathy
(C) tibial neuropathy
(D) meralgia paresthetica
(E) femoral neuropathy

Answer: (B). The common peroneal nerve mediates dorsiflexion and eversion of the foot and supplies sensation to the dorsum of the foot and ankle. It is particularly prone to compression at the level of the fibular head, whether due to trauma, sitting cross-legged, improperly applied stirrups at the time of delivery, or an ill-fitting cast. Diabetic, vasculitic, and hereditary neuropathies may also affect the peroneal nerve. (*Chapter 67, Page 578.*)

15.25 The patient is a 32-year-old man with severe headache, fever, and stiff neck. Lumbar puncture reveals the presence of leukocytes in the cerebrospinal fluid (CSF) together with an elevated CSF protein level and a decreased CSF glucose level. Empiric treatment would reasonably begin with the intravenous administration of

(A) ceftriaxone
(B) nafcillin
(C) gentamicin
(D) thiamine
(E) dexamethasone

Answer: (A). In suspected acute bacterial meningitis, antibiotic treatment is begun immediately after cultures are obtained because of the potentially dire consequences of delayed treatment. Reasonable empiric treatment of pyogenic meningitis in adults consists of ceftriaxone 2 g ql12h IV with the addition of (1) vancomycin or rifampin when penicillin resistance is suspected or (2) ampicillin when the patient is immunocompromised. (*Chapter 68, Page 583.*)

15.26 The patient is an 18-year-old high school senior with fever, mild headache, and meningeal signs. All symptoms have been present for about 36 hours. The CSF shows a lymphocytic pleocytosis, glucose of 60 mg/dl, and protein of 60 mg/dl. The patient is awake and alert. The most likely diagnosis is

(A) meningococcal meningitis
(B) *Haemophilus influenzae* meningitis
(C) viral encephalitis
(D) brain abscess
(E) meningitis associated with the second stage of Lyme disease

Answer: (C). In viral encephalitis, the CSF examination generally shows a lymphocytic pleocytosis with normal glucose and modest elevation of protein. (*Chapter 68, Page 585.*)

15.27 The patient is a 76-year-old white man who lives a solitary existence in a mountain cabin. He has not seen a doctor for almost two decades. He complains of difficulty with balance, pains that shoot down the legs, and impaired vision. He recalls being told he had a "social disease" about 50 years ago and cannot remember what treatment was given. On physical examination, he seems to have a wide-based gait and a positive Romberg sign. The most likely diagnosis in this patient is

(A) brain tumor
(B) chronic schizophrenia
(C) senile dementia
(D) tabes dorsalis
(E) advanced pernicious anemia

Answer: (D). Tabes dorsalis (myeloneuropathy) is classically described as a triad of symptoms (lightning pains, urinary incontinence, ataxia) and a triad of signs (Argyll Robertson pupils, areflexia, loss of proprioception). Other symptoms may include visceral crises, optic atrophy, ocular palsy, and Charcot's joints. A progressive ataxia with a wide-based gait and Romberg sign develop. Tabes dorsalis has the longest incubation time of the presentations of neurosyphilis. (*Chapter 68, Page 587.*)

15.28 The drug of choice for all stages of syphilis is

(A) IV ceftriaxone
(B) parenteral penicillin G
(C) IV gentamicin
(D) parenteral vancomycin
(E) rifampin by either oral or parenteral route

Answer: (B). Parenteral penicillin G is the drug of choice for all stages of syphilis and is the only therapy with documented efficacy for neurosyphilis (or for syphilis during pregnancy). Those with penicillin allergy should undergo desensitization and receive penicillin if possible. (*Chapter 68, Page 587.*)

15.29 The patient is a 30-year-old white female salesclerk with a 2-month history of weakness in both arms, impaired vision in the left eye, double vision, urinary incontinence, and fatigue. She has pain in the muscles of the back and neck that become worse with exercise. The imaging method of choice for this patient is

(A) cervical myelogram
(B) cerebral angiography
(C) plain films of the skull
(D) CT of the head
(E) MRI of the head

Answer: (E). In suspected multiple sclerosis (MS), the imaging method of choice is MRI; it is more sensitive than CT and provides better imaging of the posterior fossa. No MRI findings are specific, but typical lesions are proximal to the ventricles, infratentorial, and more than 6 mm in size. MRI can, however, yield false-positive results, as a number of normal adults display typical white matter lesions. Advances in MRI technology may provide insight into the natural history of MS and response to various treatment modalities. (*Chapter 68, Page 590.*)

15.30 The patient is a 47-year-old white woman who has had MS for about 6 years. She has recently had an exacerbation of symptoms, especially involving optic neuritis and difficulty with micturation. She is currently taking no medication. Appropriate management at this time would be

(A) anticholinergics
(B) corticosteroids
(C) levodopa
(D) isoniazide
(E) IV immunoglobulin

Answer: (B). Acute attacks are treated with short courses of corticosteroids, typically IV methylprednisolone, especially for a presentation of optic neuritis, which seems to respond fairly well. Mild sensory attacks are usually not treated. Although steroids accelerate the time to recovery from a relapse, they do not provide long-term benefit. (*Chapter 68, Page 590.*)

DIRECTIONS (Items 15.31 through 15.54): Each of the items in this section is a multiple true–false problem that consists of a stem and four lettered options. Indicate whether each of the four options is TRUE or FALSE.

15.31 In the evaluation of a headache patient, which of the following headache symptoms would prompt you to order CT or MRI?

(A) a patient with severe headache that has occurred intermittently for approximately 10 years
(B) a patient with a severe headache that has recently changed from intermittent to constant
(C) a patient with a bitemporal headache, intermittent, aching in nature, that occurs during or following times of stress
(D) a patient with a mild, intermittent, left-sided headache and whose roommate believes that he experienced a seizure during sleep a few nights ago

Answer: (A-False, B-True, C-False, D-True). Family physicians should refer a patient for CT or MRI only when the history and physical examination indicate that an intracranial lesion is the probable diagnosis. This protocol is in general agreement with the National Institutes of Health Consensus Development Panel. The panel recommended CT investigation of patients whose headaches were "severe, constant, unusual, or associated with neurological symptoms." (*Chapter 63, Page 541.*)

15.32 The patient with migraine headache is likely to describe the pain using which of the following adjectives?

(A) aching
(B) throbbing
(C) band-like
(D) aggravated by movement

Answer: (A-False, B-True, C-False, D-True). The headache of migraine is severe, usually unilateral, described as "throbbing" or "pulsating," and aggravated by movement. (*Chapter 63, Page 542.*)

15.33 True statements regarding the Lennox-Gastaut syndrome include which of the following?

(A) This syndrome occurs in older adults generally between ages 60 and 70.
(B) The syndrome includes two or more types of seizure.
(C) There may be associated absence spells.

(D) Patients with this syndrome often score highly on standardized measurements of intelligence.

Answer: (A-False, B-True, C-True, D-False). Specific generalized seizure syndromes during childhood include the Lennox-Gastaut syndrome, which begins between 1 and 10 years of age and includes two or more types of seizure, usually brief myotonic, atonic (drop), or tonic fits and associated absence spells. Behavioral problems and mental retardation are usually seen with this syndrome. (*Chapter 64, Page 549.*)

15.34 The patient is a 46-year-old white male gym teacher who had two epileptic seizures about 7 years ago and was begun on phenytoin. He asks if he might discontinue taking the medication. True statements regarding discontinuing antiepileptic therapy include which of the following?

(A) Patients rarely become seizure-free.
(B) If the patient has been taking medication for 2 years or more, the dose must be slowly tapered over 3 to 6 months.
(C) The presence or absence of risk factors for seizures has no predictive value for recurrence of seizure activity following discontinuation of medication.
(D) Predictors of success include few seizures before treatment and absence of seizures for a prolonged period.

Answer: (A-False, B-True, C-False, D-True). At least 60% of patients eventually become seizure-free. To discontinue therapy after a 2- to 5-year treatment period, the anticonvulsant dose is slowly tapered to zero over a 3- to 6-month interval. Those without risk factors fare the best. Few seizures before treatment, absence of seizures for a prolonged period, normal examinations, normal electroencephalographs (EEG), and absence of a structural brain lesion suggest success when medication is stopped. (*Chapter 64, Page 551.*)

15.35 The patient is a 22-year-old white woman with generalized seizures that will require her to take phenytoin during her pregnancy. True statements regarding anticonvulsive medication used during pregnancy include which of the following?

(A) Valproate and gabapentin are the only anticonvulsive medications safe for use during pregnancy.
(B) Fetus will be at increased risk of macrosomia.

(C) The risk of fetal malformations is increased by 1 to 2%.

(D) The fetus will be especially at risk for cleft lip or palate.

Answer: (A-False, B-False, C-True, D-True). All anticonvulsants increase the risk of fetal malformation, especially cleft lip or palate and cardiac defects, by 1 to 2%. (*Chapter 64, Page 552.*)

15.36 True statements regarding status epilepticus (SE) include which of the following?

(A) Constant neuronal stimulation may lead to cell death.

(B) SE may be followed by residual damage including hemiparesis.

(C) Intensive treatment of SE has no effect on reducing postictal morbidity.

(D) If death occurs, it is usually related to cerebral anoxia caused by the seizure.

Answer: (A-True, B-True, C-False, D-False). Because constantly stimulated neurons may die, patients with SE are at risk, albeit low, of residual damage, often hemiparesis. Evidence suggests that intensive treatment that halts seizures within 1 hour results in a marked reduction of postictal morbidity. If death occurs it is usually related to the underlying problem that produces the SE complicated by circulatory collapse, fever, or renal failure, often from rhabdomyolysis. (*Chapter 64, Page 554.*)

15.37 The emergency management of SE may include which of the following?

(A) nasal oxygen or intubation

(B) thiamine

(C) 50 ml of 50% glucose IV

(D) immediate EEG

Answer: (A-True, B-True, C-True, D-True). Despite the presence of SE, termination of the seizure within minutes is usually not mandatory. Immediate stabilization of vital signs includes airway maintenance with nasal oxygen or intubation as required, electrocardiograph (ECG) monitoring, and blood pressure control. After blood specimens are obtained, adolescents and adults are given 100 mg thiamine and 50 ml of 50% glucose IV (children, 2–4 ml/kg of 25% glucose IV) as well as naloxone (Narcan) when appropriate. An immediate EEG can confirm the diagnosis, and continuous EEG recording may aid in guiding medication dosage. (*Chapter 64, Page 554.*)

15.38 The patient is a 3-year-old child whom you saw last night in the emergency department for her first "febrile seizure." Today in the office, the child is afebrile. True statements regarding this child include which of the following?

(A) This child is too old for a diagnosis of febrile seizure.

(B) She has the most common seizure disorder seen in children of her age group.

(C) Her chance of developing epilepsy is the same as other children in her age group.

(D) If the child had a family history of epilepsy and an abnormal neurologic or development status prior to the seizure, her risk of developing eventual epilepsy increases to about 15%.

Answer: (A-False, B-True, C-False, D-True). Febrile convulsions are the most common seizure disorder between the ages of 6 months to 5 years. The chance of developing epilepsy is 3%. However, children who meet at least two of the following conditions have a 15% chance of eventual epilepsy: (1) family history of epilepsy; (2) abnormal neurologic or development status prior to the seizure; or (3) focal or atypical seizures lasting more than 15 minutes. (*Chapter 64, Page 555.*)

15.39 Daily drug therapy for prophylaxis of febrile convulsions should be considered for which of the following children?

(A) any child with a febrile seizure

(B) a 1-year-old child with multiple recurrences of febrile seizures

(C) a child with a persistent neurologic abnormality

(D) Prophylactic therapy is no longer recommended for any child with febrile convulsions.

Answer: (A-False, B-True, C-True, D-False). Only children with many recurrences at a young age, with persistent neurologic abnormality, or with demanding parents should be considered for daily drug treatment. (*Chapter 64, Page 555.*)

15.40 Isolated systolic hypertension

(A) is unrelated to the incidence of atherothrombotic infarction

(B) is an independent risk factor for stroke

(C) is a normal finding after age 65 and requires no therapy

(D) treatment in the elderly reduces the morbidity and mortality due to stroke

Answer: (A-False, B-True, C-False, D-True). Isolated systolic hypertension has been associated with an increased incidence of atherothrombotic infarction and has been identified as an independent risk factor for stroke. In the Systolic Hypertension in the Elderly Program, there was strong evidence that treatment of isolated systolic hypertension in the elderly reduced the morbidity and mortality due to stroke. (*Chapter 65, Page 556.*)

15.41 The risk of stroke is increased in patients who have

(A) MI
(B) congestive heart failure (CHF)
(C) mitral valve prolapse
(D) chronic atrial fibrillation

Answer: (A-True, B-True, C-False, D-True). Patients with cardiac dysfunction are at twice the risk of developing a stroke as patients without cardiac abnormalities. Cardiac abnormalities include MI (1.7 times the risk), CHF (9.0 times the risk), chronic atrial fibrillation (8.5 times the risk), atrial fibrillation with rheumatic valve disease (25.0 times the risk), left ventricular disease diagnosed by ECG (more than 4.0 times the risk), and coronary artery disease (2.0 times the risk). To date, there is no conclusive evidence that mitral valve prolapse is a significant risk factor for stroke. (*Chapter 65, Page 558.*)

15.42 TIA is a temporary neurologic deficit of sudden onset secondary to a vascular insult that lasts less than 24 hours. Which of the following are characteristic of TIAs?

(A) vertigo as an isolated symptom
(B) visual disturbances
(C) ataxia as the only finding
(D) amaurosis fugax

Answer: (A-False, B-True, C-False, D-True). Symptoms common to TIAs include sensory and motor deficits, visual disturbances, vertigo, aphasia, dysarthria, dysphasia, amaurosis fugax, and ataxia. If isolated vertigo, dysarthria, dysphasia, or ataxia occur, a TIA should not be diagnosed. (*Chapter 65, Page 559.*)

15.43 Symptoms common in a stroke involving the anterior circulation of the brain include

(A) amaurosis fugax
(B) homonymous hemianopia
(C) visual hallucinations
(D) contralateral hemiparesis

Answer: (A-True, B-False, C-False, D-True). The *anterior circulation* includes brain areas supplied by the middle and anterior cerebral arteries, which are major branches of the internal carotid arteries. Other important branches of the internal carotid artery include the ophthalmic artery, posterior communicating artery, and anterior choroidal artery. Symptoms may include amaurosis fugax (ophthalmic artery), contralateral hemiparesis (middle cerebral: face/upper extremity deficits; anterior cerebral: lower extremity deficits), dysphasia (if the dominant hemisphere is involved), and sensory disturbances.

The posterior cerebral artery and its branches, when occluded, commonly present with homonymous hemianopia, visual hallucinations, and visual neglect. (*Chapter 65, Page 559.*)

15.44 The Wallenberg syndrome

(A) is a specific disorder secondary to a lesion in the proximal vertebral artery
(B) may cause hoarseness, nystagmus, and vertigo
(C) may cause hiccups
(D) causes symptoms that resolve quickly on development of collateral circulation

Answer: (A-True, B-True, C-True, D-False). A specific disorder secondary to a lesion in the proximal vertebral artery is the Wallenberg syndrome. Signs and symptoms that occur in combination with some consistency are facial pain and temperature abnormalities ipsilateral to the lesion, hoarseness, nystagmus, vertigo with nausea and vomiting, ataxia, and hiccups. This syndrome is an example of a small artery occlusion with resultant major neurologic deficits. The reason is that the occluded artery, which is the posteroinferior cerebral artery, is an end artery with no collaterals. (*Chapter 65, Page 559.*)

15.45 A stroke due to subarachnoid hemorrhage is commonly caused by

(A) atherosclerosis
(B) trauma
(C) embolization from a source in a damaged heart valve
(D) ruptured aneurysm

Answer: (A-False, B-True, C-False, D-True). Approximately 5% of all strokes are due to subarachnoid hemorrhage, for which trauma or ruptured aneurysm is the most common cause. (*Chapter 65, Page 560.*)

15.46 On routine examination of a 60-year-old retired teacher, you note a bruit in the right carotid artery. She is normotensive and has no symptoms. True statements regarding asymptomatic bruits include the following:

(A) Asymptomatic bruits are more common in men than in women.
(B) As the stenosis in the artery becomes more severe, the bruit may disappear.
(C) With increasing arterial stenosis, the bruit becomes louder and its duration tends to increase.
(D) Only about one-third of patients with severe carotid stenosis have a bruit.

Answer: (A-False, B-True, C-True, D-True). What is the significance of a carotid bruit? The prevalence of asymptomatic bruits is approximately 4% in those older than age 45 years and increases with age. More women than men have asymptomatic bruits. As the stenosis in the artery becomes severe, the bruit may disappear altogether. With increasing arterial stenosis, the bruit becomes louder and its duration increases. Forty percent of neck bruits are of no clinical significance; they do not reflect the presence of stenosis. Only one in three patients with a moderate-to-severe stenosis has a bruit. (*Chapter 65, Page 560.*)

15.47 The patient is a 72-year-old white woman with a tremor involving the thumb and fingers of the right hand, some rigidity of the right side of the body, and a slowness of movement. The symptoms have been present for about 6 months. The confirmation of a diagnosis of PD should be based on

(A) history and physical examination
(B) MRI
(C) lumbar puncture and CSF analysis
(D) the patient's response to a trial of medication

Answer: (A-True, B-False, C-False, D-False). The diagnosis of PD is currently dependent on history taking and physical examination by physicians. There are currently no clinically available blood tests or imaging techniques to confirm the diagnosis of PD. (*Chapter 66, Page 566.*)

15.48 Selegiline (Eldepryl) is often used to treat PD. True statements regarding this drug include which of the following?

(A) The drug is a direct-acting dopamine receptor agonist.

(B) The drug appears to slow down progression of the disease.
(C) To optimize a neuroprotective effect, selegiline must begin early in the clinical course of PD.
(D) Patients with advanced PD can receive significant neuroprotective benefit from selegiline.

Answer: (A-False, B-True, C-True, D-False). Selegiline (Eldepryl) is unique as a dual therapeutic agent for PD in that it can be useful as an adjunct to levodopa to alleviate symptoms, and it appears to slow down the progression of the disease. Selegiline is a monamine oxidase B inhibitor that limits the breakdown of dopamine, allowing more to be available at the receptors to control symptoms. Selegiline also slows the oxidative metabolism of dopamine, which is thought to limit the formation of free radicals, which can further damage substantia nigra cells (i.e., neuroprotective effect). To optimize this neuroprotective effect, selegiline must be initiated early in the clinical course of PD to limit further substantia nigral damage. Selegiline has essentially no neuroprotective benefit to offer more advanced PD. (*Chapter 66, Page 566.*)

15.49 The most common symptoms seen with levodopa overdosage include

(A) dyskinesias
(B) dry mouth and constipation
(C) confusion
(D) pruritic macular rash

Answer: (A-True, B-False, C-True, D-False). Excessive levodopa most often manifests as dyskinesias and confusion. (*Chapter 66, Page 568.*)

15.50 The patient is a 32-year-old white female clerk-typist who reports pain in her left hand and wrist, present for about 6 weeks. Findings that would support a presumptive diagnosis of carpal tunnel syndrome include

(A) nocturnal pain
(B) weakness of the fourth and fifth fingers with hypothenar eminence atrophy
(C) pain or dysesthesia with percussion of the median nerve at the carpal tunnel
(D) pain relieved by sustained wrist flexion

Answer: (A-True, B-False, C-True, D-False). Any process that encroaches on the median nerve, either intrinsically or extrinsically, can cause a carpal tunnel syndrome. Numbness or intermittent paresthesias in the sensory distribution of the median nerve (palmer surface of thumb, index and middle fingers, radial half of the ring finger, radial two-thirds of the palm), nocturnal pain, and pain at rest, often with weakness of the thumb and thenar atrophy, are the classic symptoms of carpal tunnel syndrome. Percussion of the median nerve at the carpal tunnel may cause pain or dysesthesias (positive Tinel sign). Sustained wrist flexion, or sometimes sustained wrist extension, for 60 seconds may produce similar findings (positive Phalen test and positive reverse Phalen test, respectively). (*Chapter 67, Page 576.*)

15.51 Diabetic neuropathy is characterized by

(A) a distal symmetric polyneuropathy
(B) predominantly motor involvement
(C) pain and dysesthesias particularly involving the feet
(D) preservation of joint position sense

Answer: (A-True, B-False, C-True, D-False). Most commonly, diabetic patients experience a distal, symmetric polyneuropathy with predominantly sensory involvement and only mild motor signs. The pain and dysesthesias, particularly of the soles of the feet, may be experienced as severe burning discomfort. Involvement of large myelinated sensory fibers may cause decreased joint position sense, leading to both sensory ataxia and secondary arthropathy (Charcot joints). (*Chapter 67, Page 579.*)

15.52 A nutritional neuropathy due to vitamin B_6 (pyridoxine) may occur in patients taking which of the following drugs?

(A) streptomycin
(B) metoclopramide
(C) isoniazid
(D) dapsone

Answer: (A-False, B-False, C-True, D-True). Certain drugs, notably isoniazid and dapsone, interfere with pyridoxine metabolism and may also produce peripheral neuropathies. (*Chapter 67, Page 580.*)

15.53 True statements regarding the GBS include which of the following?

(A) Findings begin proximally and rapidly descend to the legs and feet.
(B) There is systemic paralysis with decreased or absent reflexes.
(C) Sensory symptoms are not part of the clinical picture.
(D) The disease is more common during the winter months.

Answer: (A-False, B-True, C-False, D-False). GBS, or acute inflammatory demyelinating polyradiculoneuropathy, consists of a rapidly ascending, symmetric paralysis accompanied by decreased reflexes or areflexia, sensory symptoms, and varying autonomic disturbances. Occurring worldwide, it is the most common cause of acute neuromuscular paralysis in the developed world and the most common acquired demyelinating neuropathy. There is no seasonal preponderance. (*Chapter 68, Page 588.*)

15.54 The current mainstays of therapy for GBS syndrome include

(A) plasma exchange
(B) disruption of the blood-brain barrier with administration of antiviral agents
(C) antisense therapy
(D) IV immunoglobulin

Answer: (A-True, B-False, C-False, D-True). Because GBS is probably the result of an autoimmune phenomenon, treatment is directed at suppressing the immune response. The two mainstays of therapy are plasma exchange and intravenous immunoglobulin. (*Chapter 68, Page 589.*)

16
The Eye

The questions in this chapter constitute a review of the following chapters in *Family Medicine: Principles and Practice, Fifth Edition:*

    The Red Eye (Chapter 69)
    Ocular Trauma (Chapter 70)
    Selected Disorders of the Eye (Chapter 71)

DIRECTIONS (Items 16.1 through 16.18): Each of the questions or incomplete statements in this section is followed by five suggested answers or completions. Select the ONE that is BEST in each case.

16.1 The most common cause of bacterial conjunctivitis in infants and children is

  (A) *Staphylococcus aureus*
  (B) *Chlamydia trachomatis*
  (C) *Haemophilus influenzae*
  (D) *Staphylococcus epidermidis*
  (E) *Neisseria gonorrhoeae*

Answer: (C). In infants and children *H. influenzae* is the most common isolate followed by *S. pneumoniae* and *Moraxella catarrhalis*. (*Chapter 69, Page 592.*)

16.2 Topical antimicrobial therapy is generally recommended for the treatment of bacterial conjunctivitis. In addition to topical therapy, systemic therapy is recommended for infections with which of the following organisms?

  (A) *Staphylococcus aureus*
  (B) *Streptococcus pneumoniae*
  (C) *Proteus mirabilis*
  (D) *Neisseria gonorrhoeae*
  (E) *Pseudomonas aeruginosa*

Answer: (D). Because of the frequent spread of infection, both eyes are treated, with therapy continued for 7 to 10 days. If gonococcal infection is diagnosed, systemic therapy is added to the topical therapy. (*Chapter 69, Page 594.*)

16.3 The most common cause of viral conjunctivitis in neonates is

  (A) varicella
  (B) adenovirus
  (C) respiratory syncytial virus
  (D) Epstein-Barr virus
  (E) herpes simplex virus

Answer: (E). Herpes simplex virus may cause conjunctivitis and is the most common viral cause of conjunctivitis in neonates. Primary infection and reactivation of the disease may result in keratitis. (*Chapter 69, Page 594.*)

16.4 The patient is a 24-year-old white woman with unilateral conjunctivitis manifested as irritation and redness with a watery discharge. There is some pain and photophobia. Fluorescein staining reveals a dendritic keratitis. This patient appears to have an infection with

  (A) herpes simplex virus
  (B) *Chlamydia trachomatis*
  (C) allergic conjunctivitis
  (D) *Haemophilus influenzae*
  (E) *Neisseria gonorrhoeae*

Answer: (A). Fluorescein staining may reveal a diffuse punctate keratitis with adenoviral or enteroviral infection or a typical dendritic keratitis with herpes virus infections. (*Chapter 69, Page 595.*)

16.5 In a patient with acute conjunctivitis, a Giemsa-stained smear showing numerous lymphocytes suggests that the cause of the patient's conjunctivitis is

(A) allergic
(B) viral
(C) bacterial
(D) chemical
(E) chlamydial

Answer: (B). A Giemsa-stained smear demonstrating numerous lymphocytes may be helpful for delineating a viral etiology. (*Chapter 69, Page 595.*)

16.6 The patient is a 21-day-old female infant with a conjunctivitis that has been present since day 5 and resistant to topical antibody therapy. The infant seems to have an associated vaginal discharge. The most likely type of conjunctivitis is

(A) allergic
(B) viral
(C) bacterial
(D) chemical
(E) chlamydial

Answer: (E). In the newborn, the time of onset may provide a clue to the diagnosis. Chlamydial infection usually begins at 5 to 14 days of life, although it has been reported within 24 hours of delivery. In adolescents and adults, the symptom is usually chronic bilateral irritation of the eyes. There is no change in vision, and usually a discharge is present. Symptoms of urethritis or a vaginal discharge may be present. An important clue to the diagnosis is a history of chronic conjunctivitis, often unresponsive to topical antimicrobial therapy in association with venereal symptoms. (*Chapter 69, Page 595.*)

16.7 The patient is a 36-year-old clerical worker and contact lens user whose left eye has been red and painful for 2 days. Photophobia is present, but there is no discharge. Fluorescein examination reveals a corneal ulcer in the visual axis. Treatment of this problem should be

(A) gentamicin ophthalmic drops
(B) ciprofloxacin ophthalmic drops
(C) ceftriaxone, 2 g intramuscularly
(D) patching overnight with a follow-up examination in the morning
(E) immediate referral to an ophthalmologist

Answer: (E). A corneal ulcer is an ophthalmologic emergency, and immediate referral to an ophthalmologist is indicated. (*Chapter 69, Page 597.*)

16.8 The patient is a 42-year-old white woman who has pain and photophobia in both eyes. There is intense localized vascular injection of the sclera that is tender to palpation. The cornea and pupil appear normal, and visual acuity is unaffected. It would be reasonable to screen this patient for the presence of which of the following diseases?

(A) carcinoma of the lung
(B) acute thyroiditis
(C) rheumatoid arthritis
(D) chronic urethritis
(E) herpes progenitalis

Answer: (C). Scleritis, or inflammation of the scleral tissue, is much more serious than episcleritis. In contrast to episcleritis, approximately 50% of patients with scleritis have an underlying systemic disorder. The incidence of rheumatoid arthritis in patients presenting with scleritis is 30%; it is the most common connective tissue disorder associated with the condition. (*Chapter 69, Page 597.*)

16.9 The patient is a 75-year-old man with well-controlled diabetes mellitus and hypertension. He awoke this morning with severe unilateral eye pain and redness. He has nausea and has vomited twice. The pupil of the affected eye is mildly dilated, and it does not react to light. The patient probably has

(A) anterior uveitis
(B) acute angle-closure glaucoma
(C) keratitis
(D) allergic conjunctivitis
(E) scleritis

Answer: (B). The patient with acute angle-closure glaucoma usually presents with rapidly developing, severe, unilateral eye pain and redness. The pain is typically deep and may be described as a headache. Nausea and vomiting are common owing to vagal stimulation and may be the presenting complaint. Vision is usually decreased, and the patient may see halos around lights. A medication history is important, as certain medications can precipitate an attack. The predominant feature is that the pupil of the affected eye is semidilated and does not react to light. If the pupil constricts with light, angle-closure glaucoma is not present. (*Chapter 69, Page 599.*)

16.10 The patient is a 42-year-old white female household worker brought to your office as an emergency. She splashed drain cleaner in both eyes 30 minutes ago. There is bilateral ocular redness, pain, and photophobia. Your initial treatment should be

(A) careful evaluation with fluorescein staining and slit-lamp evaluation
(B) application of a topical anesthetic agent
(C) pressure patching
(D) application of an antibiotic ointment, to be applied every two hours, day and night
(E) irrigation

Answer: (E). The initial treatment of all chemical burns is irrigation. This point cannot be emphasized strongly enough. Irrigation must be started as soon as possible—ideally in the field but certainly on initial presentation in the physician's office. The main goal is copious flushing. (*Chapter 70, Page 603.*)

16.11 The word *hyphema* describes

(A) the appearance of herpes simplex virus on fluorescein staining
(B) retinal damage due to macular degeneration
(C) an injury to the ocular orbit
(D) bleeding into the anterior chamber of the eye
(E) visual loss caused by acute angle-closure glaucoma

Answer: (D). Hyphema, or bleeding into the anterior chamber, is a serious complication of blunt or penetrating trauma to the eye. The dramatic view of layering of blood in the anterior chamber is often a sign of other associated damage. (*Chapter 70, Page 603.*)

16.12 The patient is a 17-year-old high school boy who was in a fistfight last night. He was struck in the left eye and now complains of double vision. He appears to have some difficulty with extraocular movements. There is ecchymosis of the tissue surrounding the eye. This patient is likely to have

(A) orbital cellulitis
(B) rupture of the globe of the eye
(C) blowout fracture of the orbit
(D) hyphema
(E) subjunctival hemorrhage and ecchymosis

Answer: (C). Orbital fractures are commonly seen with blunt trauma. The orbit should be palpated for step-offs or crepitus. Rupture into a sinus can cause tissue emphysema; injury to the inferior orbital nerve causes a dysesthesia below the eye. A blowout fracture constitutes entrapment of orbital fat and an extraocular muscle in the bony fragments. The weakest part of the orbit lies inferiorly and is the most common area for a blowout. The patient presents with diplopia and defective extraocular movements. The diagnosis is confirmed by computed tomography. (*Chapter 70, Page 604.*)

16.13 The patient is a 42-year-old white woman who has noticed a firm, painless nodule within the tarsus of the right eye. The nodule is about 6 mm in diameter, and the skin moves freely over the small mass. This patient appears to have which of the following?

(A) pterygium
(B) chalazion
(C) ectropion
(D) external hordeolum
(E) cicatricial entropion

Answer: (B). A chalazion (lipogranuloma) is a chronic granuloma that may follow and be secondary to inflammation of a meibomian gland. During its chronic phase, it is a firm painless nodule up to 8 mm in diameter that lies within the tarsus and over which the skin of the lid moves freely. It usually begins as an acute inflammation with pain, redness, and swelling that points to the conjunctival surface of the eyelid (internal hordeolum). Asymptomatic chalazia usually resolve spontaneously within a few months. (*Chapter 71, Page 607.*)

16.14 The patient is a 52-year-old white male truck driver. For the past 2 days, he has noted a bright red, sharply delineated area of the left eye surrounded by normal-appearing conjunctiva. There is minimal discomfort, and visual acuity is normal. There is no history of trauma. This patient's problem was probably caused by

(A) a sudden increase in intrathoracic pressure
(B) acute open-angle glaucoma
(C) a hyphema
(D) a foreign body
(E) scleritis

Answer: (A). Subconjunctival hemorrhage not caused by direct ocular trauma is usually the result of a sudden increase in intrathoracic pressure, as when sneezing, coughing, or straining to evacuate. Rupture of a conjunctival blood vessel causes a bright red, sharply delineated area surrounded by normal-appearing conjunctiva. (*Chapter 71, Page 607.*)

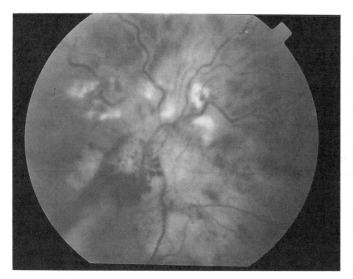

Fig. 16.1. Question 16.16.

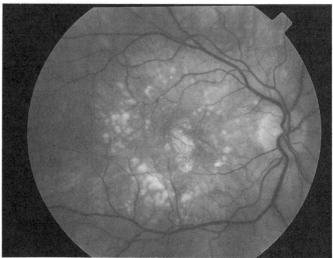

Fig. 16.2. Question 16.17.

16.15 The patient is a 4-year-old Mexican American child. He and his family have recently moved to your city from Mexico City. The parents describe a common cold with nasal drainage for 4 days. For the past day, he has had left periorbital redness, swelling, and tenderness, associated with fever. Treatment of this child must include coverage of the most likely pathogen, which is

(A) *Haemophilus influenzae*
(B) *Streptococcus pneumoniae*
(C) *Neisseria gonorrhoeae*
(D) herpes simplex virus
(E) *Klebsiella pneumoniae*

Answer: (A). Treatment of children age 5 and younger with infections of the periocular tissues has been directed toward the most common pathogen, *Haemophilus influenzae,* although since the introduction of a vaccine (HibCV) for young infants in 1990, there has been about a 90% decrease in the incidence of *H. influenzae* type B infections. A bacterial pathogen is identified as the cause of periorbital cellulitis in only 30% of cases. If there is an associated local wound, the infection pathogen is most likely *Staphylococcus aureus* or *Streptococcus pyogenes.* (*Chapter 71, Page 609.*)

16.16 The figure above represents appearance of the retina through a dilated pupil in a 74-year-old white man with hypertension, ischemic heart disease, and diabetes mellitus. This patient's examination is consistent with a diagnosis of

(A) macular degeneration
(B) central retinal vein occlusion

(C) central retinal artery occlusion
(D) chronic open-angle glaucoma
(E) proliferative diabetic retinopathy

Answer: (E). Proliferative diabetic retinopathy is diagnosed when a neovascularization is detected at the optic nerve or elsewhere in the retina. It poses a risk of retinal hemorrhage, tractional retinal detachment, fibroglial proliferation, and retinal fibrosis. With a dilated pupil, a lacy network of fine vessels is seen, indicating retinal ischemia. (*Chapter 71, Page 610.*)

16.17 The figure above is a photograph of the retinal examination of an 82-year-old white male with coronary artery disease, osteoarthritis, and peptic ulcer disease. For the past six to eight months, he has noted increased difficulty with reading, and more recently there have appeared to be some blind spots in the central part of his field of vision, especially in the left eye. This patient appears to have

(A) proliferate diabetic retinopathy
(B) dry age-related macular degeneration
(C) central retinal vein occlusion
(D) chronic open-angle glaucoma
(E) papilledema

Answer: (B). Dry age-related macular degeneration presents with slow visual loss in the central field of vision. Often the first signs are reduced reading vision and later scotoma in the central field of vision as the severity increases. (*Chapter 71, Page 611.*)

16.18 The most prevalent form of amblyopia is that seen in association with

(A) maternal diabetes
(B) retinopathy of prematurity
(C) strabismus
(D) central retinal artery occlusion
(E) retinoblastoma

Answer: (C). Amblyopia is defined as a poorly sighted eye secondary to some form of visual deprivation at an early age, normally younger than 6 to 7 years. The earlier it occurs, the more severe is the amblyopia. The most prevalent form of amblyopia is seen in association with strabismus. Treatment for amblyopia must be completed by age 7 or 8. (*Chapter 71, Page 613.*)

DIRECTIONS (Items 16.19 through 16.23): Each of the items in this section is a multiple true–false problem that consists of a stem and four lettered options. Indicate whether each of the four options is TRUE or FALSE.

16.19 The patient is a 16-year-old boy who suffered an accidental corneal abrasion while wrestling. The abrasion appears superficial, and vision is intact. True statements regarding management include which of the following?

(A) A pressure patch may be applied over the affected eye to help facilitate healing and relieve pain.
(B) The use of a cycloplegic agent is contraindicated.
(C) The cornea usually reepithelializes within 24 to 48 hours.
(D) The patient should be instructed to return for his next follow-up visit in 5 to 7 days.

Answer: (A-True, B-False, C-True, D-False). Treatment consists of topical antibiotics, pain control, and in some cases a pressure patch over the affected eye. A cycloplegic agent may be instilled into the eye to relieve ciliary spasm and dilate the pupil. Many of these patients require oral analgesia. The patient is examined daily with fluorescein staining until the abrasion resolves. The cornea usually reepithelializes within 24 to 48 hours. Vision should return to normal once healing occurs. Topical antibiotics should be continued 5 to 7 days to prevent infection and for continued lubrication. (*Chapter 70, Page 602.*)

16.20 The patient is a 12-year-old boy who was struck in the left eye by a baseball. There is a bright red subconjunctival hemorrhage involving the lateral aspect of the eye extending to the border of the iris. Vision is normal. Treatment might logically include

(A) a pressure patch
(B) applications of ice
(C) topical antibiotics
(D) watchful waiting

Answer: (A-False, B-True, C-False, D-True). Treatment of a subconjunctival hemorrhage consists of ice, pain relief as needed, and watchful waiting. A subconjunctival hemorrhage commonly goes through the stages of changing color to yellow or green and, at times, takes as long as 2 to 3 weeks to resolve. (*Chapter 70, Page 603.*)

16.21 The patient is a 78-year-old white woman with a sudden painless visual loss in the left eye. Physical examination of the eye reveals a cherry red spot in the central macula. Appropriate treatment of this condition includes which of the following?

(A) pressure patching
(B) immediate pharmacologic decompression of the eye
(C) surgery
(D) topical steroids

Answer: (A-False, B-True, C-True, D-False). Central and branch retinal artery occlusions (CRAO, BRAO) must be recognized. CRAO is a severe sudden loss of vision due to an embolic or thrombotic occlusion, or obstruction, of the central retinal artery. It is considered an ocular emergency, usually painless, and is always monocular. Occasionally, it is preceded by symptoms of amaurosis fugax, lasting 5 to 20 minutes. A cherry red spot is often seen in the central macula. Treatment consists of immediate decompression of the eye by pharmacologic or surgical intervention. (*Chapter 71, Page 609.*)

16.22 True statements regarding chronic open-angle glaucoma (COAG) include which of the following?

(A) COAG is much less common than angle-closure glaucoma.
(B) There is an obstruction of aqueous outflow at the level of the trabecular meshwork.
(C) A family history of glaucoma is a predisposing factor.
(D) The incidence of COAG in those older than age 80 is 1 to 2%.

Answer: (A-False, B-True, C-True, D-False). COAG is a relatively common disorder whose incidence increases with advancing age. There is an obstruction of aqueous outflow at the level of the trabecular meshwork. Predisposing factors include a family history of glaucoma, severe blunt trauma to the eye, and possibly high myopia. The incidence of COAG is 10% in those older than age 80. (*Chapter 71, Page 612.*)

16.23 The patient is a 26-year-old white woman who works as a department store model. She has myopia and uses contact lenses. She asks about your opinion of radial keratotomy. True statements regarding radial keratotomy include which of the following?

(A) The procedure has not been proved to be effective.
(B) The outcome of radial keratotomy is relatively predictable.
(C) Complications can include glare.
(D) Progressive hyperopia following surgery has not been reported.

Answer: (A-False, B-True, C-True, D-False). Radial keratotomy is the most common procedure performed today to correct myopia. Radial 90% corneal incisions are made to relax the cornea and create a new focal point of the eye. This procedure is effective and relatively predictable. Complications can include glare, fluctuating vision, and progressive hyperopia. (*Chapter 71, Page 614.*)

The Ear, Nose, and Throat

The questions in this chapter constitute a review of the following chapters in *Family Medicine: Principles and Practice, Fifth Edition:*

Otitis Media and Otitis Externa (Chapter 72)
Oral Cavity (Chapter 73)
Selected Disorders of the Ear, Nose, and Throat (Chapter 74)

DIRECTIONS (Items 17.1 through 17.9): Each of the questions or incomplete statements in this section is followed by five suggested answers or completions. Select the ONE that is BEST in each case.

17.1 Most instances of acute otitis media (AOM) in children are related to

(A) trauma
(B) eustachian tube (ET) dysfunction
(C) acute sinusitis
(D) immunodeficiency
(E) swimming

Answer: (B). The most probable cause of AOM in children is ET dysfunction. In infants and small children, because of the ET's increased flexibility or the swelling of lymphoid tissue underneath the lining, fluid accumulates in the middle ear. Children have short small ETs; the same volume of nasopharyngeal secretions that may be cleared by the adult ET may accumulate in children. (*Chapter 72, Page 616.*)

17.2 The patient is an 8-year-old girl with left-sided AOM. The antibiotic choice for this patient is

(A) erythromycin
(B) sulfamethoxazole
(C) amoxicillin
(D) cefixime
(E) azithromycin

Answer: (C). The antibiotic of choice for AOM is amoxicillin. Amoxicillin is active against many strains of *H. influenzae* and *S. pneumonia*, is not affected by food intake, and is relatively inexpensive. Amoxicillin had the highest levels of penetration into middle ear fluid in one study, making it the preferred treatment for AOM. (*Chapter 72, Page 619.*)

17.3 The patient is a 4-year-old white girl whom you have treated for chronic serous otitis media (CSOM) for 3 to 4 months. She continues to have a bilateral hearing deficit of 20 to 25 decibels (dB). Your management for this child should be

(A) oral corticosteroids for 4 weeks
(B) myringotomy with tube placement
(C) oral antihistamines for 3 months
(D) tonsillectomy and adenoidectomy
(E) adenoidectomy (only)

Answer: (B). Myringotomy with tube placement is indicated in a child with bilateral CSOM for 3 months with a bilateral hearing deficit of at least 20 dB threshold loss or worse. Steroids, antihistamines, adenoidectomy, and tonsillectomy are not recommended. (*Chapter 72, Page 621.*)

17.4 The most common pathogen in acute inflammatory otitis externa is

(A) *Pseudomonas aeruginosa*
(B) *Staphylococcus epidermidis*

(C) *Haemophilus influenzae*
(D) *Staphylococcus aureus*
(E) *Moraxella catarrhalis*

Answer: (A). *Pseudomonas aeruginosa*, the universal inhabitant of moist environments, is the most likely bacterial cause of external otitis. Other pathogens include *E. coli*, *Aerobacter*, *S. aureus*, streptococci, and some *Proteus* species. (*Chapter 72, Page 622.*)

17.5 The first sign of oral cancer is likely to be

(A) infection
(B) weight loss
(C) tooth abscess
(D) erythroplasia
(E) ulceration

Answer: (D). The earliest, most consistent marker of oral cancer is erythroplasia. Later signs of oral cancer include tissue retraction, raised lesions, palpable thickening, and ulceration. (*Chapter 73, Page 626.*)

17.6 The most common cause of conductive hearing loss in adults is

(A) maternal rubella infection
(B) CSOM
(C) ET dysfunction
(D) cerumen impaction
(E) acoustic trauma

Answer: (D). By far the most common cause of conductive hearing loss in adults is cerumen impaction. It can be relieved by curet or irrigation using warm water or water and peroxide. (*Chapter 74, Page 633.*)

17.7 The patient is a 6-year-old child with a nosebleed that began this morning. The bleeding is probably coming from

(A) the anteroinferior aspect of the nasal septum
(B) the maxillary sinus
(C) the ethmoid sinus
(D) adenoidal tissue
(E) the posterior pharynx

Answer: (A). Epistaxis in children is usually from an anterior site on the nasal septum, generally in Kesselbach's area (also called Little's area) on the anteroinferior aspect of the nasal septum. Bleeding from this area can be arterial or venous. (*Chapter 74, Page 633.*)

17.8 The patient is a 30-month-old white boy who has had recurrent nosebleeds from the left nostril for 1 week. On examination, you note some purulent malodorous discharge in the involved nostril. The most likely diagnosis is

(A) chronic allergic rhinitis
(B) chronic maxillary sinusitis
(C) von Willebrand's disease
(D) sarcoidosis
(E) foreign body

Answer: (E). In young children, foreign bodies may cause epistaxis with a malodorous discharge. (*Chapter 74, Page 634.*)

17.9 Xerostomia may be caused by all EXCEPT which of the following?

(A) therapeutic radiation
(B) Sjögren syndrome
(C) pilocarpine
(D) antihistamines
(E) antidepressants

Answer: (C). The three most common causes are medications, therapeutic radiation, and Sjögren syndrome. Medications causing xerostomia include sedatives, antipsychotics, antidepressants, antihistamines, and antireflux drugs with anticholinergic effects. Pilocarpine appears effective in management and is pending U.S. Food and Drug Administration approval for postirradiation-induced xerostomia. (*Chapter 74, Page 635.*)

DIRECTIONS (Items 17.10 through 17.20): Each of the items in this section is a multiple true–false problem that consists of a stem and four lettered options. Indicate whether each of the four options is TRUE or FALSE.

17.10 The patient is a 4-year-old white boy who has had four episodes of AOM in the past 12 months. True statements regarding the management of this child include which of the following?

(A) Daily prophylactic antibiotics should be considered.
(B) Sulfisoxazole is safe for long-term use in prophylaxis of AOM.
(C) The patient should be treated with diphenhydramine (Benadryl) taken three times daily.
(D) Tetracycline is a safe and effective choice for prophylaxis of AOM.

Answer: (A-True, B-True, C-False, D-False). Daily prophylactic antibiotics should be considered if there are three to four episodes within 6 to 18 months. Sulfisoxazole has been proved effective for preventing recurrent symptomatic AOM and is safe for long-term use. (*Chapter 72, Page 620.*)

17.11 Factors that may contribute to the development of CSOM include which of the following?

(A) ET dysfunction
(B) allergies
(C) passive smoke inhalation
(D) upper respiratory infections (URI)

Answer: (A-True, B-True, C-True, D-True). The etiology of serous otitis media (SOM) is complex and not completely understood. ET dysfunction, AOM, allergies, passive smoke inhalation, and URIs can contribute to CSOM. Serous effusions are found in as many as 40% of children after AOM. There is a higher incidence of CSOM in children with allergy, URIs, and smoking in the home. In one study, up to 76% of children with SOM had prior URIs. (*Chapter 72, Page 621.*)

17.12 Swimmers who develop acute inflammatory otitis externa (swimmer's ear) are likely to have which of the following characteristics?

(A) They are more likely to have been swimming in pool or ocean water than in fresh water.
(B) They are more likely to have engaged in surface swimming than in frequent submersion of the head.
(C) They have been swimming in a hot humid climate.
(D) Their episodes of swimming have been relatively brief and infrequent.

Answer: (A-False, B-False, C-True, D-False). Swimmers who developed otitis media were more likely to have swum longer, more frequently, and with more frequent submersion of their head than swimmers without otitis media, independent of the type of water. Otitis media was more likely associated with swimming in fresh water rather than in the ocean and a pool; it increased with 1 month of exposure, but only in those who swam frequently. Swimmer's ear is more likely in hot humid climates and 10 to 20 times more likely during the summer. (*Chapter 72, Page 622.*)

17.13 The treatment of acute inflammatory otitis externa (swimmer's ear) generally includes which of the following?

(A) systemic antibiotics
(B) topical medication given 3 or 4 times daily
(C) insertion of a wick if the external canal is swollen
(D) return to swimming as soon as itching and pain subside

Answer: (A-False, B-True, C-True, D-False). Topical medication should be given three or four times a day. If the canal is too swollen to allow easy access for the drops, a wick of 0.25-inch gauze or cotton may be inserted into the swollen external canal for 24 to 36 hours. Medication can then be dropped onto the wick. Treatment should be continued 7 to 10 days and ear canal protected from water for 2 weeks. Systemic antibiotics are seldom needed. (*Chapter 72, Page 622.*)

17.14 Risk factors for oral and pharyngeal squamous cell cancers include the frequent use of

(A) unrefined carbohydrates
(B) tobacco
(C) alcohol
(D) fluoride-containing toothpaste

Answer: (A-False, B-True, C-True, D-False). Oral and pharyngeal squamous cell cancers constitute a potentially lethal disease that is highly curable with early diagnosis. A high-risk group exists, defined by regular use of tobacco or alcohol. (*Chapter 73, Page 626.*)

17.15 Temporomandibular arthralgia is related to internal joint derangements, which may be accompanied by crepitus on jaw movement. Causes of these internal joint derangements and temporomandibular arthralgia include which of the following?

(A) bruxism
(B) exaggerated jaw opening during dental procedures
(C) generalized joint hypomobility
(D) male gender

Answer: (A-True, B-True, C-False, D-False). Causes of these internal joint derangements include forceful jaw trauma, bruxism, malocclusion, exaggerated jaw opening during dental procedures, generalized joint hypermobility, female gender, and inflammatory arthritis. (*Chapter 73, Page 628.*)

17.16 Drugs that may cause tinnitus include which of the following?

(A) antihistamines
(B) aspirin

(C) loop diuretics
(D) antimalarials

Answer: (A-False, B-True, C-True, D-True). Drugs and other chemical exposures may be linked to tinnitus. Most well known is the association with aspirin; other offenders are loop diuretics, arsenic, and antimalarials. (*Chapter 74, Page 630.*)

17.17 Risk factors that help identify the child at risk for hearing loss include which of the following?

(A) hearing loss in blood relatives that began following age 60
(B) pregnancy complicated by toxoplasmosis
(C) pregnancy complicated by cytomegalovirus infection
(D) maternal exposure to aminoglycoside antibiotics

Answer: (A-False, B-True, C-True, D-True). During well-baby visits, specific questions concerning the family and pregnancy history help identify the child at risk for hearing loss. These factors include a family history of hearing loss in blood relatives younger than 5 years old, pregnancy complicated by TORCH (toxoplasmosis, other agents, rubella, cytomegalovirus, herpes simplex) or other infections accompanied by rash, and exposure to medications such as aminoglycoside antibiotics. (*Chapter 74, Page.*) 632

17.18 Saliva has a number of functions that include which of the following?

(A) lubrication of the mouth and upper pharynx
(B) remineralize teeth
(C) augment the acidity of gastric acid
(D) help protect against infection

Answer: (A-True, B-True, C-False, D-True). Saliva is a complex secretion that lubricates the mouth and upper pharynx, modulates the oral flora, aids in initial digestion of food, and facilitates speech and swallowing. Saliva also helps remineralize teeth and buffers gastric acid, thereby protecting the esophagus. High levels of immunoglobulin A are present, suggesting a role in host defense. The normal adult produces up to 1.5 L daily. (*Chapter 74, Page 634.*)

17.19 True statements regarding cancer of the larynx include which of the following?

(A) Cancer of the larynx is most common on the vocal folds.
(B) Symptoms occur late in the course of laryngeal cancer.
(C) Most vocal cord cancers are adenocarcinomas.
(D) The carcinogen responsible for most cases is alcohol.

Answer: (A-True, B-False, C-False, D-False). Cancer may occur anywhere in the larynx but is most common on the vocal folds. Because vocal cord cancer gives rise to symptoms early in its course, it is potentially curable when diagnosed. More than 95% of vocal cord cancers are squamous cell carcinomas. Cigarette smoke is the chief carcinogen responsible for most of the cases. (*Chapter 74, Page 636.*)

17.20 The patient is a 52-year-old overweight white woman. Her chief complaint today is hoarseness of about 4 months' duration. She has known hypertension, coronary artery disease, and hypothyroidism. Current medications include a diuretic for hypertension, thyroid replacement therapy, and sublingual nitroglycerin for use as needed. Her diabetes is currently diet-controlled. She has never smoked. Diagnostic considerations today include

(A) autoimmune disease affecting the vocal cords
(B) fungal infections of the larynx
(C) vocal cord edema
(D) neuropathy with vocal cord weakness or paralysis

Answer: (A-False, B-False, C-True, D-True). Several endocrine disorders may present with hoarseness. Acromegaly results in irreversible laryngeal changes and hoarseness. Hypothyroidism causes vocal cord edema and weakness with resultant hoarseness. Hypoparathyroidism may result in hypocalcemia, and subsequent tetany may cause laryngospasm. Diabetic neuropathy may cause vocal cord weakness or paralysis. (*Chapter 74, Page 636.*)

18

The Cardiovascular System

The questions in this chapter constitute a review of the following chapters in *Family Medicine: Principles and Practice, Fifth Edition:*

Hypertension (Chapter 75)
Ischemic Heart Disease (Chapter 76)
Cardiac Arrhythmias (Chapter 77)
Heart Sounds, Murmurs, and Valvular Heart Disease (Chapter 78)
Heart Failure (Chapter 79)
Cardiovascular Emergencies (Chapter 80)
Venous Thromboembolism (Chapter 81)
Selected Disorders of the Cardiovascular System (Chapter 82)

DIRECTIONS (Items 18.1 through 18.41): Each of the questions or incomplete statements in this section is followed by five suggested answers or completions. Select the ONE that is BEST in each case.

18.1 According to current recommendations the diastolic blood pressure measurement should be based on

(A) a change in the quality of the sound heard while recording the blood pressure
(B) careful palpation of the radial artery
(C) measurement taking with the patient seated with the arm positioned at about shoulder level
(D) the first appearance of sound
(E) the disappearance of sound

Answer: (E). Measurement of the diastolic blood pressure should be based on the disappearance of sound (phase V Korotkoff sound). (*Chapter 75, Page 640.*)

18.2 The patient is a 46-year-old white male truck driver. On performing a physical examination related to his job, you find his blood pressure to be 126/88. What should your recommendation for this patient be?

(A) Begin diuretic therapy.
(B) Begin treatment with a beta-blocker.
(C) Evaluate further with electrocardiogram (ECG) and chest radiograph.
(D) Recheck the blood pressure in 1 week.
(E) Recheck the blood pressure in 1 year.

Answer: (E). In general, individuals with diastolic blood pressure ranges considered borderline high (i.e., 85 to 89 mm Hg) should have their blood pressures rechecked within 1 year. (*Chapter 75, Page 642.*)

18.3 The calcium-entry antagonists are useful drugs in the treatment of high blood pressure. They are good choices for patients with all the following EXCEPT

(A) heart block
(B) diabetes mellitus
(C) angina pectoris
(D) chronic obstructive pulmonary disease
(E) supraventricular arrhythmias

Answer: (A). The calcium-entry antagonists are contraindicated in patients with heart block, cardiogenic shock, or acute myocardial infarction (MI). Common adverse effects include peripheral edema, dizziness, headache, asthenia, nausea, constipation, flushing, and tachycardia. Calcium-entry antagonists have no significant impact on lipid profiles or glucose metabolism. These agents are effective at all ages and in all races. They are good choices for patients with diabetes, angina pectoris, migraine, chronic obstructive pulmonary disease/asthma, peripheral vascular disease, renal insufficiency, and supraventricular arrhythmias. (*Chapter 75, Page 645.*)

18.4 Of the centrally acting antiadrenergic antihypertensive agents, methyldopa (Aldomet) has a distinctive adverse effect in that the drug may cause

(A) renal failure
(B) autoimmune disorders
(C) hypermagnesemia
(D) cluster headaches
(E) sarcoidosis

Answer: (B). Methyldopa exhibits a unique adverse effect profile as it induces autoimmune disorders, such as those with positive Coombs' and antinuclear antibody tests, hemolytic anemia, and hepatic necrosis. (*Chapter 75, Page 647.*)

18.5 The patient is a 60-year-old white male who reports chest pain that occurs at rest and often during the night. Symptoms also occasionally occur after exercise. He has noted sporadic episodes with long pain-free intervals. His blood pressure is 120/78. The pulse is 72. The ECG shows an ST segment elevation. This patient appears to have

(A) classical angina
(B) esophageal chest pain
(C) anginal equivalent
(D) variant (Prinzmetal's) angina
(E) syndrome X (microvascular angina)

Answer: (D). Variant (Prinzmetal's) angina occurs at rest and may manifest in stereotyped patterns, such as nocturnal symptoms or symptoms that appear only after exercise. It is thought to be caused by coronary artery spasm. Its symptoms often occur periodically, with characteristic pain-free intervals, and are associated with typical ECG changes, most commonly ST segment elevation. (*Chapter 76, Page 652.*)

18.6 The patient is a 72-year-old black man who has had periodic chest pain for several months. His pain is sharp and stabbing, and is located in the substernal area. It occasionally radiates to the jaw or down the left arm. The pain is sometimes related to exertion and relieved by rest. According to the history, this patient appears to have

(A) classic angina
(B) atypical angina

(C) angina equivalent
(D) variant (Prinzmetal's) angina
(E) esophageal spasm

Answer: (B). With atypical angina, similar symptoms are experienced but with the absence of one or more of the criteria for classic angina. For example, the pain may not be consistently related to exertion or relieved by rest. Conversely, the pain may have an atypical character (sharp, stabbing), but the precipitating factors are clearly anginal. (*Chapter 76, Page 652.*)

18.7 You are writing a prescription for a long-acting nitrate for your 62-year-old white male patient with angina pectoris. Which of the following might concern you about the use of long-acting nitrates for this indication?

(A) anaphylaxis
(B) tolerance
(C) postural hypotension
(D) flushing
(E) fatigue

Answer: (B). The most significant concern about the long-acting nitrates is tolerance. Most studies have shown that tolerance develops rapidly when long-acting nitrates are given for anginal prophylaxis. (*Chapter 76, Page 655.*)

18.8 The patient is a 58-year-old white male salesman with known stable angina for 2 to 3 years. Although his angina occurs only once or twice monthly, he has been aware of some palpitations and you have ordered a Holter monitor. The report of the Holter monitor includes some "palpitation" episodes accompanied by 1.2 mm of downsloping ST segment depression lasting 1 to 2 minutes, separated from other episodes by 5 to 10 minutes of a normal baseline. These findings appear to represent

(A) gastroesophageal reflux
(B) heart block
(C) sinus arrhythmia
(D) myocardial ischemia
(E) a normal variation in the tracing

Answer: (D). For Holter monitoring, when ST segment changes that meet strict criteria are seen in a patient with known ischemic heart disease, it is generally accepted that they represent episodes of myocardial ischemia. Ischemic criteria include at least 1.0 mm of horizontal or downsloping ST segment depression that lasts for at least 1 minute and is separated from other

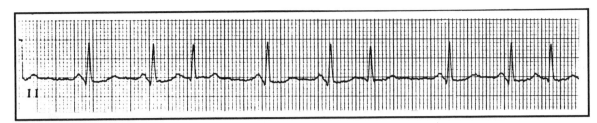

Fig. 18.1. Question 18.11.

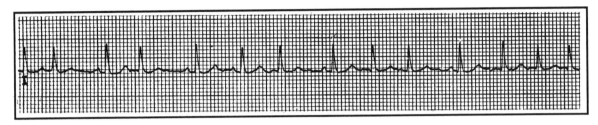

Fig. 18.2. Question 18.12.

discrete episodes by at least 1 minute of a normal base-line. (*Chapter 76, Page 658.*)

18.9 The patient is a 59-year-old white woman, concerned about a "skipped heart beat." As part of your examination, you plan an ECG. The best single lead for evaluation of cardiac rhythm in most patients is

(A) lead I
(B) lead II
(C) lead III
(D) lead V1
(E) lead V6

Answer: (B). The ECG is necessary to establish a specific diagnosis and may be the point at which evaluation of arrhythmia begins for asymptomatic patients. Lead II is the best single lead for evaluation of cardiac rhythm in most patients, as the P and QRS electrical vectors in patients without axis deviation are most positive in this lead. (*Chapter 77, Page 666.*)

18.10 In some patients, a cardiac arrhythmia problem may be eliminated by stopping the ingestion of

(A) aspartame
(B) aspirin
(C) nonsteroidal anti-inflammatory drugs (NSAID)
(D) alcohol
(E) caffeine

Answer: (E). Medication use or ingestions (e.g., caffeine) are the most commonly seen reversible causes of arrhythmias; and changing or discontinuing medications or discontinuing use of caffeine or other substances may eliminate the problem. (*Chapter 77, Page 667.*)

18.11 The ECG tracing above is consistent with a diagnosis of

(A) sinus arrest
(B) premature atrial complexes (PAC)
(C) sinus tachycardia
(D) multifocal atrial tachycardia (MAT)
(E) atrial fibrillation (AF)

Answer: (B). The terms *premature atrial complexes* and *atrial premature beats* are both used, although they represent the same phenomenon. Cardiac impulses are initiated in one or more ectopic atrial foci but are otherwise conducted as for a normal beat. (*Chapter 77, Page 672.*)

18.12 The ECG tracing above is consistent with a diagnosis of

(A) sinus tachycardia
(B) MAT
(C) atrioventricular (AV) nodal reentrant tachycardia
(D) Wolff-Parkinson-White syndrome (WPW)
(E) AF

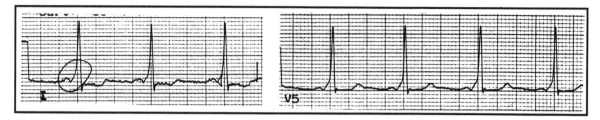

Fig. 18.3. Question 18.13.

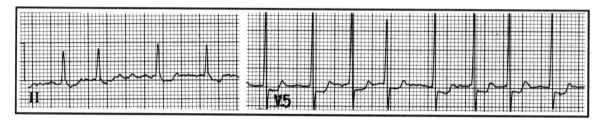

Fig. 18.4. Question 18.14.

Answer: (B). MAT is characterized by the appearance of multiple ectopic atrial foci, with a rapid and slightly irregular rhythm the result of transmission of these multiple foci through the AV node. (*Chapter 77, Page 672.*)

18.13 The tracing above is taken from a 32-year-old woman who reports occasional bursts of rapid heartbeat. This tracing is consistent with

(A) PACs
(B) atrial tachycardia
(C) MAT
(D) WPW
(E) atrial flutter

Answer: (D). The classic ECG appearance of WPW is a short PR interval (less than 0.12 second) and a widened QRS complex with a slurred upsloping initial component called the delta wave. The heart rate is usually normal between episodes of tachycardia, and the tachycardia itself may have an ECG appearance indistinguishable from other types of supraventricular tachycardia. Delta waves can be present during tachycardia and, if large, can cause a widened QRS complex easily mistaken for ventricular tachycardia. (*Chapter 77, Page 674.*)

18.14 The above tracing is consistent with a diagnosis of

(A) AF with rapid ventricular response
(B) atrial flutter

(C) PACs
(D) sinus tachycardia
(E) WPW

Answer: (A). In AF, the ECG is characterized by an irregular wavy baseline representing chaotic atrial depolarization, the absence of P waves, and irregularly appearing QRS complexes. A ventricular rate of more than 100 beats per minute (bpm) is labeled a "rapid" ventricular response, between 60 and 100 bpm a "moderate" response, and less than 60 bpm a "slow" response. (*Chapter 77, Page 675.*)

18.15 The ECG tracing at the top of the next page is consistent with a diagnosis of

(A) AF
(B) preexcitation syndrome
(C) AV nodal reentrant tachycardia
(D) MAT
(E) atrial flutter with a 4:1 AV conduction

Answer: (E). Atrial flutter is now believed to be caused by a reentry circuit in the right atrium associated with underlying cardiac disease such as myocarditis, MI, coronary artery disease, or acute ischemia. The underlying atrial rate is approximately 300 bpm (250 to 350 bpm, although it can be higher), with the ventricular rate dependent on the degree of AV block present. If an AV bypass is present, 1:1 conduction occurs for a ventricular rate of about 300 bpm; and conduction through a healthy AV node results in a 2:1 block and ventricular rate of about 150 bpm. A higher degree of block (3:1 or

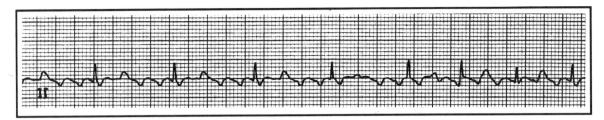

Fig. 18.5. Question 18.15.

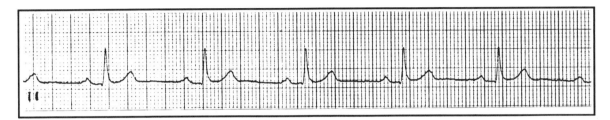

Fig. 18.6. Question 18.16.

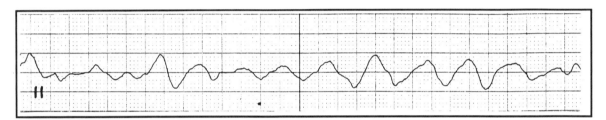

Fig. 18.7. Question 18.17.

4:1) may occur with a diseased or fibrotic AV node, resulting in a ventricular rate of 70 to 100 bpm. (*Chapter 77, Page 676.*)

18.16 The ECG tracing above is consistent with a diagnosis of

(A) atrial flutter
(B) first-degree AV block
(C) AF
(D) third-degree AV block
(E) ventricular premature beats

Answer: (B). First-degree block is commonly caused by increased vagal tone or as a drug side effect (digoxin). It is characterized by a prolonged PR interval of more than 0.2 second, with an otherwise normal ECG. Unless it is accompanied by significant bradycardia, treatment is not necessary. (*Chapter 77, Page 677.*)

18.17 The tracing above is consistent with a diagnosis of

(A) ventricular premature beats
(B) nonsustained ventricular tachycardia
(C) sustained ventricular tachycardia
(D) ventricular fibrillation (VF)
(E) torsade de pointes

Answer: (D). VF is a state of chaotic ventricular activity caused by the random firing of multiple ectopic foci, probably due to a complex reentry mechanism. (*Chapter 77, Page 681.*)

18.18 The fourth heart sound (S4) is a sign of

(A) ischemic heart disease (IHD)
(B) ventricular arrhythmia
(C) AF
(D) VF
(E) loss of ventricular compliance

Answer: (E). The S4 is a sign of loss of ventricular compliance. Rarely is an S4 detected in the absence of heart disease. (*Chapter 78, Page 684.*)

18.19 The most common cause of mitral valve regurgitation is

(A) rheumatic fever
(B) mitral valve prolapse
(C) syphilis
(D) atrial myxoma
(E) bacterial endocarditis

Answer: (B). Mitral valve prolapse is the most common cause of mitral valve regurgitation. (*Chapter 78, Page 686.*)

18.20 The first symptom of mitral regurgitation is usually

(A) dyspnea
(B) orthopnea
(C) paroxysmal nocturnal dyspnea
(D) fatigue
(E) dependent edema

Answer: (D). Mitral regurgitation may progress for decades without causing symptoms. Symptoms usually occur insidiously because of the ability of the left atrium to distend and the left ventricle to increase cardiac output. The first symptom is usually fatigue because of decreased cardiac output. Later dyspnea, orthopnea, and paroxysmal nocturnal dyspnea occur as the left atrial pressure and pulmonary vascular pressure rise. Edema is a late finding. (*Chapter 78, Page 686.*)

18.21 The mitral valve prolapse syndrome is defined as mitral valve prolapse associated with

(A) subclinical mitral regurgitation
(B) chest pain
(C) occurrence in patients younger than age 30
(D) occurrence in young women
(E) increased autonomic tone

Answer: (E). The mitral valve prolapse syndrome has been defined as mitral valve prolapse associated with increased autonomic tone. Studies have shown increased catecholamine levels and changes in diurnal variation of catecholamine levels in patients with mitral valve prolapse. In addition, these patients have abnormalities of beta-adrenergic receptors and evidence of decreased intravascular volume. Patients with this syndrome often complain of anxiety and show signs of increased adrenergic tone, such as unexplained elevations of the resting pulse. (*Chapter 78, Page 687.*)

18.22 The cases of mitral stenosis a family physician is likely to encounter during a practice lifetime will be caused by which of the following?

(A) congenital heart disease
(B) myxomatous heart disease
(C) ischemic heart disease
(D) rheumatic heart disease
(E) hypertrophic cardiomyopathy

Answer: (D). Mitral stenosis has a single cause: rheumatic heart disease. Although only 50% of patients with mitral stenosis can recall an episode of rheumatic fever, the surgical pathology of stenotic mitral valves virtually always reveals the changes associated with rheumatic heart disease. There is no inherited component and only 60 reported cases of congenital mitral stenosis. (*Chapter 78, Page 687.*)

18.23 Which of the following heart and vascular findings is characteristic of mitral stenosis?

(A) water-hammer pulse
(B) a sustained point of maximum impulse
(C) opening snap
(D) holosystolic murmur
(E) soft first heart sound

Answer: (C). One of the characteristic heart sounds of mitral stenosis is the opening snap, which occurs after S2 and is sharper and higher pitched than an S3. The shorter the time between S2 and the opening snap, the higher is the atrium pressure and the more severe the stenosis. (*Chapter 78, Page 688.*)

18.24 The patient is a 42-year-old white woman who complains of some fatigue and occasional shortness of breath. Her blood pressure is 142/62. The first heart sound is soft, and the second heart sound is normal. There is a grade 3/6 high-pitched, soft, blowing diastolic murmur best heard along the left sternal border. The most likely diagnosis in this patient is

(A) mitral valve prolapse
(B) mitral stenosis
(C) aortic insufficiency
(D) aortic stenosis
(E) hypertrophic cardiomyopathy

Answer: (C). The first heart sound is soft with aortic insufficiency. Although S2 is normal, the aortic component may be lost, so S2 can sound single. Because of elevated diastolic pressure before the atrial contraction, S4 is rare until the ventricle is markedly dilated and failing, but an S3 is common. The murmur of aortic insufficiency is a high-pitched, soft, blowing diastolic murmur heard best with the diaphragm. It is most audible along the left sternal border (Erb's point) with the patient leaning forward and holding expiration. (*Chapter 78, Page 688.*)

18.25 In the evaluation of valvular heart disease, the finding of a carotid pulse that seems "weak and slow" (*parvus et tardus*) is characteristic of which of the following disorders?

(A) aortic stenosis
(B) mitral regurgitation
(C) mitral stenosis
(D) aortic insufficiency
(E) hypertrophic cardiomyopathy

Answer: (A). The carotid pulse provides the best clue to the presence and severity of aortic stenosis. Called *parvus et tardus* (weak and slow), the carotid pulse rises slowly and often with a shudder. The changes in the carotid pulse are highly correlated to the severity of the valvular gradient and the severity of the disease. (*Chapter 78, Page 689.*)

18.26 The patient is a 58-year-old white woman with exercise-related substernal pain. Her blood pressure is 98/62; the pulse is 70. There is a loud, coarse, crescendo-decrescendo murmur best heard at the second right intercostal space and radiating to the neck. The most likely diagnosis in this patient is

(A) mitral stenosis
(B) mitral regurgitation
(C) aortic stenosis
(D) aortic insufficiency
(E) hypertrophic cardiomyopathy

Answer: (C). The murmur of aortic stenosis is best heard at the second right intercostal space and often radiates to the neck. It is coarse and usually loud. It is described as a crescendo-decrescendo murmur or a diamond-shaped murmur; the later the peak of the crescendo, the more severe is the gradient. (*Chapter 78, Page 689.*)

18.27 The patient is a 55-year-old white man with a characteristic murmur of aortic stenosis. Over the past 3 months, he has developed exercise-related angina pectoris, and there have been three episodes of syncope. There have also been a few times in which he has noted some weight gain associated with ankle edema. The optimum treatment at this time would be

(A) digitalis
(B) angina prophylaxis with nitrates

(C) loop diuretics
(D) calcium-entry blockers
(E) surgery

Answer: (E). During the asymptomatic phase of aortic stenosis, no medical intervention is indicated. Once symptoms occur, surgery should be considered quickly. (*Chapter 78, Page 690.*)

18.28 At a 4-week examination of a newborn infant, you notice a continuous "machinery" murmur present throughout systole and diastole, with a palpable thrill in the area of the second left intercostal space. Your physical findings are consistent with a diagnosis of

(A) tetralogy of Fallot
(B) ventricular septal defect
(C) Eisenmenger complex
(D) Down syndrome
(E) patent ductus arteriosus (PDA)

Answer: (E). The murmur of a PDA is a continuous, "machinery" murmur that is present during systole and diastole; it peaks at or near S2. There is often a thrill palpable at the area of the pulmonary artery, the second left intercostal space. (*Chapter 78, Page 691.*)

18.29 The cornerstone of pharmacologic management of systolic heart failure (HF) is which of the following classes of drugs?

(A) diuretics
(B) calcium channel blockers
(C) coronary vasodilators
(D) angiotensin converting enzyme (ACE inhibitors)
(E) beta-blockers

Answer: (D). ACE inhibitors are the cornerstone of the pharmacologic management of systolic HF, and contemporary therapy of systolic HF mandates an ACE inhibitor unless contraindicated. (*Chapter 79, Page 698.*)

18.30 The patient is a 70-year-old white man whose hobby is carpentry. He reports that three times over the past month, syncope has occurred following heavy exertion using the arms. This finding may be the tipoff to which of the following diagnoses?

(A) transient ischemic attack
(B) subclavian steal syndrome
(C) hyperventilation
(D) mitral stenosis
(E) primary pulmonary hypertension

Answer: (B). Syncope with arm exertion suggests sub-clavian steal syndrome. (*Chapter 80, Page 705.*)

18.31 The leading cause of cardiogenic shock is

(A) aortic stenosis
(B) ruptured cordae tendinae
(C) cocaine overdose
(D) acute MI
(E) cardiac arrhythmia

Answer: (D). The leading cause of cardiogenic shock is acute MI. Both the onset and severity are closely related to the quantitative loss of functional myocardium. (*Chapter 80, Page 708.*)

18.32 The diagnosis of cardiogenic shock is based on

(A) serial ECG findings
(B) clinical findings
(C) echocardiography
(D) chest roentgenogram
(E) continuous cardiac monitoring

Answer: (B). The diagnosis of cardiogenic shock is based on the clinical syndrome of tissue hypoperfusion in the setting of adequate intravascular volume and a primary or secondary cause of cardiac dysfunction. (*Chapter 80, Page 708.*)

18.33 The patient is a 71-year-old white man, admitted to the intensive care unit of your rural hospital in cardiogenic shock. You have initiated invasive monitoring with bedside hemodynamic measurements. With cardiogenic shock, you expect to find the pulmonary artery occlusion pressure to be

(A) too low to measure
(B) less than 1 to 2 mm Hg
(C) greater than 18 mm Hg
(D) greater than 200 mm Hg
(E) too high to measure

Answer: (C). In cardiogenic shock, routine bedside hemodynamic measurements demonstrate increases in left ventricular filling pressure, as reflected in pulmonary artery occlusion pressure, to levels of more than 18 mm Hg in combination with a decline in the cardiac index to less than 2.2 L/m^2. (*Chapter 80, Page 708.*)

18.34 Which of the following diagnostic tests is NOT useful in the diagnosis of deep vein thrombosis (DVT)?

(A) Doppler evaluation
(B) contrast venography
(C) impedance plethysmography
(D) real-time ultrasonography
(E) radiofibrinogen leg scanning

Answer: (A). Clinical suspicion of DVT necessitates further investigation. Familiarity with diagnostic options locally available is necessary to take a logical, cost-effective approach. Four diagnostic techniques—contrast venography, impedance plethysmography (IPG), real-time ultrasonography, and radiofibrinogen leg scanning—are widely available and useful. Duplex scanning should not be confused with a Doppler study. Doppler evaluation of the lower extremity requires only a small hand-held unit and does not use B-mode ultrasonography. It detects only venous occlusion, so significant mural thrombi may be missed. The test has poor sensitivity and no role as a definitive diagnostic test. (*Chapter 81, Page 714.*)

18.35 The patient is a 58-year-old white woman being treated with heparin for DVT. She has developed gastrointestinal bleeding with a drop in her hematocrit. To counteract the effects of heparin, you will give the patient an intravenous injection of

(A) vitamin K
(B) vitamin C
(C) fibrinogen
(D) antithrombin III
(E) protamine sulfate

Answer: (E). The effects of heparin can be terminated by intravenous injection of protamine sulfate. (*Chapter 81, Page 717.*)

18.36 You are treating a 58-year-old white woman for DVT of the left lower extremity. Following initial care with heparin, anticoagulation is being continued with warfarin. Following her discharge from the hospital, you will plan to maintain her prothrombin time at an international normalized ratio (INR) of

(A) less than 1.5
(B) 2.0 to 3.0
(C) 4.0 to 6.0
(D) 8.0 to 11.0
(E) 15.0 to 20.0

Answer: (B). Early initiation of warfarin therapy, started within 3 days of the initial heparinization, shortens hospital stays and is safe and effective. Warfarin is continued for at least 3 months in all patients and for at least 6 months in patients with clinical risk factors, recurrent disease, or pulmonary embolism. The dosage of warfarin is adjusted to maintain a prothrombin time approximately 1.5 times control or an INR of 2.0 to 3.0. (The INR is a worldwide system used to standardize prothrombin times among laboratories.) (*Chapter 81, Page 717.*)

18.37 The patient is a 36-year-old white man who awoke in the early morning hours with retrosternal chest discomfort radiating to the neck that is aggravated by deep breathing, swallowing, or lying down. The pain seems to be relieved by sitting and leaning forward. Based on this history, the most likely diagnosis is

(A) acute MI
(B) unstable angina
(C) acute pericarditis
(D) atrial flutter
(E) costosternal arthralgia

Answer: (C). Acute pericarditis must always be considered when evaluating a patient with chest pain. Retrosternal discomfort that is worsened by lying down, deep breathing, swallowing, or moving is characteristic. There may be crushing retrosternal chest pain or pain radiating to the neck or arms. The pain is usually relieved by leaning forward or sitting. (*Chapter 82, Page 720.*)

18.38 The patient is a 32-year-old white man who is under your care for dilated cardiomyopathy. He is currently treated with sodium restriction, digitalis, and diuretics. Today, he complains of fatigue. His fatigue is most likely due to which of the following?

(A) hyponatremia
(B) low cardiac output
(C) depression
(D) digitalis toxicity
(E) hyperkalemia

Answer: (B). Fatigue associated with dilated cardiomyopathy is due to a low cardiac output state. (*Chapter 82, Page 721.*)

18.39 Which of the following cardiac diseases is genetically transmitted as an autosomal dominant?

(A) hypertrophic cardiomyopathy
(B) restrictive cardiomyopathy
(C) dilated cardiomyopathy

(D) pulmonary hypertension
(E) myocarditis

Answer: (A). Also known as idiopathic hypertrophic subaortic stenosis, asymmetric septal hypertrophy, obstructive cardiomyopathy, and muscular subaortic stenosis, hypertrophic cardiomyopathy is obstruction of the outflow tract. Transmission is genetic: autosomal dominant with variable but high penetrance. (*Chapter 82, Page 722.*)

18.40 The diagnosis of rheumatic fever involves use of the revised Jones criteria. The *major* Jones criteria include all EXCEPT which of the following?

(A) carditis
(B) polyarthritis
(C) chorea
(D) fever
(E) erythema marginatum

Answer: (D). The revised Jones criteria are used to help diagnose the patient with rheumatic fever. The presence of two major or one major and two minor criteria form the basis for the diagnosis. The major Jones criteria are carditis, polyarthritis, chorea, erythema marginatum, and subcutaneous nodules. Minor criteria (manifestations) include fever, arthralgia, previous acute rheumatic fever, or evidence of pre-existing rheumatic heart disease. (*Chapter 82, Page 723.*)

18.41 The patient is a 68-year-old white man who has a 5-month history of shortness of breath, substernal chest pain, and occasional fainting. There are murmurs consistent with tricuspid insufficiency and pulmonic regurgitation, associated with a loud P_2. The radiograph shows right heart enlargement, and the ECG is consistent with right ventricular hypertrophy. The most likely diagnosis in this patient is

(A) pulmonary hypertension
(B) mitral regurgitation
(C) patent foramen ovale
(D) restrictive cardiomyopathy
(E) hypertrophic cardiomyopathy

Answer: (A). The patient with pulmonary hypertension usually develops dyspnea, angina, and syncope. On physical examination, the patient may exhibit murmurs due to tricuspid and pulmonic regurgitation. A loud P_2 is common, as is a left parasternal systolic lift. The ECG is consistent with right ventricular hypertrophy. (*Chapter 82, Page 723.*)

DIRECTIONS (Items 18.42 through 18.90): Each of the items in this section is a multiple true–false problem that consists of a stem and four lettered options. Indicate whether each of the four options is TRUE or FALSE.

18.42 When evaluating a patient for hypertension, you are aware that certain drugs can increase blood pressure. These include which of the following?

(A) diuretics
(B) nasal decongestants
(C) NSAIDs
(D) oral contraceptives

Answer: (A-False, B-True, C-True, D-True). It is important to ensure that the patient is not on medications that may result in increased blood pressure, such as oral contraceptives, nasal decongestants, appetite suppressants, NSAIDs, and steroids. (*Chapter 75, Page 640.*)

18.43 The patient is a 46-year-old white man with high blood pressure who is currently taking no medication. You are considering prescribing an ACE inhibitor. True statements regarding this class of drugs include which of the following?

(A) These drugs generally increase renin levels.
(B) These drugs generally increase potassium levels.
(C) These drugs generally decrease renal blood flow.
(D) These drugs generally increase blood glucose levels.

Answer: (A-True, B-True, C-False, D-False). ACE inhibitors block the conversion of angiotensin I to angiotensin II, resulting in decreased aldosterone production with subsequent increased sodium and water excretion. Renin and potassium levels are usually increased as a result of this medication. The hemodynamic response includes decreased peripheral resistance, increased renal blood flow, and minimal changes in cardiac output and glomerular filtration rate. There is little change in insulin and glucose levels or in the lipid fractions. (*Chapter 75, Page 643.*)

18.44 The ACE inhibitors are an appropriate initial drug choice prescribed for hypertension in patients who also have

(A) diabetes mellitus
(B) congestive HF
(C) peripheral vascular disease
(D) renal insufficiency

Answer: (A-True, B-True, C-True, D-True). The ACE inhibitors are good first-line agents for patients with diabetes, congestive HF, peripheral vascular disease, elevated lipids, and renal insufficiency. This class is effective in all races and ages, although black patients respond better with addition of a diuretic. (*Chapter 75, Page 643.*)

18.45 The physiologic effects of angiotensin receptor blockers include which of the following?

(A) an increase in plasma renin
(B) a decrease in angiotensin II levels
(C) an increase in aldosterone production
(D) an increase in plasma potassium levels

Answer: (A-True, B-False, C-False, D-False). The physiologic effects of losartan include a rise in plasma renin and angiotensin II levels and a decrease in aldosterone production. There is no significant change in plasma potassium levels and no effect on glomerular filtration rate, renal plasma flow, heart rate, triglycerides, total cholesterol, high-density lipoprotein cholesterol, or glucose. Losartan use does produce a small uricosuric effect with lowering of plasma uric acid levels. (*Chapter 75, Page 643.*)

18.46 The physiologic effects of thiazide diuretics, when used in the treatment of hypertension, include which of the following?

(A) increased renal excretion of sodium and chloride
(B) increased plasma volume
(C) increased renal blood flow
(D) decreased potassium excretion

Answer: (A-True, B-False, C-False, D-False). Thiazide diuretics increase renal excretion of sodium and chloride at the distal segment of the renal tubule, resulting in decreased plasma volume, cardiac output, and renal blood flow and increased renin activity. Potassium excretion is increased, and calcium and uric acid elimination is decreased. (*Chapter 75, Page 646.*)

18.47 Spironolactone is a potassium-sparing diuretic sometimes used in the treatment of hypertension and various causes of edema. Adverse effects of this drug include

(A) gynecomastia
(B) nausea and vomiting
(C) muscle cramps
(D) hypokalemia

Answer: (A-True, B-True, C-True, D-False). Adverse reactions associated with spironolactone include gynecomastia, nausea, vomiting, diarrhea, muscle cramps, lethargy, and hyperkalemia. (*Chapter 75, Page 646.*)

18.48 The physiologic effects of antihypertensive direct vasodilators (e.g., hydralazine and minoxidil) include which of the following?

(A) peripheral vasoconstriction
(B) sympathetic reflex decrease in heart rate
(C) increased renin release
(D) sodium and water retention

Answer: (A-False, B-False, C-True, D-True). The two direct vasodilators, hydralazine (Apresoline) and minoxidil (Loniten), dilate peripheral arterioles, resulting in a significant fall in blood pressure. A sympathetic reflex increase in heart rate, renin and catecholamine release, and venous constriction occur. The renal response includes sodium and water retention. The patient often experiences tachycardia, flushing, and headache. (*Chapter 75, Page 647.*)

18.49 The patient is a 46-year-old black man with hypertension and asthma. Appropriate antihypertensive medications for this patient include

(A) calcium channel blockers
(B) central alpha$_2$-agonists
(C) alpha$_1$-blockers
(D) beta-blockers

Answer: (A-True, B-True, C-True, D-False). Asthma and chronic obstructive pulmonary disease patients may be effectively treated with calcium-entry antagonists, central alpha$_2$-agonists, and alpha$_1$-blockers. Beta-blockers and possibly diuretics should be avoided because they might exacerbate bronchospasm. (*Chapter 75, Page 648.*)

18.50 The patient is a 38-year-old married white man who participates in an active sports program. His blood pressure is 156/102. Appropriate therapeutic options for this patient include which of the following?

(A) ACE inhibitor
(B) beta-blocker
(C) calcium channel blocker
(D) diuretic

Answer: (A-True, B-False, C-True, D-False). An active young man would be better served with an ACE inhibitor, calcium-entry antagonist, or alpha-blocker, as

beta-blockers and diuretics may cause impotence and exercise intolerance. (*Chapter 75, Page 648.*)

18.51 The patient is a 56-year-old businessman who has recurrent chest pain and a history of epigastric distress in the past. You are interested in differentiating between cardiac and esophageal chest pain. Features suggesting esophageal origin include

(A) brief episodes of pain
(B) pain that interrupts sleep or is meal-related
(C) pain relieved by antacids
(D) absence of dysphagia

Answer: (A-False, B-True, C-True, D-False). The clinical history frequently does not differentiate between cardiac and esophageal chest pain, although certain features may be helpful in this process. Features suggesting esophageal origin include pain that continues for hours, pain that interrupts sleep or is meal-related, pain relieved by antacids, or the presence of other esophageal symptoms (heartburn, dysphagia, regurgitation). Conversely, it is well documented that gastroesophageal reflux may be triggered by heavy exercise and may produce exertional chest pain mimicking angina even during treadmill testing. (*Chapter 75, Page 651.*)

18.52 In exercise treadmill testing (ETT), factors that may lead to false-positive results include

(A) use of nitrates
(B) use of digoxin
(C) use of beta-blockers
(D) a submaximal effort

Answer: (A-False, B-True, C-False, D-False). Many factors influence the results of an ETT and can lead to false-positive or false-negative findings. Factors leading to false-positive results include (1) the use of medications such as digoxin, estrogens, and diuretics; and (2) conditions such as mitral valve prolapse, cardiomyopathy, and hyperventilation. Factors leading to false-negative results include (1) the use of medications such as nitrates, beta-blockers, and calcium channel blockers and (2) conditions such as a prior MI or a submaximal effort. (*Chapter 76, Page 653.*)

18.53 True statements regarding nitroglycerin use in IHD include which of the following?

(A) Most patients with recurrent angina-like chest pain who exhibit a prompt response to nitroglycerin have IHD.

(B) Patients who do not have IHD will generally see no change in their chest pain after taking nitroglycerin.

(C) Patients with unusually severe IHD may not respond to nitroglycerin.

(D) Failure to respond to nitroglycerin effectively excludes the diagnosis of IHD.

Answer: (A-True, B-True, C-True, D-False). It was concluded that 90% of patients with recurrent, angina-like chest pain who exhibit a prompt response to nitroglycerin (within 3 minutes) have IHD; however, a delayed or absent response paradoxically indicates either an absence of IHD or unusually severe disease. Therefore, failure to respond to nitroglycerin should not be used to exclude the diagnosis of IHD. (*Chapter 76, Page 654.*)

18.54 Nitrates, beta-blockers, and calcium channel blockers are all used in the treatment of angina pectoris. True statements regarding the actions of these drugs in angina pectoris include which of the following?

(A) Of the three, nitrates are the most effective in relieving chest pain.

(B) Of the three, calcium channel blockers are the most effective in decreasing exercise-induced ischemia.

(C) Each reduces myocardial oxygen demand.

(D) Only nitrates increase coronary blood flow to ischemic areas.

Answer: (A-False, B-False, C-True, D-False). Three classes of antianginal drugs are commonly used: nitrates, beta-blockers, and calcium channel blockers. Each reduces myocardial oxygen demand and may improve blood flow to the ischemic regions. The mechanisms by which these agents reduce myocardial oxygen demand or increase coronary blood flow to ischemic areas differ from one class of drug to another. No greater efficacy in relieving chest pain or decreasing exercise-induced ischemia has been shown for one or another group of drugs. (*Chapter 76, Page 654.*)

18.55 True statements regarding the antianginal effect of beta-blockers include which of the following?

(A) The effect of beta-blockers on angina pectoris is controversial.

(B) In patients with angina pectoris, beta-blockers can improve exercise tolerance.

(C) In patients with angina pectoris, beta-blockers do not reduce myocardial ischemia.

(D) In patients with angina pectoris, beta-blockers produce a reduction in myocardial oxygen demand.

Answer: (A-False, B-True, C-False, D-True). The antianginal effect of beta-blockers is well established. These agents improve exercise tolerance and reduce myocardial ischemia. The effect produces a reduction in myocardial oxygen demand through a reduction in heart rate and contractility. (*Chapter 76, Page 655.*)

18.56 In the treatment of a patient with angina pectoris, calcium channel blockers may be preferred in patients who also have

(A) obstructive airway disease

(B) constipation

(C) congestive HF

(D) peripheral vascular disease

Answer: (A-True, B-False, C-False, D-True). Calcium channel blockers may be preferred in patients with obstructive airway disease, hypertension, peripheral vascular disease, or supraventricular tachycardia. In general, they are well tolerated. The most troublesome side effects include constipation, edema, headache, and aggravation of congestive HF. (*Chapter 76, Page 655.*)

18.57 The patient is a 60-year-old white man who has had stable angina pectoris for about four years. Recently, there has been an increase in the frequency, severity, and duration of chest pain as well as an increasing incidence of symptoms occurring at rest or with multiple effort. In addition to other management, you are considering antiplatelet therapy. True statements regarding antiplatelet therapy in this clinical setting include which of the following?

(A) Antiplatelet therapy is contraindicated in this clinical setting.

(B) Antiplatelet therapy would be an important addition to other therapy for this patient.

(C) This patient's angina may be related to platelet aggregation and thrombus formation on the surface of an ulcerated plaque.

(D) The addition of aspirin in a dose of 325 mg/day may reduce this patient's risk of subsequent death from MI.

Answer: (A-False, B-True, C-True, D-True). Antiplatelet therapy is an important addition for patients with unstable angina. A number of studies have demonstrated that a common cause of crescendo angina is platelet aggregation and thrombus formation on the surface of an ulcerated plaque. In the Veterans Administration Cooperative Study, men with unstable angina who received aspirin (325 mg/day) had a 50% reduction in subsequent death from MI. (*Chapter 76, Page 657.*)

18.58 Silent ischemia presents difficulties in the diagnosis of ischemic heart disease (IHD). True statements regarding silent ischemia include which of the following?

(A) Silent ischemia occurs uncommonly.
(B) Silent ischemia is prevalent.
(C) Silent ischemia can be noted on 24-hour Holter monitoring.
(D) Patients with unstable angina rarely manifest painless ST segment depression.

Answer: (A-False, B-True, C-True, D-False). Silent ischemia is prevalent. Seventy percent of ischemic episodes in patients with IHD are estimated to be asymptomatic. Among patients with stable angina who undergo 24-hour Holter monitoring, 40 to 72% of the episodes are painless. Among patients with unstable angina, more than half manifest painless ST segment depression. (*Chapter 76, Page 658.*)

18.59 The patient is a 57-year-old black man who has a 1 hour history of substernal crushing chest pain radiating to the shoulder, associated with dyspnea. The ECG shows changes consistent with an acute MI. In this patient, signs that would suggest left ventricular dysfunction include which of the following?

(A) elevated blood pressure
(B) peripheral vasoconstriction
(C) pulse rate of 62
(D) elevated jugular venous pressure

Answer: (A-False, B-True, C-False, D-True). For the patient with an "uncomplicated MI," there are few physical examination findings. The main purpose of the examination is to assess the patient for evidence of complications from the MI and to establish a baseline for future comparisons. Signs of severe left ventricular dysfunction include hypotension, peripheral vasoconstriction, tachycardia, pulmonary rates, an S3, and elevated jugular venous pressure. (*Chapter 76, Page 659.*)

18.60 ECG changes typically associated with an acute MI include which of the following?

(A) the new appearance of Q waves
(B) prolongation of the QRS interval
(C) ST segment elevation
(D) T wave inversions

Answer: (A-True, B-False, C-True, D-True). Changes associated with an infarction are (1) the fresh appearance of Q waves or the increased prominence of preexisting ones; (2) ST segment elevations; and (3) T wave inversions. It is important to recognize that with acute MI, the ECG may be entirely normal or contain only "soft" ECG evidence of infarction. (*Chapter 76, Page 659.*)

18.61 True statements regarding the role of creatine kinase MB (CK-MB) in the diagnosis of acute MI include which of the following?

(A) Elevation of CK-MB is not essential for the diagnosis of acute MI.
(B) Acute elevations of CK-MB are generally due to myocardial necrosis.
(C) Noncardiac causes of an elevated CK-MB include trauma or surgery.
(D) In an acute MI, the peak level appearance of CK-MB occurs within 1 to 2 hours after the onset of symptoms.

Answer: (A-False, B-True, C-True, D-False). Elevation of the CK-MB isoenzyme is essential for the diagnosis of acute MI. In general, acute elevations of this enzyme are accounted for by myocardial necrosis. Detectable CK-MB from noncardiac causes is rare except during trauma or surgery. The peak level appearance of CK-MB is expected within 12 to 24 hours after the onset of symptoms. (*Chapter 76, Page 659.*)

18.62 You have just been called at home from the emergency department, where your patient has been brought by ambulance. The patient is a 57-year-old white man with the acute onset of severe substernal pain and dyspnea and with ECG changes consistent with an acute MI. His symptoms have been present for about 1 hour. The emergency department physician asks your feeling about thrombolytic therapy for your patient. True statements regarding thrombolytic therapy in this setting include which of the following?

(A) This patient may be a good candidate for thrombolytic therapy.
(B) It is already too late for thrombolytic therapy to be of value to this patient.
(C) Thrombolytic therapy can cause a reduction in mortality with early administration.
(D) When compared with placebo, administration of thrombolytic therapy within 6 hours from the onset of MI symptoms has shown no advantage over placebo.

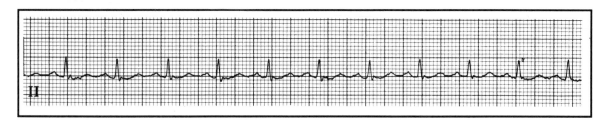

Fig. 18.8. Question 18.65.

Answer: (A-True, B-False, C-True, D-False). Early administration of thrombolytic therapy, within 6 hours from the onset of symptoms, has been associated with a reduction in mortality from acute MI. (*Chapter 76, Page 660.*)

18.63 The patient is a 44-year-old white woman who has the subjective sensation of palpitations, especially when in bed at night. A physical examination and ECG in your office are both normal. True statements regarding this patient include which of the following?

   (A) The patient appears to have a cardiac neurosis, and no further diagnostic studies are warranted.
   (B) Continuous ambulatory ECG monitoring for 24 to 48 hours may clarify the diagnosis.
   (C) Cardiac event monitoring may identify occasional episodes of cardiac arrhythmia.
   (D) There is generally close correlation between patient symptoms and events on the monitoring tracing.

Answer: (A-False, B-True, C-True, D-False). If the clinical history is suspicious for arrhythmia but the physical examination and ECG do not confirm its presence, 24- or 48-hour continuous ambulatory ECG monitoring or cardiac event monitoring may be performed to capture occasional periods of cardiac arrhythmia. However, studies have shown that rhythm abnormalities noted in the monitor tracing often have little temporal correspondence with patient symptoms as recorded in a symptom diary, and the clinical significance of this pattern of results is not clear. (*Chapter 77, Page 666.*)

18.64 The patient is a 42-year-old white man who has had some vague chest pain and a suspicion of palpitations. His blood pressure is 126/72. His pulse rate is noteworthy at 50 bpm. Further history should include questioning regarding which of the following?

   (A) athletic conditioning
   (B) hyperthyroidism

   (C) cocaine use
   (D) use of beta-blockers

Answer: (A-True, B-False, C-False, D-True). Sinus bradycardia consists of normally conducted cardiac impulses originating in the sinus node at a rate less than 60 bpm. It occurs in individuals at a high level of athletic conditioning, with vagal hyperactivity or pain, and during sleep. It can be a symptom of hypothyroidism and is often associated with medication use (e.g., narcotic analgesics, calcium channel antagonists, beta-blockers, digoxin, quinidine, procainamide). It can also occur in the setting of an inferior wall MI. (*Chapter 77, Page 670.*)

18.65 The ECG above is recorded from a 43-year-old white male laboratory worker. This patient should be questioned regarding which of the following possible causes?

   (A) hyperthyroidism
   (B) anemia
   (C) theophylline
   (D) propranolol

Answer: (A-True, B-True, C-True, D-False). Sinus tachycardia consists of normally conducted cardiac impulses originating in the sinus node at a rate of greater than 100 bpm. It may be asymptomatic or symptomatic, often described by patients as "palpitations" or a "racing heart." This rhythm is an appropriate response to the need for increased cardiac output and can be a normal finding in distressed or exercising individuals. However, its occurrence at rest is not normal and should lead to a search for an underlying cause. Possible causes include hyperthyroidism, fever, anemia, hypoxia, congestive HF, hypovolemia, anxiety, caffeine or other stimulants, and medication use (common nonprescription medications such as cold preparations with sympathomimetic effects, as well as tricyclic antidepressants, prazosin, and theophylline). (*Chapter 77, Page 672.*)

18.66 True statements about AF include which of the following?

(A) AF is the most common sustained supra-ventribular arrhythmia.
(B) The disease occurs chiefly in young and middle-aged persons.
(C) Approximately 9% of persons older than age 70 have AF.
(D) Although troublesome to the patient, it is rarely a cause for morbidity or mortality.

Answer: (A-True, B-False, C-True, D-False). AF is the most common sustained supraventricular arrhythmia and is primarily a disease of elderly patients, by one estimate affecting more than 3% of those older than 60 years of age and 9% of those older than 70. It represents a major cause of morbidity and mortality in the United States, particularly due to its association with embolic stroke. (*Chapter 77, Page 675.*)

18.67 The patient is a 62-year-old white woman with chronic AF. Appropriate medications for this patient include which of the following?

(A) digoxin
(B) beta-blockers
(C) calcium channel blockers
(D) none of the above

Answer: (A-True, B-True, C-True, D-False). Three types of antiarrhythmic drugs can be used to block AV node conduction and slow a rapid ventricular rate: digoxin, beta-blockers, and calcium channel blockers. (*Chapter 77, Page 675.*)

18.68 True statements regarding warfarin in stroke prevention in AF patients include which of the following?

(A) Warfarin is no longer recommended for primary stroke prevention in AF patients.
(B) Warfarin is recommended for primary stroke prevention in AF patients older than 60 years of age who are not at high risk for bleeding complications.
(C) Warfarin is recommended for primary stroke prevention in AF patients younger than 60 who have no additional risk factors for stroke.
(D) The use of warfarin for prevention of stroke is especially cost-effective in AF patients aged 75 and older.

Answer: (A-False, B-True, C-False, D-False). At present, warfarin is recommended for primary stroke prevention in AF patients older than 60 years of age who are not at high risk for bleeding complications

and in patients younger than 60 with additional risk factors for stroke. The higher risk of bleeding complications in those older than 75 years of age makes prevention far less cost-effective in this age group, and decisions regarding warfarin use must be individualized. (*Chapter 77, Page 675.*)

18.69 In auscultation of the heart, the third heart sound (S_3)

(A) is heard late during diastole
(B) occurs immediately after the opening of the tricuspid and mitral valves
(C) occurs when ventricular filling is most rapid
(D) is best heard with the patient seated in the upright position

Answer: (A-False, B-True, C-True, D-False). The third heart sound (S_3) is heard early during diastole, immediately after the opening of the tricuspid and mitral valves, when ventricular filling is most rapid. The S_3 is a low-pitched sound, usually soft. It is best heard with the patient in the left lateral decubitus position and the bell of the stethoscope placed lightly over the cardiac apex. (*Chapter 78, Page 683.*)

18.70 A third heart sound (S_3) heard in a 62-year-old patient may be caused by which of the following?

(A) AF
(B) ventricular diastolic overload
(C) ventricular dysfunction
(D) constrictive pericarditis

Answer: (A-False, B-True, C-True, D-True). An S_3 heard after age 40 can be caused by three types of cardiac disease: ventricular diastolic overload, ventricular dysfunction, and constrictive pericarditis. (*Chapter 78, Page 684.*)

18.71 The fourth heart sound (S_4)

(A) is sometimes called the "atrial gallop"
(B) occurs during atrial filling
(C) is related to vibration of the ventricles at the time of atrial contraction
(D) is best heard with the patient sitting and using the diaphragm of the stethoscope

Answer: (A-True, B-False, C-True, D-False). The fourth heart sound (S_4) is known as the "atrial gallop." It is caused by the sudden distension and vibration of the ventricles at the time of atrial contraction. S_4 is best heard with the patient in the left lateral decubitus position and the bell of the stethoscope placed lightly over the cardiac apex. (*Chapter 78, Page 684.*)

18.72 Approximately 90% or more of murmurs identified by family physicians are physiologic murmurs. Examples of physiologic murmurs include those associated with which of the following?

(A) anemia
(B) mitral valve regurgitation
(C) increased blood volume of normal pregnancy
(D) patent foramen ovale

Answer: (A-True, B-False, C-True, D-False). Murmurs are physiologic when there is an identifiable cause but the heart is normal. Examples of physiologic murmurs include the murmurs heard with anemia, thyrotoxicosis, the increased blood volume of normal pregnancy, and the high output state caused by fever. (*Chapter 78, Page 685.*)

18.73 True statements regarding the characteristics of innocent murmurs include which of the following?

(A) These murmurs are generally best heard at the apex.
(B) Innocent murmurs are always systolic.
(C) Innocent murmurs are rarely louder than grade 2/6.
(D) Innocent murmurs are typically short in duration.

Answer: (A-False, B-True, C-True, D-True). Innocent murmurs are usually best heard along the left sternal border, between the second and the fourth intercostal spaces. Innocent murmurs are always systolic and are rarely louder than grade 2/6. They begin shortly after Sl. The intensity of innocent murmurs is early peaking, and the murmur is typically short, ending early enough that S2 is clearly heard. Innocent murmurs are not heard well at the apex. (*Chapter 78, Page 685.*)

18.74 The murmur of mitral regurgitation is often described as

(A) an atrial gallop
(B) presystolic
(C) "plateau" in intensity
(D) "blowing" in quality

Answer: (A-False, B-False, C-True, D-True). The murmur of mitral regurgitation is a holosystolic murmur. It is described as "plateau" in intensity and "blowing" in quality. (*Chapter 78, Page 686.*)

18.75 The patient is a 23-year-old female graduate student with occasional mild palpitations and chest pain. On cardiac examination, the first and second heart sounds are normal, and there is a high-pitched midsystolic click and a mid- to late systolic murmur that follows the click and ends before the second heart sound. True statements regarding this patient and her findings include which of the following?

(A) The physical findings noted are likely to be constant from visit to visit.
(B) An increase in afterload or preload will make the click and murmur occur later.
(C) An increase in the preload will make the murmur louder.
(D) Following a compensatory pause after a premature beat, the click and murmur of mitral valve prolapse should occur later and may be softer.

Answer: (A-False, B-True, C-False, D-True). The findings in mitral valve prolapse are inconstant. There may be no click or murmur one day, but the next day these findings are obvious. An increase in afterload or preload makes the click and murmur occur later, and a decrease in preload makes the click earlier and the murmur louder. The click and murmur of mitral valve prolapse should occur later and may be softer during the beat following the compensatory pause after a premature beat. (*Chapter 78, Page 687.*)

18.76 True statements regarding patients with aortic insufficiency include which of the following?

(A) These patients are sometimes described as flushed and sweaty.
(B) A normal blood pressure in the presence of normal ventricular function is common in moderate or severe disease.
(C) With severe regurgitation, a wide pulse pressure is common.
(D) In patients with moderate to severe disease, the peripheral pulses are often soft and difficult to palpate.

Answer: (A-True, B-False, C-True, D-False). Patients with aortic insufficiency are often described as flushed and sweaty. Their skin is warm, and until the late stages of the disease, they look healthy. Blood pressure can be normal in aortic insufficiency, but a normal blood pressure in the presence of normal ventricular function virtually rules out moderate or severe disease. With severe regurgitation, there is a wide pulse pressure, and the width of the pulse pressure correlates with the severity of the disease until the left ventricle starts to fail. The fourth Korotkoff sound, muffling, is a more valid indicator of diastolic pressure than the fifth sound, which can sometimes be heard down to 0 mm Hg. The peripheral pulses are bounding and collapsing in nature. (*Chapter 78, Page 688.*)

18.77 The patient is a 78-year-old white female with valvular heart disease who has arrived in the emergency department with cardiogenic pulmonary edema. As part of your emergency management, you plan to use morphine. True statements regarding the use of morphine in this situation include which of the following?

(A) The drug is a potent venoconstrictor.
(B) Part of morphine's action on pulmonary edema is its tendency to reduce anxiety.
(C) Morphine can cause or worsen hypotension.
(D) The starting dose in acute pulmonary edema is 10 to 15 mg intramuscularly.

Answer: (A-False, B-True, C-True, D-False). Morphine has long had a role in the treatment of cardiogenic pulmonary edema but must be used with caution. It is a potent venodilator and also reduces anxiety. However, it can cause or worsen hypotension and may mask symptoms and signs that are important for the clinician to observe when assessing these patients. The starting dose is 1 to 3 mg intravenously; subsequent doses can be titrated according to the patient's response. (*Chapter 79, Page 694.*)

18.78 The patient is a 76-year-old white woman whom you are treating for chronic HF, which has become worse despite appropriate medication. The patient and her family have some questions regarding prognosis. True statements regarding the outlook in HF include which of the following?

(A) The outlook for this patient achieving a near-normal life expectancy remains good with adequate therapy.
(B) With optimal treatment, there is a 10% annual mortality.
(C) Many persons with chronic congestive HF die suddenly.
(D) The mortality risk from HF is greater among African Americans than among whites.

Answer: (A-False, B-True, C-True, D-True). Despite medical and surgical advances in the treatment of HF, the prognosis generally remains grim. Overall mortality for optimally treated HF is about 10% annually, with a 5-year mortality of 50%. Approximately 30 to 50% of these deaths are sudden. Data from the Framingham Study suggest that this 5-year mortality has not changed appreciably since the 1930s. African Americans have about a 1.5-fold higher risk of mortality from HF than whites. (*Chapter 79, Page 696.*)

18.79 True statements regarding diuretic therapy in patients with heart failure (HF) include which of the following?

(A) Diuretics are appropriate only for HF patients who demonstrate evidence of fluid volume overload.
(B) Diuretics promote renal excretion of sodium and water.
(C) Diuretics block the renin-angiotensin-aldosterone axis.
(D) Diuretics may decrease cardiac output, especially in patients with diastolic dysfunction.

Answer: (A-True, B-True, C-False, D-True). Diuretic therapy is used only in patients with HF who demonstrate symptoms or signs of fluid volume overload ("congestive" HF). Diuretics improve the clinical status of patients with congestive HF by promoting renal excretion of sodium and water, but they also activate the renin-angiotensin-aldosterone axis, potentiate the hypotensive effect of ACE inhibitors, and may decrease cardiac output, especially in patients with diastolic dysfunction. Therefore, diuretics should not be used "routinely" in all patients with HF. (*Chapter 79, Page 699.*)

18.80 Metozalone (Zaroxolyn) is a diuretic commonly used in patients with refractory HF. True statements regarding metolazone include which of the following?

(A) The typical starting dose is 25 mg once daily.
(B) Volume depletion and hypotension may occur.
(C) Hypokalemia may occur.
(D) Hypermagnesemia may occur.

Answer: (A-False, B-True, C-True, D-False). Metolazone is a diuretic commonly reserved for patients with severe or refractory HF because of its potency. It must be used with great caution. A typical starting dose of metolazone is 2.5 mg once daily. The major side effects are similar to those of other diuretic agents: volume depletion, hypotension, hypokalemia, and hypomagnesemia. (*Chapter 79, Page 700.*)

18.81 The patient is a 46-year-old white woman who has had several episodes of syncope over the past few months. The episodes are not related to position change or to meals, and there have been no headaches, chest pains, or other suspicious symptoms. As part of your evaluation, you will do a drug history, searching for medications that commonly cause syncope. These include which of the following?

(A) nitrates
(B) corticosteroids
(C) vasodilators
(D) beta-blockers

Answer: (A-True, B-False, C-True, D-True). The most common drugs causing syncope include nitrates, vasodilators, and beta-blockers. (*Chapter 80, Page 705.*)

18.82 The patient is an 82-year-old white woman who has had several syncopal episodes. Her supine blood pressure is 110/70, which drops to 82 over 66 with standing. The cardiac examination is normal. Appropriate management of this patient's problem might include

(A) wearing supportive stockings from toe to thigh
(B) raising the head of the bed at night
(C) increasing periods of prolonged standing, which can help to develop pressor reflexes
(D) use of fludrocortisone

Answer: (A-True, B-True, C-False, D-True). Elderly patients who become syncopal with positional changes and who demonstrate orthostatic hypertension are encouraged to wear supportive stockings (to the thigh), raise the head of the bed at night, rise from the bed or chair slowly, avoid prolonged standing, and maintain an appropriate electrolyte balance. They should avoid medications that may cause syncope. Fludrocortisone (0.1 to 1.0 mg/day) in conjunction with increased salt intake has been shown to be effective. Various adrenergic agents have been used, including ephedrine, phenylephrine, and others. (*Chapter 80, Page 707.*)

18.83 Vasopressors are often used in the treatment of cardiogenic shock if volume infusion is contraindicated (in the setting of pulmonary edema) or ineffectual. The initial vasopressor used is usually dopamine. True statements regarding dopamine use in the setting of cardiogenic shock include which of the following?

(A) The effects of dopamine are dose-dependent.
(B) At low doses, dopamine constricts renal and mesenteric vessels.
(C) At intermediate doses (2 to 10 μg/kg/min), dopamine has significant inotropic effects that increase cardiac output.
(D) At high doses, dopamine causes peripheral vasoconstriction.

Answer: (A-True, B-False, C-True, D-True). The effects of dopamine are dose-dependent. At low doses (1 to 2 μg/kg/min IV), dopamine dilates renal and mesenteric vessels. At intermediate doses (2 to 10 μg/kg/min IV), it maintains splanchnic effects but has significant beta-adrenergic receptor (inotropic) effects, which result in increased cardiac output. At high doses (greater than 10 mg/kg/min IV) increasing alpha-adrenergic receptor effects and peripheral vasoconstriction occur. (*Chapter 80, Page 709.*)

18.84 The greatest risk of DVT in hospitalized patients occurs in which of the following settings?

(A) surgery of the pelvis or lower extremities
(B) young patients undergoing surgery
(C) early ambulation following surgery
(D) anesthesia lasting more than 30 minutes

Answer: (A-True, B-False, C-False, D-True). The Worcester DVT study, a regional survey of hospital discharge diagnoses, reported a diagnosis of DVT in 0.9% of all hospital discharges. The incidence rates increased exponentially with age, rising by a factor of approximately 200 between ages 20 and 80 years. Studies using screening techniques to evaluate hospitalized patients identified surgery of the pelvis or lower extremity and anesthesia lasting more than 30 minutes as the highest risk events. More patients hospitalized for medical reasons experience an episode of DVT than surgical patients because of the greater number of total admissions. (*Chapter 81, Page 713.*)

18.85 Impedance plethysmography (IPG) can be useful in the diagnosis of DVT. True statements regarding this technique include which of the following?

(A) The technique measures venous filling following extrinsic venous compression.
(B) The test has a sensitivity of only 60% in the diagnosis of proximal DVT.
(C) The test is limited in that it is invasive and cannot be performed at the bedside.
(D) IPG cannot accurately diagnose thrombi below the knee.

Answer: (A-True, B-False, C-False, D-True). IPG measures maximal filling of the venous system in the leg after extrinsic venous compression with a thigh cuff and venous emptying during the first 3 seconds after its release. Several large studies have shown it to be an accurate test for proximal DVT, with sensitivity of 95% and specificity of 96%. It is noninvasive and can be performed at the bedside. IPG cannot be used to accurately diagnose thrombi below the knee because venous outflow obstruction is less impaired by thrombi in the calf. (*Chapter 81, Page 715.*)

18.86 The major complications of heparin therapy include

(A) disseminated intravascular coagulation
(B) thrombocytopenia
(C) osteoporosis
(D) anaphylaxis

Answer: (A-False, B-True, C-True, D-True). The major complications of heparin therapy include hemorrhage, thrombocytopenia, osteoporosis, and anaphylaxis. The risk of hemorrhage is increased with increased age, significant coexistent illness, and the presence of known bleeding sites. (*Chapter 81, Page 717.*)

18.87 Prophylaxis against bacterial endocarditis is recommended in which of the following clinical situations?

(A) a 62-year-old white woman with a prosthetic heart valve
(B) an 8-year-old child with a functional heart murmur
(C) a 26-year-old white man with mitral stenosis of rheumatic origin
(D) a 25-year-old white woman with a midsystolic click

Answer: (A-True, B-False, C-True, D-False). Endocarditis prophylaxis is recommended when treating patients with the following high-risk cardiac conditions: previous endocarditis, prosthetic heart valves, congenital cardiac malformations, rheumatic and other acquired valvular disorders, a history of valvular surgery, hypertrophic cardiomyopathy, and mitral valve prolapse with valvular regurgitation. (*Chapter 82, Page 719.*)

18.88 In a 38-year-old white female with mitral regurgitation secondary to rheumatic heart disease, prophylaxis against bacterial endocarditis is indicated for which of the following procedures?

(A) urethral catheterization
(B) dilation and curettage
(C) insertion of an intrauterine contraceptive device
(D) uncomplicated vaginal delivery

Answer: (A-False, B-False, C-False, D-False). In the absence of infection, urethral catheterization, dilation and curettage, uncomplicated vaginal delivery, therapeutic abortion, sterilization procedures, and insertion or removal of an intrauterine device do not require prophylaxis. (*Chapter 82, Page 720.*)

18.89 Pericarditis can be caused by ingestion of certain medications, including which of the following?

(A) isoniazid (INH)
(B) indomethacin (Indocin)
(C) procainamide (Procan)
(D) hydralazine (Apresoline)

Answer: (A-True, B-False, C-True, D-True). Pericarditis is inflammation of the parietal and visceral pericardium. Causes of pericarditis include infection (viral agents most commonly), postcardiac injury, collagen vascular disease, uremia, tumor, myxedema, irradiation, and medications such as INH, procainamide, and hydralazine. (*Chapter 82, Page 720.*)

18.90 Which of the following clinical findings is/are characteristic of pericarditis?

(A) leukopenia
(B) pericardial friction rub
(C) deep Q waves on the ECG
(D) diffuse ST elevations on the ECG

Answer: (A-False, B-True, C-False, D-True). The diagnosis of pericarditis is based on clinical suspicion (i.e., the presence of sharp anterior chest pain, leukocytosis, a pericardial friction rub, and diffuse ST segment elevation). Further diagnostic workup includes echocardiography to rule out pericardial effusion. (*Chapter 82, Page 720.*)

19

The Respiratory System

The questions in this chapter constitute a review of the following chapters in *Family Medicine: Principles and Practice, Fifth Edition:*

    Obstructive Airway Disease (Chapter 83)
    Pulmonary Infections (Chapter 84)
    Lung Cancer (Chapter 85)
    Selected Disorders of the Respiratory System
      (Chapter 86)

DIRECTIONS (Items 19.1 through 19.18): Each of the questions or incomplete statements in this section is followed by five suggested answers or completions. Select the ONE that is BEST in each case.

19.1 The patient is an 18-year-old white man who has had a few episodes of expiratory wheezing over the past year, and occasionally has wheezing during exercise. In addition to avoidance therapy, the medication of choice (if medication is needed) would be

    (A) beta$_2$-adrenergic agonist
    (B) steroid inhaler
    (C) oral steroids
    (D) oral theophylline
    (E) cromolyn sodium

Answer: (A). Beta$_2$s are the treatment of choice for episodic or mild asthmatics and for exercise-induced bronchospasm. Once the need is established for continual usage, as for moderate and severe asthmatics, some authorities use these agents as first-line treatment whereas others reserve their use for rescue efforts, preferring to use anti-inflammatory drugs first. Certainly, every patient with significant obstructive disease should always have this medication on hand. (*Chapter 83, Page 730.*)

19.2 You have just accepted a position with an inner-city medical center in an area with a relatively high acquired immunodeficiency syndrome (AIDS) prevalence. In this setting, the leading cause of community-acquired pneumonia (CAP) hospital admissions is likely to be

    (A) *Streptococcus pneumoniae*
    (B) *Mycoplasma pneumoniae*
    (C) *Chlamydia pneumoniae*
    (D) *Haemophilus influenzae*
    (E) *Pneumocystis carinii*

Answer: (E). If the AIDS prevalence is one or more per 1,000 hospital discharges, *P. carinii* pneumonia can be the leading cause of CAP hospital admissions. (*Chapter 84, Page 734.*)

19.3 In a patient with pneumonia, which of the following five symptoms is *most* likely to be present?

    (A) cough
    (B) dyspnea
    (C) sputum production
    (D) chest pain
    (E) hemoptysis

Answer: (A). The signs and symptoms of pneumonia are well recognized. In a study of 453 patients with pneumonia, cough was present in 88%, dyspnea in 71%, sputum production in 69%, chest pain in 64%, hemoptysis in 17%, and confusion in 17%. (*Chapter 84, Page 734.*)

19.4 The patient is a 68-year-old white male smoker with fever, left-sided chest pain, shortness of breath, and rusty sputum. The chest radiograph confirms the presence of a left lower lobe pneumonia. Gram stain of the sputum shows gram-positive diplococci. The treatment of choice for this patient is

(A) a macrolide
(B) a tetracycline
(C) a cephalosporin
(D) penicillin
(E) vancomycin

Answer: (D). If the Gram stain shows the classic picture of pneumococci with abundant gram-positive lancet-shaped diplococci, both extracellularly and intracellularly, penicillin is the treatment of choice if resistance is not an issue. (*Chapter 84, Page 736.*)

19.5 The laboratory finding characteristic of patients with *Mycoplasma* pneumonia is

(A) an elevated sedimentation rate
(B) an elevated cold agglutinin titer
(C) leukopenia
(D) eosinophilia
(E) lymphocytosis

Answer: (B). The most common laboratory finding with *Mycoplasma* pneumonia patients is an elevated cold agglutinin titer, seen in up to 75%. This test, however, also has many false-positives, and cold agglutinins are also present in up to 25% of patients with a viral pneumonia. (*Chapter 84, Page 738.*)

19.6 Legionnaire's disease is most likely to be contracted by

(A) ingesting contaminated food
(B) inhalation of aerosolized water particles
(C) fecal contamination
(D) exposure to droplet infection spread by coughing
(E) exposure to an infected dog or cat

Answer: (B). *Legionella* bacteria are found in water, and institutional water systems (e.g., cooling towers, condensers, showers, nebulizers) are an important source for infection. Transmission seems to be exclusively from the environment, not person to person. Inhalation or ingestion of aerosolized particles is a likely means of lung infection. (*Chapter 84, Page 739.*)

19.7 In the United States, histoplasmosis is most likely to be found in which of the following areas?

(A) tropical areas of south Florida
(B) the Southwest United States including the San Joaquin Valley

(C) the Pacific Northwest
(D) the Rocky Mountain region, especially in the higher elevations
(E) the Ohio and Mississippi River valleys

Answer: (E). Histoplasmosis is caused by a fungus found in moist soil throughout the temperate zones of the world (in the United States especially in the Ohio and Mississippi River valleys). (*Chapter 84, Page 739.*)

19.8 The patient is a 43-year-old farmer who until recently lived in northwest Ohio. He has had a mild recurrent cough for 6 to 8 months. His histoplasmosis skin test is positive, and the chest radiograph shows bilateral patchy lower lobe densities with some hilar lymph node enlargement. This patient should be treated with

(A) erythromycin
(B) rifampin
(C) ciprofloxacin
(D) itraconazole
(E) no treatment is necessary

Answer: (E). In a normal host, no treatment is usually needed. Therapy of life-threatening chronic or disseminated histoplasmosis requires high-dose intravenous amphotericin given over 8 to 12 weeks. In patients with less life-threatening situations, such as those with progressive disseminated histoplasmosis, or AIDS patients needing chronic suppressive therapy, itraconazole is the drug of choice. (*Chapter 84, Page 740.*)

19.9 The term *valley fever* is a synonym for

(A) tuberculosis
(B) coccidioidomycosis
(C) byssinosis
(D) *Pneumocystis carinii* pneumonia
(E) histoplasmosis

Answer: (B). *Coccidioides,* a fungus, is found in the soil of the semiarid Southwest. Dust storms, outdoor recreation, and new construction are associated with an increased risk of infection. The primary infection, which results from inhaling the arthrospore, is usually asymptomatic, although up to 40% have symptoms of acute "valley fever" with cough, low-grade fever, and often arthralgias or erythema nodosum. (*Chapter 84, Page 740.*)

19.10 Most active tuberculosis (TB) is reactivation of an earlier primary infection. Which of the following is most likely to cause reactivation to occur?

(A) Parkinson's disease
(B) *Mycoplasma* pneumonia
(C) emotional stress
(D) AIDS
(E) Type II diabetes mellitus under good control

Answer: (D). Between 70 and 90% of active TB is reactivation, that is, a breakdown of these foci years later. Why it happens is poorly understood. Risk factors for active TB include recent weight loss (associated with malnutrition or alcoholism), poorly controlled diabetes, and immunosuppression (from steroids, AIDS, or cancer). Human immunodeficiency virus (HIV) has been called the most potent activator of TB ever detected. (*Chapter 84, Page 740.*)

19.11 The leading concern in the use of INH for the chemoprophylaxis of tuberculosis is

(A) fatigue
(B) drug-induced renal disease
(C) drug-induced leukopenia
(D) drug-induced hepatitis
(E) vasospasm causing angina pectoris

Answer: (D). The most common concern about INH is drug-induced hepatitis. The overall incidence is about 1%, although it is age-related. In persons younger than age 20, hepatitis is rare, whereas in those older than age 50 it occurs in more than 2%. (*Chapter 84, Page 742.*)

19.12 Carcinogens found in cigarette smoke include all EXCEPT which of the following?

(A) benzopyrene
(B) cadmium
(C) hydrazine
(D) vinyl chloride
(E) nicotine

Answer: (E). Cigarette smoke with its identified carcinogens, such as benzopyrene, dibenzanthracene, nitrosamines, nickel, cadmium, hydrazine, vinyl chloride, and others, account for 80% of lung cancer in men and 75% of lung cancer in women. Nicotine is not considered carcinogenic but, rather, a highly addictive substance that leads to continued exposure to cigarette carcinogens. (*Chapter 85, Page 746.*)

19.13 The patient is a 58-year-old with a 60 pack/year history of smoking. He has a 6-month history of hemoptysis, cough, and dyspnea. The patient has shoulder pain radiating down the left arm. The chest radiograph shows a tumor, 6 cm in diameter, in the apex of the left lung. This patient appears to have

(A) squamous cell tumor of the lung
(B) a small-cell carcinoma of the lung
(C) a mediastinal tumor
(D) a Pancoast tumor of the lung
(E) sarcoidosis

Answer: (D). Pancoast tumors originate in the apex of the lung and present with shoulder pain that can radiate down the arm, caused by invasion of the brachial plexus. Routine chest radiographs are often normal, and apical lordotic views of the lung or a computed tomography scan is often needed to detect Pancoast tumors. (*Chapter 85, Page 748.*)

19.14 The patient is a 72-year-old white male retired shipyard worker with a long history of smoking one pack of cigarettes daily. For the past 5 months, he has had shortness of breath and some swelling of the right arm. You note some venous distension in the neck, distension of veins in the chest, and a hint of cyanosis. This patient is most likely to have which of the following diagnoses?

(A) pulmonary embolus from a thrombosis in the lower extremity
(B) lung cancer involving the mediastinum
(C) syphilitic aortitis
(D) primary pulmonary hypertension
(E) pulmonary TB

Answer: (B). Blood flow through the superior vena cava can be obstructed by bulky tumors in the mediastinum, producing the superior vena cava syndrome. These patients can have venous distension in the neck (66%), dyspnea (63%), distension of the veins on the chest wall (54%), facial edema (46%), cyanosis (20%), and arm swelling (18%). Of all patients who present with the superior vena cava syndrome, 65% have lung cancer. (*Chapter 85, Page 748.*)

19.15 The patient is a 56-year-old white man retired tunnel worker whom you treated in the office yesterday for an acute left lower lobe pneumonia. This morning, the patient went to the emergency department. The nurse at the emergency department calls and reports that the patient has dyspnea and a pulse of 106. Blood gases show a decreased PO_2 and a normal PCO_2. She administered oxygen by mask, and although improving initially, the patient has become more dyspneic. Based on this telephone conversation, this patient appears to have

(A) acute pulmonary embolism
(B) sepsis
(C) acute pneumothorax
(D) acute pneumoconiosis
(E) acute respiratory distress syndrome (ARDS)

Answer: (E). ARDS should be considered when any patient with one or more known causative factors develops dyspnea and tachypnea. Blood gases show decreased PO_2, with the PCO_2 normal or decreased. After initially responding to supplemental O_2, the patient becomes more dyspneic, and the hypoxia can no longer be corrected by giving O_2. Rales and bilateral interstitial infiltrates develop. At this point the patient requires ventilator management in an intensive care unit setting with Swan-Ganz monitoring and involvement of a pulmonary or intensivist consultant if available. (*Chapter 86, Page 753.*)

19.16 Most pulmonary emboli originate from

(A) deep veins of the calf
(B) superficial veins of the lower extremity
(C) deep veins of the thigh and pelvis
(D) deep veins of the upper extremity
(E) right atrial thrombi

Answer: (C). Most pulmonary emboli originate from the deep veins of the thigh and pelvis. Thrombi usually develop from vein bifurcations or valve cusps; they may also arise in the calf but rarely embolize. Deep vein thrombosis (DVT) may arise in the upper extremity, with most cases seen in patients with central venous catheters, although spontaneous DVT of the upper extremity does occur. Right atrial thrombus during atrial fibrillation is also a potential source. (*Chapter 86, Page 754.*)

19.17 The patient is a 17-year-old white boy who suffered a cramp while swimming in a lake and was pulled to shore, where he briefly received cardiopulmonary resuscitation. He has been brought to the emergency department, where he is alert and coherent. He complains of severe left-sided chest pain and shortness of breath. The respiratory rate is 42, and his pulse rate is 112 bpm. Based on this evidence, you suspect that this patient may have

(A) aspiration of lake water
(B) anoxia-induced angina pectoris
(C) flail chest
(D) ARDS
(E) traumatic pneumothorax

Answer: (E). A traumatic pneumothorax can result from penetrating or nonpenetrating chest trauma as well as from such invasive procedures as bronchoscopy, thoracentesis, central line placement, mechanical ventilation, and cardiopulmonary resuscitation. (*Chapter 86, Page 756.*)

19.18 The patient is a 70-year-old white woman with a cough, shortness of breath, and a right pleural effusion. On tapping the effusion, you find pleural fluid characteristics of a transudative effusion. The most common cause of a transudative effusion is

(A) pulmonary embolus
(B) neoplasm
(C) collagen vascular disease
(D) congestive heart failure
(E) acute pancreatitis

Answer: (D). The major causes of a transudative effusion are congestive heart failure (most common), cirrhosis, nephrotic syndrome, and hypoalbuminemia. The most common groups causing exudative effusions are infection (most commonly bacterial pneumonia and tuberculosis), pulmonary embolism, neoplasms, collagen vascular diseases, pancreatitis, and other intra-abdominal diseases. (*Chapter 86, Page 756.*)

DIRECTIONS (Items 19.19 through 19.34): Each of the items in this section is a multiple true–false problem that consists of a stem and four lettered options. Indicate whether each of the four options is TRUE or FALSE.

19.19 While performing pulmonary function testing for the diagnosis of asthma, it is sometimes useful to use provocative testing. Stimulators that may be used for provocative testing include which of the following?

(A) exercise
(B) terbutaline
(C) histamine
(D) methacholine

Answer: (A-True, B-False, C-True, D-True). With asthma, a useful test is to observe the change in FEV_1 following treatment with a bronchodilator. An increase of 15% is indicative of reversible airway disease. Three stimulators—exercise, histamine, and methacholine—may be used for provocative testing. A decrease in FEV_1 of 20% is considered positive. (*Chapter 83, Page 727.*)

19.20 Cromolyn is often used as a prophylactic agent in asthma; it is an anti-inflammatory drug with an almost complete lack of side effects. True statements regarding cromolyn include which of the following?

(A) The drug is available in syrup, tablet, and injectable forms.
(B) The initial dosage frequency is four times daily.
(C) This prophylactic medication should be discontinued during an acute episode.
(D) Cromolyn may be useful in the prevention of exercise-induced bronchospasm.

Answer: (A-False, B-True, C-False, D-True). Cromolyn (Intal) is available for multiple dose inhaler or nebulizer. Its onset of action can be as long as 1 to 2 months. Dosage is two inhalations q.i.d.; tapering to less frequent dosage can be attempted. Once in usage this medication should be used throughout an acute episode so as not to lose the prophylaxis. Along with beta$_2$s and inhaled steroids, cromolyn is useful for exercise-induced bronchospasm. (*Chapter 83, Page 731.*)

19.21 The patient is a 23-year-old primigravida at 15 weeks' gestation. She has asthma that antedated her pregnancy and now has expiratory wheezing and cough. In the setting of asthma during pregnancy, which of the following medications are generally considered safe for use?

(A) theophylline
(B) beta$_2$-adrenergic agonists
(C) iodides
(D) cromolyn

Answer: (A-True, B-True, C-False, D-True). Pregnancy is complicated by asthma about 1% of the time, with a potentially large risk to the fetus if hypoxia develops. The use of theophylline, beta$_2$s, cromolyn, and steroids is generally considered safe. Some antibiotics and decongestants, live virus vaccines, and iodides must be avoided. (*Chapter 83, Page 732.*)

19.22 True statements regarding asthma include which of the following?

(A) The disease may cause death.
(B) Preventable hospitalization may occur because of the patient's or family's inability to recognize the severity of an attack.
(C) Preventable death may occur because of the physician's inadequate assessment of the severity of an attack.
(D) Peak flow meters have not been useful as an objective guide to the severity of an asthma attack.

Answer: (A-True, B-True, C-True, D-False). Asthma is usually viewed as a nonfatal disease, but it does carry the potential for death. Most studies show that preventable deaths and hospitalizations have been the result of delayed treatment due primarily to two factors: the patient's or family's inability to recognize the severity of an attack, or the physician's poor assessment of the severity of an attack. Suggestions for prevention include frequent use of peak flow meters as an objective guide to severity, establishing effective maintenance therapy, and emphasizing patient and family education. (*Chapter 83, Page 732.*)

19.23 True statements regarding the use of pneumococcal vaccine include which of the following?

(A) The vaccine should be recommended to patients with chronic obstructive pulmonary disease (COPD).
(B) Because of the immunodeficiency, pneumococcal vaccine is contraindicated in HIV-positive patients.
(C) The vaccine is indicated in patients who have undergone splenectomy.
(D) In very elderly patients, revaccination is advisable every 6 to 7 years.

Answer: (A-True, B-False, C-True, D-True). The use of pneumococcal vaccine in the elderly or those with underlying conditions (e.g., COPD, transplants, HIV-positive, splenectomy) probably reduces the chances of pneumococcal pneumonia by 60 to 80%. It is less effective in the very old and the institutionalized, in whom revaccination every 6 to 7 years is indicated. (*Chapter 84, Page 737.*)

19.24 Legionnaire's disease often presents like a bacterial pneumonia with a high fever, shaking chills, and a minimally productive cough. The physical examination is often similar to that for other pneumonias. Some features that may be helpful in the diagnosis of Legionnaire's disease include which of the following?

(A) Leukopenia is common.
(B) Hyponatremia may occur in more than half of all patients.
(C) The chest radiography may show a patchy infiltrate that progresses to involve contiguous lobes.
(D) Pleural effusions are rare.

Answer: (A-False, B-True, C-True, D-False). A high index of suspicion is needed, as few findings are characteristic. Leukocytosis (up to 30,000/ml) is common, as is hyponatremia (seen in more than 50% of patients). The chest radiograph typically shows a patchy infiltrate that rapidly progresses to involve contiguous lobes. Pleural effusions are common. (*Chapter 84, Page 739.*)

19.25 Common symptoms of active pulmonary TB include

(A) progressive cough, productive of mucopurulent sputum
(B) hemoptysis
(C) malaise, low-grade fever, and weight loss
(D) dyspnea and chest pain

Answer: (A-True, B-False, C-True, D-False). Pulmonary TB usually presents with a progressive cough, productive of mucopurulent sputum. Hemoptysis is not common but when present can be massive. Malaise, low-grade fever, and weight loss are often present. Dyspnea and chest pain are uncommon. (*Chapter 84, Page 741.*)

19.26 True statements regarding the TB skin test include which of the following?

(A) The recommended test is the Mantoux test using 0.1 ml of PPD-T injected subcutaneously.
(B) Multiple puncture tests are recommended for mass screening.
(C) The TB skin test is positive in 90 to 95% of AIDS patients who have TB.
(D) All patients with a positive TB skin test should have a chest radiograph.

Answer: (A-True, B-False, C-False, D-True). The TB skin test is one of the oldest diagnostic tests still in use today, having been initially developed by Koch more than 100 years ago. The Mantoux test is recommended using 0.1 ml of PPD-T injected subcutaneously, with the result (induration, not erythema) read in 48 to 72 hours. Multiple-puncture tests are not recommended. A positive reaction indicates past exposure (at least 2 to 3 months ago). Unfortunately, it is often negative in the elderly and those with HIV. (Up to 60% of patients with AIDS and TB have a false-negative test.) All patients with a positive test should have a chest radiograph to rule out active disease. (*Chapter 84, Page 742.*)

19.27 The most common pulmonary infection seen in AIDS patients is *Pneumocystis carinii* pneumonia. The drug of choice for the management of *Pneumocystis carinii* pneumonia is

(A) prednisone
(B) trimethoprim-sulfamethoxazole (TMP-SMX)
(C) dapsone
(D) clindamycin
(E) primaquine

Answer: (B). TMP-SMX is the drug of choice. It can be given orally or intravenously, but the latter route is usually chosen for the first episode because of the potential for acute deterioration. (*Chapter 84, Page 744.*)

19.28 The patient is a 74-year-old white woman with a long history of cigarette smoking. Four months ago, you diagnosed lung cancer, and she comes today with signs and symptoms of hyponatremia. True statements regarding hyponatremia in lung cancer patients include which of the following?

(A) The most likely cancer type is adenocarcinoma.
(B) Hyponatremia is due to inappropriate secretion of antidiuretic hormone (SIADH).
(C) The initial treatment is administration of fluids sufficient to reverse the abnormality.
(D) Demeclocycline may help reverse the hyponatremia.

Answer: (A-False, B-True, C-False, D-True). Several paraneoplastic syndromes can be seen in lung cancer patients. Small-cell carcinoma can cause hyponatremia due to SIADH. The initial treatment is fluid restriction. Demeclocycline, which causes a mild nephrogenic diabetes insipidus, can also help to reverse hyponatremia. The SIADH often resolves as the tumor responds to chemotherapy and radiation therapy. (*Chapter 85, Page 749.*)

19.29 The patient is a 68-year-old white man with metastatic non–small-cell lung carcinoma (NSCLC). You have found him to have a high serum calcium level. True statements regarding hypercalcemia as a complication of metastatic NSCLC include which of the following?

(A) The elevated calcium may be due to a paraneoplastic phenomenon.
(B) The use of intravenous saline and furosemide (Lasix) may be helpful in treatment.
(C) Pamidronate (Aredia), an intravenous diphosphonate, has been found to increase serum calcium levels.
(D) Mithramycin may be effective but has greater toxicity than pamidronate.

Answer: (A-True, B-True, C-False, D-True). Hypercalcemia is a frequent complication of metastatic NSCLC. It may be due to widespread bone metastases, but it also can be a paraneoplastic phenomenon caused by secretion of substances that act like parathyroid hormone. In addition to intravenous saline and furosemide (Lasix), hypercalcemia can be readily treated with one dose of pamidronate (Aredia), an intravenous diphosphonate. Calcitonin, gallium nitrate, and mithramycin are also effective treatments for hypercalcemia, but these agents have more toxicity than pamidronate. (*Chapter 85, Page 751.*)

19.30 ARDS is characterized by which of the following findings?

(A) left heart failure
(B) severe hypoxemia
(C) diffuse pulmonary infiltrates
(D) poor lung compliance

Answer: (A-False, B-True, C-True, D-True). First described by Ashbauh et al. in 1967 as ARDS, this condition of acute respiratory failure is marked by severe hypoxemia, diffuse pulmonary infiltrates, poor lung compliance, and the absence of left heart failure. (*Chapter 86, Page 752.*)

19.31 True statements regarding the clinical diagnosis of pulmonary emboli include which of the following?

(A) The most common symptoms include dyspnea, pleuritic pain, apprehension, and cough.
(B) The most common signs of pulmonary embolus are tachypnea, rales, increased P_2 heart sound, tachycardia, and fever.
(C) Hemoptysis occurs in about 90% of patients.
(D) Clinically evident lower extremity thrombophlebitis is found in most patients.

Answer: (A-True, B-True, C-False, D-False). Signs and symptoms of pulmonary emboli are inconsistent, and no finding or combination of findings is diagnostic. The most common symptoms are dyspnea, pleuritic pain, apprehension, and cough. Hemoptysis occurs in about one-third of patients. The most common signs are tachypnea, rales, increased P_2 heart sound, tachycardia, and fever. Only one-third of patients have clinically evident lower extremity phlebitis. (*Chapter 86, Page 754.*)

19.32 Pulmonary angiography or pulmonary-ventilation perfusion scanning is important in establishing the diagnosis of pulmonary embolism. Pulmonary angiography should be the initial test order in which of the following clinical settings?

(A) patients at high risk of complications from anticoagulation
(B) patients suspected of minimal pulmonary embolism
(C) patients in whom thrombolytic therapy might be undertaken
(D) all patients suspected of pulmonary embolus

Answer: (A-True, B-True, C-False, D-False). Pulmonary ventilation-perfusion scanning or pulmonary angiography must be performed to establish the diagnosis of pulmonary embolism. Angiography should be used at the outset in patients at high risk of complications from anticoagulation, when massive pulmonary embolism is suspected, or when thrombolytic therapy might be undertaken. Ventilation-perfusion scanning may be used initially in other patients, but results must be interpreted carefully. (*Chapter 86, Page 754.*)

19.33 Pulmonary hypertension may develop in the setting of which of the following conditions?

(A) athletic training
(B) surgical loss of pulmonary tissue
(C) chronic atrial fibrillation
(D) chronic obstructive lung disease

Answer: (A-False, B-True, C-False, D-True). Pulmonary hypertension develops when local physiologic conditions such as hypoxia and acidosis occur, leading to vasoconstriction and elevated pulmonary pressure. These and other mechanisms may play a role in the development of pulmonary hypertension secondary to other conditions, including surgical loss of pulmonary tissues, ventricular septal defect, left heart failure, obesity-hypoventilation syndrome, mitral valve disease, chronic obstructive lung disease, bronchial asthma, chronic thromboembolism, and interstitial fibrosis. (*Chapter 86, Page 755.*)

19.34 Up to 95% of patients with pulmonary sarcoidosis have some abnormality on the chest radiogram. The characteristic abnormalities are

(A) cavitary disease in the lung apex
(B) bilateral hilar lymphadenopathy
(C) pleural effusion
(D) diffuse infiltrates

Answer: (A-False, B-True, C-False, D-True). The most common radiographic findings are bilateral hilar lymphadenopathy and diffuse infiltrates. (*Chapter 86, Page 758.*)

20

The Digestive System

The questions in this chapter constitute a review of the following chapters in *Family Medicine: Principles and Practice, Fifth Edition*:

Gastritis, Esophagitis, and Peptic Ulcer Disease (Chapter 87)
Diseases of the Large and Small Bowel (Chapter 88)
Pancreatic Diseases (Chapter 89)
Diseases of the Liver (Chapter 90)
Diseases of the Rectum and Anus (Chapter 91)
Colorectal Cancer (Chapter 92)
Surgical Problems of the Digestive System (Chapter 93)
Selected Disorders of the Digestive System and Nutrition (Chapter 94)

DIRECTIONS (Items 20.1 through 20.36): Each of the questions or incomplete statements in this section is followed by five suggested answers or completions. Select the ONE that is BEST in each case.

20.1 The most characteristic symptom of gastroesophageal reflux disease (GERD) is

(A) laryngitis
(B) heartburn
(C) cough
(D) chest pain
(E) wheezing

Answer: (B). The most reliable symptom of GERD is heartburn, a retrosternal burning sensation that may radiate from the epigastrium to the throat. Patients may also complain of pyrosis or water brash, the regurgitation of bitter-tasting material into the mouth. GERD can cause respiratory problems including laryngitis, chronic cough, aspiration pneumonia, and wheezing. Atypical chest pain can also be caused by GERD. Finally, patients may complain of odynophagia (pain with swallowing) or dysphagia. (*Chapter 87, Page 762.*)

20.2 Most gastric cancers are

(A) adenocarcinoma
(B) non-Hodgkin's lymphoma
(C) leiomyosarcoma
(D) small-cell carcinoma
(E) metastatic carcinoma

Answer: (A). The incidence of gastric cancer has declined significantly since the 1930s, but it still causes thousands of deaths each year. Ninety percent of the lesions are adenocarcinomas; non-Hodgkin's lymphomas and leiomyosarcomas comprise the remainder. (*Chapter 87, Page 766.*)

20.3 The patient is a 22-year-old white woman with the acute onset of fever and malaise yesterday, followed this morning by nausea, vomiting, diarrhea, and abdominal cramps. The diarrhea is profuse and watery. Although no obvious blood is present, a test for occult blood on a fecal specimen is positive. This patient most likely has an acute infectious diarrheal syndrome caused by

(A) *Salmonella*
(B) *Camplyobacter jejuni*
(C) *Escherichia coli*
(D) *Shigella*
(E) *Clostridium difficile*

Answer: (B). *Campylobacter jejuni is* probably the most common cause of inflammatory diarrhea in developed countries. Infection can vary from asymptomatic clinical cases to severe enterocolitis. A typical episode begins with fever and malaise, followed within 24 hours by nausea, vomiting, diarrhea, and abdominal pain. The diarrhea is profuse and watery and contains blood and leukocytes. The illness is self-limited, usually lasting less than 1 week. (*Chapter 88, Page 768.*)

20.4 Pseudomembranous colitis is a form of bacterial toxin-mediated colitis that is characteristically associated with

    (A) *H. pylori*
    (B) *Yersinia*
    (C) intestinal parasites
    (D) inadequately treated *Salmonella* infection
    (E) prior antibiotic use

Answer: (E). Several forms of acute diarrhea illness have been associated with the presence of *Clostridium difficile* toxin in the stool. Pseudomembranous colitis is the best described form of this bacterial toxin-mediated colitis. It is associated with blood and white blood cells in the stool. Almost all antibiotics have been implicated in the etiogenesis of pseudomembranous colitis. Time between onset of diarrhea symptoms and prior antibiotic use varies from 2 days to 6 weeks. (*Chapter 88, Page 769.*)

20.5 The patient is a 36-year-old white man with a 6-month history of recurrent, colicky abdominal pain, diarrhea, weight loss, and fever. The pain most often occurs in the right lower quadrant (RLQ). Endoscopic examination reveals a cobblestone appearance to the mucosa. A perianal fissure is present. This patient's most likely diagnosis is

    (A) diverticular disease
    (B) irritable bowel syndrome (IBS)
    (C) ulcerative colitis (UC)
    (D) Crohn's disease
    (E) pseudomembranous colitis

Answer: (D). Common presenting symptoms of Crohn's disease include colicky abdominal pain, diarrhea, weight loss, and fever. Pain most often occurs in the RLQ and is occasionally associated with an inflammatory mass. When the disease is confined to the colon, presenting symptoms are usually rectal bleeding and diarrhea. Involvement of the terminal ileum, colon, or both is common, but any site within the alimentary tract can be affected. Transmural involvement by the inflammatory process is common and extensive, and deep ulceration with relatively preserved inter-

vening tissue ("skip areas") may cause a cobblestone appearance in the mucosa. Involvement is typically segmental and frequently spares the rectum. The inflammatory process may extend beyond the gastrointestinal tract by formation of fistulas. Perianal disease, such as fissures, fistulas, abscesses, and "blind" sinus tracts, are a prominent feature of Crohn's disease. (*Chapter 88, Page 770.*)

20.6 Diverticulosis of the right colon, when symptomatic, characteristically causes

    (A) bleeding
    (B) infection
    (C) perforation
    (D) obstruction
    (E) infarction

Answer: (A). The right colon is the site of bleeding in more than 70% of cases of diverticulosis, although diverticula are more numerous in the left colon. The blood is usually bright red and the bleeding self-limiting, although it may be massive and even fatal. Chronic occult blood loss should not be attributed to diverticula until colonic cancer has been ruled out. (*Chapter 88, Page 772.*)

20.7 The patient is a 38-year-old white male computer programmer with a 3-month history of crampy lower abdominal pain, often relieved by defecation. There has been an increased frequency of bowel movements, associated with alternating constipation and loose stools with the passage of mucus. He notes several small-volume diarrheal stools that occur during the early morning and do not recur later that day. Based on this history, the probable diagnosis is

    (A) UC
    (B) Crohn's disease
    (C) infectious diarrhea syndrome
    (D) IBS
    (E) malabsorption

Answer: (D). Classically, patients with IBS present with a history of cramping pain poorly localized to the lower half of the abdomen, rather than a specific location. Usually the pain is relieved by defecation or is associated with a change in the frequency or consistency of stools. Patients also have a history of disturbed defecation that may involve constipation, loose stools, passage of mucus, straining, urgency, or a feeling of incomplete evacuation. Frequently, several small-volume diarrheal stools occur during the early morning and do not recur that day. (*Chapter 88, Page 772.*)

20.8 The physiologic event that occurs at the beginning of pancreatitis is

(A) release of insulin into the pancreatic parenchyma
(B) conversion of trypsinogen to trypsin
(C) development of an acute deficiency of glucagon
(D) blockage of the conversion of indirect to direct-acting bilirubin
(E) development of intolerance to carbohydrates

Answer: (B). Pancreatitis develops when trypsinogen is activated to trypsin by an inciting event. Trypsin subsequently activates other pancreatic enzymes, including chymotrypsin, elastase, carboxypeptidase, and phospholipase A. These activated enzymes cause local and systemic manifestations ranging from local pain to adult respiratory distress syndrome. (*Chapter 89, Page 774.*)

20.9 The patient is a 58-year-old white man with a long history of heavy alcohol use. Almost a year ago, you diagnosed type II diabetes mellitus, which has been diet-controlled. Now for the past 5 to 6 months, he has had vague upper abdominal pain, lower thoracic back pain, and weight loss of 8 to 10 pounds. While sitting in your office with the patient, you noticed that his skin appears slightly jaundiced. This clinical picture is most characteristic of

(A) chronic cholecystitis
(B) chronic pancreatitis
(C) acute pancreatitis
(D) pancreatic cancer
(E) cancer of the cecum

Answer: (D). The clinical features of pancreatic cancer are initially vague and nonspecific and frequently contribute to a delay in diagnosis. Jaundice is the most common physical finding, although weight loss, epigastric pain, or incapacitating back pain may be the presenting complaint. Glucose intolerance may develop 6 to 12 months prior to the diagnosis in 10 to 15% of patients. (*Chapter 89, Page 777.*)

20.10 The finding of a palpable gallbladder in the absence of cholangitis (Courvoisier's sign) suggests which of the following?

(A) large gallstones
(B) cancer of the hepatic flexure of the colon
(C) amebiasis of the gallbladder
(D) a malignant obstruction of the common bile duct
(E) torsion of the gallbladder

Answer: (D). A palpable gallbladder (Courvoisier's sign) in the absence of cholangitis suggests a malignant obstruction of the common bile duct until proved otherwise. (*Chapter 89, Page 777.*)

20.11 Hepatitis A begins with a prodrome phase 1 to 2 weeks before the onset of jaundice, consisting of fatigue, anorexia, nausea, vomiting, and myalgias. Following the onset of jaundice, these symptoms generally subside, with the EXCEPTION of

(A) fatigue
(B) anorexia
(C) nausea
(D) vomiting
(E) myalgias

Answer: (A). Most of the prodromal symptoms of hepatitis A usually resolve quickly after jaundice occurs. The exception is lethargy, which may continue for weeks. If the case is severe, nausea, vomiting, and weight loss may also carry over into the icteric phase. (*Chapter 90, Page 780.*)

20.12 The patient is a 21-year-old white woman who has had fatigue, loss of appetite, and muscle aches for several weeks and has noticed that the whites of her eyes have appeared yellow for the past 2 days. She is not a drug user and is not sexually active. You suspect hepatitis A virus (HAV) infection. The diagnosis will be confirmed on detecting which of the following in her blood?

(A) HAV antigen
(B) serum bilirubin greater than 15 mg/dl
(C) elevated serum aspartate aminotransferase
(D) immunoglobulin G (IgG)-specific anti-HAV
(E) IgM-specific anti-HAV antibody

Answer: (E). Diagnosis of acute HAV infection depends on identification of the IgM-specific anti-HAV antibody. This antibody is usually present at the onset of jaundice and clears within 4 to 6 months after the acute infection. IgG-specific anti-HAV is present throughout the patient's life after acute infection. (*Chapter 90, Page 781.*)

20.13 Worldwide, the most common mode of hepatitis B virus (HBV) transmission is

(A) parenteral drug use
(B) homosexual activity
(C) heterosexual activity
(D) vertical or perinatal transmission
(E) transfusion of blood products

Answer: (D). In the United States, heterosexual activity is the most common mode of transmission, followed by injection drug use and homosexual activity. Vertical or perinatal transmission is the most common mode of transmission worldwide. This method of spread commonly results in chronic infection in the recipient. Post-transfusion spread in Western industrialized countries is unusual because products are now screened for HBV. (*Chapter 90, Page 781.*)

20.14 In HBV virus infection, which of the following serologic tests is detected early in the course of the disease?

(A) HBsAg
(B) HBeAg
(C) HBcAg
(D) anti-HBc
(E) anti-HBs

Answer: (A). HBsAg is detectable early in the course of the disease, usually before jaundice appears, and usually clears 6 months after the acute infection. If it persists past 6 months, it usually remains detectable indefinitely and most likely indicates a chronic infection. The core antigen (HBcAg) is found in all patients with acute infection. Core antibody usually persists for years, even in patients without a chronic infection. The HBeAg indicates that the whole virus is circulating in the blood, and so the serum is contagious. (*Chapter 90, Page 781.*)

20.15 The treatment of choice for chronic HBV infection is

(A) interferon
(B) monthly injections of immune serum globulin (ISG)
(C) *N*-acetyl cysteine
(D) high-dose vitamin therapy
(E) none of the above

Answer: (A). The treatment of choice for chronic HBV or hepatitis C virus (HCV) is interferon alpha-2b. Because of its expense, side effects, and the need for liver biopsy, it is often administered by specialists with experience in its use. Approximately 30 to 40% of patients with chronic HBV respond to therapy, as do 40 to 50% of patients with chronic HCV or hepatitis D virus. (*Chapter 90, Page 783.*)

20.16 According to recommendations of the Centers for Disease Control, hepatitis B vaccine is recommended for newborn infants in which ONE of the following settings?

(A) not recommended
(B) infants born to mothers with positive HBsAg
(C) infants born to mothers with positive HBcAg
(D) infants born to mothers with positive HBeAg
(E) all infants regardless of maternal HBsAg status

Answer: (E). Hepatitis B vaccination is recommended for all infants regardless of maternal HBsAg status. (*Chapter 90, Page 784.*)

20.17 Which of the following drugs has a dose-dependent direct hepatotoxic effect that can result in drug-induced hepatitis?

(A) halothane
(B) methyldopa
(C) isoniazid
(D) acetaminophen
(E) phenytoin

Answer: (D). Many drugs are known to have potential for acute hepatotoxicity, with ethanol being the most well-known example. Acetaminophen has a direct hepatotoxic effect that is dose-dependent. Most other drugs result in an idiosyncratic drug reaction that is infrequent and unpredictable in that it may occur at any time during or shortly after exposure. (*Chapter 90, Page 785.*)

20.18 A 52-year-old white woman has had painless rectal bleeding for about 1 week. The most likely diagnosis is

(A) external hemorrhoids
(B) internal hemorrhoids
(C) rectal fissure
(D) cancer of the rectum
(E) spousal abuse

Answer: (B). Most patients with internal hemorrhoids present with painless rectal bleeding. (*Chapter 91, Page 788.*)

20.19 The patient is a 50-year-old white woman. Yesterday, you treated internal hemorrhoids with rubber band ligation. Today she returns with fever, pelvic pain, and inability to urinate. This patient should be evaluated for

(A) cystitis
(B) thrombosed hemorrhoid
(C) proctitis
(D) pelvic sepsis
(E) strangulation of the ligated hemorrhoid

Answer: (D). The rubber band ligation technique effectively strangulates the internal hemorrhoid. A small rubber band is loaded onto a hollow applicator, the hemorrhoid is pulled inside the applicator, and the rubber band is released to the base of the hemorrhoid. The hemorrhoid sloughs off during the following 1 to 2 weeks. Moderate pain can follow this procedure, as can the rare but significant complication of pelvic sepsis. Any patient with pelvic pain, fever, and inability to urinate following rubber band ligation must be immediately evaluated for this potentially fatal complication. (*Chapter 91, Page 788.*)

20.20 An anal fissure is usually caused by

(A) the passage of hard stool
(B) Crohn's disease
(C) an anorectal abscess
(D) UC
(E) bacterial infection

Answer: (A). A fissure is a crack or tear in the anal mucosa, usually produced by the passage of hard stool. The lesion classically is associated with bleeding and intense pain at defecation. Patients often complain of a sharp, cutting, or tearing sensation; nearly half of the patients present with the complaint of hemorrhoids. (*Chapter 91, Page 790.*)

20.21 Anal fissures are most usually located at which of the following sites?

(A) laterally at 3 and 9 o'clock
(B) in the posterior midline
(C) in the anterior midline
(D) at the site of an anorectal abscess
(E) at no specific location

Answer: (B). Anal fissures most commonly appear in the midline of the anal canal, with 90% in the posterior midline. Fissures outside the midline can be associated with other disease states such as Crohn's disease, tuberculosis, or syphilis. A search for associated pathology should be initiated whenever a fissure is found outside the midline. (*Chapter 91, Page 790.*)

20.22 Anal fistulas most often develop following

(A) pyogenic abscesses
(B) rectal surgery
(C) gonorrheal proctitis
(D) use of rectal steroids
(E) an exacerbation of inflammatory bowel disease

Answer: (A). Anal fistulas most commonly develop following pyogenic abscesses. Small crypt abscesses along the dentate line may serve as a reservoir for repeated infection from enteric bacteria. (*Chapter 91, Page 791.*)

20.23 You have received a call from the nursing home. One of your regular patients, a 90-year-old white woman, has had some rectal pain for about 1 week associated with incontinence of feces and flatus. The most likely diagnosis is

(A) anorectal abscess
(B) cancer of the rectum
(C) bowel obstruction
(D) diabetic neuropathy affecting the autonomic nervous system
(E) fecal impaction

Answer: (E). Incontinence frequently is associated with fecal impaction in the elderly. Fecal impaction occurs when a large, firm, immovable mass of stool develops in the rectum owing to incomplete evacuation of stool. (*Chapter 91, Page 792.*)

20.24 The patient is a 28-year-old unmarried white male salesman. He complains of rectal pain and discharge. On examination, the rectal mucosa is red and friable, and you note a mucopurulent discharge. The most likely cause of this patient's proctitis is

(A) UC
(B) Crohn's disease
(C) *Neisseria gonorrhoeae*
(D) overuse of rectal steroids
(E) a yeast infection related to antibiotic overuse

Answer: (C). Proctitis describes an inflammation limited to the distal 10 cm of the rectum. Infectious proctitis usually is caused by sexually transmitted diseases such as *Neisseria gonorrhoeae* and *Chlamydia trachomatis*. Proctitis is considered when patients complain of rectal discomfort, tenesmus, rectal discharge, and constipation. The anorectal mucosa may appear red and friable, and a mucopurulent discharge often is noted. (*Chapter 92, Page 793.*)

20.25 The patient is a 26-year-old white male with anal condylomas. The most likely etiology is

(A) human immunodeficiency virus (HIV)
(B) human papillomavirus (HPV)
(C) *Treponema pallidum*
(D) Bowen's disease
(E) Herpes simplex virus

Answer: (B). Anal condylomas are caused by HPV, usually types 6 and 11. Anal warts appear to be most common in young men, especially those engaging in anal intercourse. Women with anal warts often have coexisting warts on the cervix and labia. (*Chapter 91, Page 793.*)

20.26 The patient is a 39-year-old white man whose brother developed colorectal cancer (CRC) at age 48. According to American Cancer Society recommendations, this patient should have

(A) yearly flexible sigmoidoscopy
(B) digital rectal examination with fecal occult blood testing every 6 months
(C) colonoscopy or air contrast barium enema (ACBE) every 3 to 5 years
(D) annual determination of carcinoembryonic antigen
(E) colonoscopy or ACBE yearly beginning at age 50

Answer: (C). The American Cancer Society recommends colonoscopy or ACBE every 3 to 5 years starting at age 35 to 40 for patients with a first-degree relative having CRC with an age of onset of 55 or younger. (*Chapter 92, Page 799.*)

20.27 The patient is a 42-year-old white woman who awakened this morning with dull periumbilical pain and loss of appetite. The pain is now right-sided, and physical examination of the abdomen reveals some tenderness and muscle guarding in the right lower abdomen. The most likely diagnosis is

(A) pelvic inflammatory disease
(B) mittelschmerz
(C) appendicitis
(D) ovarian torsion
(E) ectopic pregnancy

Answer: (C). "Typical" appendicitis begins as a dull, periumbilical pain accompanied by anorexia and nausea. Within a few hours, the pain becomes sharper, more intense, and localized to the RLQ. Physical examination reveals a low-grade fever, rebound tenderness, and muscle guarding. (*Chapter 93, Page 804.*)

20.28 The patient is a 62-year-old white female retiree with RLQ abdominal pain on and off for several days. There is a slight leukocytosis. The patient has noted no change in her appetite, which is usually not robust. Her temperature is normal. Sensing that this may be an atypical presentation of appendicitis, you decide to seek diagnostic imaging. The preferred procedure would be

(A) flat plate of the abdomen
(B) computed tomography (CT)
(C) magnetic resonance imaging
(D) ACBE
(E) graded compression ultrasonography

Answer: (E). Graded compression ultrasonography—because of its ready availability, low cost, high patient acceptance, safety, and overall high diagnostic accuracy—is widely accepted as the imaging procedure of choice for diagnosing atypical appendicitis. Radiography is not diagnostic but may help to rule out other conditions. CT, although expensive, has a sensitivity of 98%, and complications such as perforation or abscess formation may be easily seen. Barium enema may show a nonfilling appendix but is not used for the acute presentation. (*Chapter 93, Page 805.*)

20.29 The patient is a 28-year-old white woman with fever, anorexia, and RLQ abdominal pain. Because of these findings and a leukocytosis, laparotomy is performed. At surgery, the appendix appears normal. In this setting, the cause of the symptoms is probably

(A) terminal ileitis
(B) pelvic inflammatory disease
(C) pyelonephritis
(D) ureteral calculus
(E) pancreatitis

Answer: (B). Several conditions may mimic appendicitis. Pelvic inflammatory disease accounts for 35 to 45% of the negative laparotomies for presumed appendicitis. Others include terminal ileitis, pyelonephritis, diverticulitis, ureteral calculus, pancreatitis, and subphrenic abscess. Mesenteric adenitis, a self-limited condition, may also masquerade as appendicitis. (*Chapter 93, Page 805.*)

20.30 The patient is a 48-year-old white woman with a 3-hour history of steady, right upper quadrant (RUQ) pain associated with nausea and vomiting that began at 4 AM last night. The most likely cause of this pain is

(A) biliary colic
(B) pancreatitis
(C) subphrenic abscess
(D) mesenteric adenitis
(E) pyelonephritis

Answer: (A). Typical biliary colic is a steady RUQ or epigastric pain that lasts 1 to 5 hours and may be associated with nausea and vomiting. It commonly occurs at night, usually around the same time. (*Chapter 93, Page 805.*)

20.31 The most frequent complication of inguinal hernia repair is

(A) wound infection
(B) hemorrhage
(C) nerve entrapment
(D) recurrence
(E) testicular infarction and atrophy

Answer: (D). Recurrence is the most frequent complication of inguinal hernia repair, with failure rates averaging 10%. Faulty technique, rather than type of repair, may be the cause of most failures. Minor complications of hernia repair include hemorrhage, wound infection, and injury to the bowel, bladder, testicles, vas deferens, and nerves. The mortality from elective hernia repair is negligible. (*Chapter 93, Page 807.*)

20.32 The patient is an 80-year-old white male resident of a care home. For the past 5 to 7 days, there have been no bowel movements. For 2 to 3 days, he has had vomiting and crampy intermittent abdominal pain. Examination of the abdomen reveals mild distension. The most likely diagnosis in this patient is

(A) perforated ulcer
(B) appendicitis
(C) bowel obstruction
(D) acute cholecystitis
(E) perirectal abscess

Answer: (C). Vomiting, obstipation, abdominal pain, and distension are the main characteristics of mechanical intestinal obstruction. The pain is typically cramping and intermittent. (*Chapter 93, Page 807.*)

20.33 In a patient with suspected small bowel obstruction (SBO), the most useful diagnostic test is likely to be

(A) upright and supine abdominal radiographs
(B) serial determinations of the white blood count
(C) electrolyte determinations
(D) CT
(E) ACBE

Answer: (A). Upright and supine abdominal radiographs continue to be the most helpful diagnostic adjunct. The distribution of air in the bowel is the most important finding. In patients with high complete SBO, there is little air in the bowel. More distal SBO produces a "stepladder" pattern of air-fluid levels within bowel loops. (*Chapter 93, Page 808.*)

20.34 Which of the following patients is most likely to have lactose intolerance?

(A) a 46-year-old immigrant from Norway
(B) a 58-year-old woman of Vietnamese ancestry
(C) a 47-year-old man of Mediterranean ancestry
(D) a 50-year-old African American man
(E) no significant difference would be expected among the four individuals described

Answer: (B). The ability to digest lactose varies with age and race. In the United States, it is estimated that 22% of Caucasians, 65% of African Americans, and almost 100% of Vietnamese ancestry are lactose malabsorbers. (*Chapter 94, Page 812.*)

20.35 The patient is a 10-year-old boy who has had grossly bloody diarrhea for 2 days. The most likely infectious cause of his complaint is

(A) *Campylobacter* species
(B) *Staphylococcus aureus*
(C) *Salmonella typhi*
(D) *Shigella* species
(E) *Escherichia coli*

Answer: (E). Food-borne enterohemorrhagic *E. coli* is most commonly caused by the serotype 0157:H7. Hemolytic-uremic syndrome, hemorrhagic colitis, and idiopathic thrombocytopenic purpura are seen in association with enterohemorrhagic *E. coli* infections. Outbreaks in the United States have been most often associated with the ingestion of undercooked ground beef. *E. coli* 0157:H7 is the most common infectious cause of grossly bloody diarrhea in the United States. (*Chapter 94, Page 813.*)

20.36 Botulism is caused by toxins produced by *Clostridium botulinum* under anaerobic conditions. The disease occasionally occurs in infants and in this setting is most often associated with the ingestion of

(A) unpasteurized milk
(B) well water
(C) homemade grain cereals
(D) honey
(E) applesauce made from contaminated apples

Answer: (D). Infant botulism, rare in the United States, is most often associated with honey ingestion. (*Chapter 94, Page 814.*)

DIRECTIONS (Items 20.37 through 20.58): Each of the items in this section is a multiple true–false problem that consists of a stem and four lettered options. Indicate whether each of the four options is TRUE or FALSE.

20.37 Cisapride (Propulsid) can be useful in the management of GERD. True statements regarding this medication include which of the following?

(A) Cisapride increases the release of acetylcholine from the myenteric plexus.
(B) Erosive esophagitis undergoes healing with cisapride therapy.
(C) Side effects include headaches, nausea, and diarrhea.
(D) The usual starting dose is 150 mg four times daily.

Answer: (A-True, B-False, C-True, D-False). Cisapride works through serotonin receptors to increase the release of acetylcholine from the myenteric plexus. Symptomatic relief has been documented, but healing of erosive esophagitis has not been demonstrated in trials in the United States. Side effects are uncommon but include headache, nausea, and diarrhea. The starting dose of cisapride is 10 mg, taken at least 15 minutes before each meal and at bedtime. The maximum dose is 20 mg four times a day. (*Chapter 87, Page 763.*)

20.38 The association of *H. pylori* with peptic ulcer disease (PUD) has revolutionized the way we view and treat PUD. True statements include which of the following?

(A) Only 10 to 20% of ulcers are thought to be caused by either *H. pylori* or nonsteroidal anti-inflammatory drugs (NSAIDs).
(B) Most individuals with *H. pylori* develop PUD.
(C) Empiric treatment of individuals with *H. pylori* is recommended even in the absence of a documented ulcer.
(D) Because of the prevalence of *H. pylori,* treatment is recommended for individuals with nonulcer dyspepsia.

Answer: (A-False, B-False, C-False, D-False). The association of *H. pylori* with PUD has revolutionized the way we view and treat PUD. Most peptic ulcers are thought to be caused by either *H. pylori* or NSAIDs. Although infection with *H. pylori* appears to be common, most individuals with *H. pylori* do not develop ulcers. For this reason, empiric treatment of individuals with *H. pylori* is not recommended in the absence of a documented ulcer. (*Chapter 87, Page 763.*)

20.39 Misoprostol (Cytotec) is a prostaglandin used to prevent ulcers due to NSAIDs. True statements regarding misoprostol include which of the following?

(A) The drug appears to act by enhancing mucosal blood flow.
(B) Misoprostol may heal ulcers at approximately the same rate as histamine-2 receptor antagonists (H₂RA).
(C) The drug is safe for use during pregnancy.
(D) A common side effect is diarrhea.

Answer: (A-True, B-True, C-False, D-True). Prostaglandins protect the gastric mucosa, possibly by enhancing mucosal blood flow. Misoprostol, a prostaglandin E₁ analog, has been used to prevent ulcers due to NSAIDs. Misoprostol also heals ulcers at approximately the same rate as H₂RAs, but severe diarrhea may limit patient compliance. Stimulation of uterine contractions and induction of abortions are the most serious side effects of misoprostol. (*Chapter 87, Page 765.*)

20.40 Four common causes of upper gastrointestinal (UGI) bleeding are peptic ulceration, gastritis, esophageal varices, and esophagogastric mucosal tears (Mallory-Weiss syndrome). True statements regarding these causes of UGI bleeding include which of the following?

(A) Bleeding due to peptic ulceration is almost always associated with acute pain.
(B) Bleeding due to varices is usually abrupt and massive.
(C) An esophagogastric mucosal tear is characterized by chronic, relentless blood loss over days and weeks.
(D) Lymphoma can be a cause of UGI bleeding.

Answer: (A-False, B-True, C-False, D-True). Because bleeding due to peptic ulceration may present without pain, peptic ulceration should always be considered. Bleeding due to varices is usually abrupt and massive, and chronic blood loss is unusual. Varices may be due to alcohol cirrhosis or any other cause of portal hypertension such as portal vein thrombosis. Mallory-Weiss syndrome classically presents with retching followed by hematemesis. Other causes of UGI bleeding include gastric carcinoma, lymphoma, polyps, and diverticula. (*Chapter 87, Page 766.*)

20.41 True statements regarding the treatment of *Salmonella* gastroenteritis include which of the following?

(A) Antibiotic treatment is recommended if there is laboratory confirmation of *Salmonella* intestinal infection.
(B) Antibiotic therapy will significantly increase the rate of recovery.
(C) Antibiotic therapy may increase the incidence and duration of intestinal carriage of the organisms.
(D) Antibiotic treatment should be considered in patients who are immunocompromised, very young, or debilitated.

Answer: (A-False, B-False, C-True, D-True). No treatment is required unless the infection is systemic. Among several clinical trials, no antimicrobial treatment has convincingly altered the rate of recovery. In addition, antibiotic therapy may increase the incidence and duration of intestinal carriage of the organisms. However, treatment should be considered in immunocompromised patients, the very young, debilitated elderly patients, or when there is evidence of sepsis, high fever, rigors, hypotension, and decreased renal function. (*Chapter 88, Page 768.*)

20.42 Nutrients absorbed in the proximal small intestine include

(A) calcium
(B) vitamin B$_{12}$
(C) iron
(D) bile acids

Answer: (A-True, B-False, C-True, D-False). The small intestine is involved in nutrient absorption. Calcium, iron, fats, and folic acid are absorbed in the proximal small intestine. Disorders that disrupt intraluminal or mucosal absorption in this area (e.g., celiac sprue, Whipple's disease, eosinophilic gastroenteritis) can result in microcytic anemia, osteomalacia, and fat malabsorption. The ileum is involved in the absorption of vitamin B$_{12}$ and bile acids. Surgical resection of this area or involvement with Crohn's disease or lymphoma can result in macrocytic anemia, diarrhea, and weight loss. (*Chapter 88, Page 769.*)

20.43 The patient is a 48-year-old white man with UC. A worrisome complication of his disease is toxic megacolon. This complication can be precipitated by

(A) a barium enema examination in the setting of an acute flare-up
(B) potassium supplementation
(C) anticholinergic medication
(D) narcotic analgesics

Answer: (A-True, B-False, C-True, D-True). A wide variety of complications are associated with both UC and Crohn's disease. One particularly dangerous complication is toxic megacolon, which can be precipitated by a barium enema (including the preparation) in the presence of severe colitis, potassium depletion, and anticholinergic, antidiarrheal, or narcotic medications. (*Chapter 88, Page 771.*)

20.44 Sulfasalazine (Azulfidine) is used in the treatment of UC and Crohn's disease. True statements regarding this medication include which of the following?

(A) Sulfasalazine is safe for use during pregnancy and nursing.
(B) The drug reduces the frequency and severity of recurrence of ulcerative colitis.
(C) The drug will maintain remission of Crohn's disease.
(D) Possible adverse effects include hemolytic anemia and aplastic anemia.

Answer: (A-True, B-True, C-False, D-True). Sulfasalazine (Azulfidine 500 mg, two tablets orally t.i.d.–q.i.d.) is highly effective in inducing remission in mild-to-moderately active UC and Crohn's colitis and ileocolitis; it is less effective for isolated ileitis. It can be used during pregnancy and is safe for nursing mothers. It reduces the frequency and severity of recurrence of UC but has not been conclusively proved to maintain remission of Crohn's disease. Adverse effects are experienced by about 25% of patients (including anorexia, headache, rash, reversible oligospermia, urticaria, fever, leukopenia, hepatotoxicity, hemolytic anemia, and aplastic anemia). (*Chapter 88, Page 771.*)

20.45 Synonyms for IBS include which of the following?

(A) irritable colon
(B) inflammatory bowel disease
(C) spastic colon
(D) mucous colitis

Answer: (A-True, B-False, C-True, D-True). Synonymous terms include irritable colon, spastic colon, and mucous colitis, but IBS is now generally believed to be related to motor disturbance of the entire gut as a result of various stimuli, including stress and meals. (*Chapter 88, Page 772.*)

20.46 Eighty percent of the cases of acute pancreatitis in the United States can be traced to which of the following causes?

(A) diabetes mellitus
(B) cholelithiasis
(C) obesity
(D) chronic excessive alcohol use

Answer: (A-False, B-True, C-False, D-True). Cholelithiasis and chronic excessive alcohol use are the leading causes of acute pancreatitis and account for 80% of the cases in the United States. (*Chapter 89, Page 774.*)

20.47 Acute pancreatitis may lead to hemorrhagic necrosis of the pancreas. Physical signs of this uncommon condition include

(A) Murphy's sign
(B) Cullen's sign
(C) Grey Turner's sign
(D) McBurney's sign

Answer: (A-False, B-True, C-True, D-False). Periumbilical ecchymoses (Cullen's sign) or flank ecchymoses (Grey Turner's sign) are uncommon but when present serve as evidence of hemorrhagic necrosis of the pancreas. (*Chapter 89, Page 775.*)

20.48 You are the medical director for a local nursing home where there have recently been three cases of HAV infection. ISG should be administered to

(A) nursing home staff
(B) other nursing home patients
(C) persons who have visited the nursing home since the time the first case was discovered
(D) none of the above

Answer: (A-True, B-True, C-False, D-False). Preventing the spread of HAV depends on an accurate diagnosis followed by the appropriate use of ISG for prophylaxis. ISG 0.02 ml/kg intramuscularly should be administered within 2 weeks of exposure to close household contacts of infected individuals, children at daycare centers where HAV is occurring, staff and patients of long-term care institutions where HAV is occurring, co-workers of food handlers with HAV, and individuals exposed during a common-source outbreak. (*Chapter 90, Page 783.*)

20.49 The patient is a 64-year-old white man with a long history of heavy alcohol use whom you have been treating for chronic alcoholic hepatitis. Following a recent episode of UGI bleeding, he has shown evidence of hepatic encephalopathy. Management of this patient's hepatic encephalopathy is likely to include the use of

(A) leukotrienes
(B) protein restriction
(C) interferon
(D) lactulose

Answer: (A-False, B-True, C-False, D-True). Management of hepatic encephalopathy begins with the identification and correction of factors that may precipitate this condition, such as UGI bleeding, spontaneous bacterial peritonitis, or the use of sedatives. Protein restriction to 40 to 60 g daily and the use of lactulose by mouth or nasogastric tube are the cornerstones of therapy. (*Chapter 90, Page 785.*)

20.50 In the patient with acute alcoholic hepatitis, adverse prognostic markers include which of the following?

(A) a prothrombin time international normalized ratio of 4.8
(B) a blood urea nitrogen level of 90 mg/dl
(C) a serum bilirubin level of 3.6 mg/dl
(D) encephalopathy

Answer: (A-True, B-True, C-False, D-True). The prognosis of acute alcoholic hepatitis is not as grim as was once thought, depending on the degree of underlying chronic disease and the coexistence of other medical conditions. Adverse prognostic markers include abnormal coagulation studies, azotemia, a bilirubin level greater than 15 mg/dl, and encephalopathy. (*Chapter 90, Page 785.*)

20.51 The patient is a 56-year-old white man with chronic HBV infection who—despite your best advice—takes a drink or two of alcoholic beverages each day. You are concerned about the development of hepatocellular carcinoma and decide to undertake periodic screening. A reasonable approach would be twice yearly

(A) liver ultrasonography
(B) determination of AFP
(C) serologic testing
(D) determination of carcinoembryonic antigen

Answer: (A-True, B-True, C-False, D-False). Early detection in asymptomatic patients at risk for developing hepatocellular carcinoma is possible. Screening with liver ultrasonography and determination of alpha-fetoprotein (AFP) twice yearly in these patients is the most widely practiced approach for early detection. Serum AFP is elevated in 50 to 90% of symptomatic patients. (*Chapter 90, Page 786.*)

20.52 The patient is a 62-year-old white man who has recently been found on colonoscopy to have two adenomatous polyps. True statements regarding the significance of this finding include which of the following?

(A) Polyps are not a risk factor for CRC.
(B) The type of polyp is not significant as a risk factor for CRC.
(C) Siblings of patients with adenomatous polyps have an increased risk for developing CRC.
(D) There is a greater risk of CRC in patients with polyps greater than 2 cm.

Answer: (A-False, B-False, C-True, D-True). Polyps are a risk factor for CRC, particularly if they are adenomatous in type. Siblings and parents of patients with adenomatous colorectal polyps have a 1.78 relative risk for developing CRC. The age at the time of polyp diagnosis is an important prognostic factor for the risk of cancer development. Siblings of patients with adenomatous polyps diagnosed before age 60 have a 2.59 relative risk for developing CRC. Polyp size and histology are directly related to the risk of CRC, with villous polyps larger than 2 cm having a 50% greater chance of containing cancer than smaller or nonvillous polyps. (*Chapter 92, Page 796.*)

20.53 True statements regarding the prognosis for patients with CRC include which of the following?

(A) Younger age seems associated with a shorter survival time.
(B) Women generally have a better prognosis than men.
(C) The prognosis is worse for cancers of the left side of the colon when compared with those of the right side of the colon.
(D) Histologic grading has not been found to be a useful prognostic factor.

Answer: (A-False, B-True, C-True, D-False). Increased age may be associated with a shorter survival time. Women have a better prognosis than men in general. The CRC prognosis worsens when moving from the right to the left side of the colon. Histologic grading and operative findings are important prognostic factors for CRC. (*Chapter 92, Page 798.*)

20.54 Laparoscopic surgery allows physicians to perform intra-abdominal operations through small incisions. However, the technique involves some unique complications. These include

(A) perforation of a viscus by a trochar
(B) sepsis
(C) hypercarbia
(D) gas embolism

Answer: (A-True, B-False, C-True, D-True). Complications that are unique to the laparoscopic approach include perforation of visceral or vascular structures by a trochar or needle and harmful effects of the pneumoperitoneum such as hypercarbia, decreased cardiac output, pneumothorax, and gas embolism. (*Chapter 93, Page 803.*)

20.55 Following abdominal trauma, CT is useful in the evaluation of injuries to which of the following organs?

(A) liver
(B) pancreas
(C) adrenal glands
(D) spleen

Answer: (A-True, B-False, C-False, D-True). CT is especially useful for evaluating liver and spleen injuries, which are common with blunt trauma. It also detects retroperitoneal bleeding missed by diagnostic peritoneal lavage and fractures of the ribs, spine, and pelvis. Diaphragmatic injuries and intestinal rupture are easily missed by CT, making it less ideal for the evaluation of penetrating trauma. CT is also insensitive for pancreatic and adrenal injuries. (*Chapter 93, Page 804.*)

20.56 Gallbladder perforation can be a complication of acute cholecystitis. Patients at greatest risk of this complication include

(A) those with diabetes
(B) patients aged 40 and younger
(C) overweight patients
(D) immunocompromised patients

Answer: (A-True, B-False, C-False, D-True). Gallbladder perforation occurs in 3 to 10% of patients with acute cholecystitis. Diabetic patients, the elderly, the immunocompromised, and patients with systemic vascular disease are at higher risk for perforation. (*Chapter 93, Page 806.*)

20.57 The patient is a 44-year-old African American man who reports abdominal bloating and cramping after eating that especially seems to occur if he takes foods containing milk products. You decide to seek testing to confirm a diagnosis of lactose intolerance. Tests to support such a diagnosis include

(A) UGI endoscopy with gastric fluid analysis
(B) examination of a stool specimen for reducing substances
(C) ACBE
(D) breath hydrogen test

Answer: (A-False, B-True, C-False, D-True). The diagnosis of lactose intolerance can be supported by evaluating the stool for a pH less than 5.8 and reducing substances and by the breath hydrogen test. (*Chapter 94, Page 812.*)

20.58 True statements regarding paralytic shellfish poisoning include which of the following?

(A) Symptoms generally begin 6 to 8 hours after ingestion.

(B) The initial symptoms may include parasthesias of the mouth and extremities.
(C) Cranial nerve dysfunction and paralysis may occur as the disease progresses.
(D) Death due to paralytic shellfish poisoning has been reported only rarely.

Answer: (A-False, B-True, C-True, D-False). Patients with paralytic shellfish poisoning can develop symptoms within 30 minutes of ingestion. Initial symptoms include paresthesias of the mouth and extremities, headache, vertigo, a floating sensation, and less frequently, gastrointestinal symptoms. The patient progresses to ataxia, cranial nerve dysfunction, and paralysis. The mortality rate is 9%, predominantly due to respiratory failure. (*Chapter 94, Page 815.*)

21

The Renal, Urinary, and Male Genital Systems

The questions in this chapter constitute a review of the following chapters in *Family Medicine: Principles and Practice, Fifth Edition:*

Urinary Tract Infections (Chapter 95)
Fluid, Electrolyte, and Acid–Base Disorders (Chapter 96)
Diseases of the Kidney (Chapter 97)
Prostate Disease (Chapter 98)
Surgery of the Male Genital Tract (Chapter 99)
Selected Disorders of the Genitourinary System (Chapter 100)

DIRECTIONS (Items 21.1 through 21.32): Each of the questions or incomplete statements in this section is followed by five suggested answers or completions. Select the ONE that is BEST in each case.

21.1 The most common cause of urinary tract infection (UTI) during pregnancy is

(A) *Escherichia coli*
(B) *Enterobacter* species
(C) *Klebsiella* species
(D) *Proteus* species
(E) enterococci

Answer: (A). As in nonpregnant females, *E. coli* is the most common cause of UTI during pregnancy, accounting for more than 80% of isolates. Other organisms include *Enterobacter* species, *Klebsiella* species, *Proteus* species, enterococci, and *Staphylococcus saprophyticus*. (*Chapter 95, Page 818.*)

21.2 Your patient is a 36-year-old white man who has a spinal cord injury that occurred 4 years ago following an automobile accident. He is paralyzed below T8, and

bladder care is a problem. The most appropriate management is likely to be

(A) an indwelling catheter with no prophylactic medication
(B) an indwelling catheter with daily doses of trimethoprim-sulfamethazole (TMP-SMX)
(C) cystostomy drainage
(D) intermittent catheterization
(E) use of oral propantheline

Answer: (D). Special considerations for increased risk of UTI with spinal cord injuries include bladder overdistension, vesicoureteral reflux, high-pressure voiding, large postvoid residuals, stones in the urinary tract, and outlet obstruction. Management of infection risks focuses primarily on proper drainage of the bladder. A turning point that occurred during the 1960s was the understanding of the value of intermittent catheterization in reducing the risk of significant bacteriuria. Development of bacteriuria is certain with an indwelling catheter and suprapubic catheter. Although not fully understood, bacteriuria and the incidence of symptomatic UTIs are reduced by intermittent catheterization. (*Chapter 95, Page 821.*)

21.3 The patient is a 76-year-old white woman who has been in the hospital for the past 2 days because of a stroke. During her 48-hours of hospitalization, she has had an indwelling catheter and now has signs of UTI. The organism most likely to be the cause of her UTI is

(A) *Pseudomonas aeruginosa*
(B) *Klebsiella pneumoniae*
(C) *Proteus mirabilis*
(D) *Escherichia coli*
(E) enterococci

202 Taylor's Family Medicine Review

Answer: (D). Mortality from UTIs is increased three-fold in hospitalized patients with an indwelling catheter. With short-term catheterization, *E. coli* is the most common organism, followed by *Pseudomonas aeruginosa*, *Klebsiella pneumoniae*, *Proteus mirabilis*, *Staphylococcus epidermidis*, and enterococci. (*Chapter 95, Page 821.*)

21.4 Pyuria represents measurable evidence of host injury. The most accurate method of defining significant pyuria is

   (A) microscopic examination of unspun urine in a counting chamber
   (B) the leukocyte excretion rate
   (C) urine culture and sensitivity
   (D) urine colony count
   (E) urine antigen testing

Answer: (B). The most accurate method, or gold standard, of defining significant pyuria is the leukocyte excretion rate. There is evidence that the significant rate is 400,000 white blood cells/hour. Obviously, this measurement is cumbersome—hence the popularity of quicker, simpler, but less accurate screening tests. (*Chapter 95, Page 822.*)

21.5 The primary event in metabolic acidosis is

   (A) hypobicarbonatemia
   (B) hypochloremia
   (C) hyponatremia
   (D) hyperchloremia
   (E) hypokalemia

Answer: (A). Hypobicarbonatemia [(HCO_3) less than 28 mEq/L] is the primary event in metabolic acidosis or the compensatory event in respiratory acidosis. (*Chapter 96, Page 825.*)

21.6 Which of the following is most often the cause of diuretic-induced volume depletion and hyponatremia?

   (A) hydrochlorothiazide
   (B) bumetamide
   (C) furosemide
   (D) amiloride
   (E) triamterene

Answer: (A). Diuretic-induced volume depletion and hyponatremia are most often caused by thiazide diuretics because these drugs do not impair the renal concentrating mechanism, as is the case with medullary loop diuretics. (*Chapter 96, Page 833.*)

21.7 The treatment of hyponatremia and hypoosmolality caused by true volume depletion is

   (A) hypotonic volume repletion via the oral or intravenous route
   (B) isotonic volume repletion via the oral or intravenous route
   (C) hypertonic volume repletion via the oral or intravenous route
   (D) administration of aqueous vasopressin
   (E) administration of furosemide intravenously

Answer: (B). Treatment of hyponatremia and hypoosmolality caused by true volume depletion is isotonic volume repletion via the oral or intravenous route; only in severe cases of hyponatremia caused by hypovolemia is water restriction or infusion of hypertonic saline (or both) required. (*Chapter 96, Page 834.*)

21.8 The most common symptom associated with hypokalemia is

   (A) decreased appetite
   (B) nausea and vomiting
   (C) palpitations
   (D) generalized weakness
   (E) muscle cramps

Answer: (D). Generalized weakness is the most common symptom associated with hypokalemia. Other symptoms include polyuria, polydipsia, anorexia, nausea, vomiting, constipation, palpitations, muscle cramps, and muscle tenderness (e.g., hypokalemia-induced rhabdomyolysis). (*Chapter 96, Page 835.*)

21.9 The patient is a 16-year-old white high school girl brought to the emergency department with a 3-day history of fever with no nausea, vomiting, or diarrhea. Her mother has been treating her fever with medications at home. The patient complains of ringing in the ears, and there is a rapid heart rate. Blood electrolytes are consistent with a metabolic acidosis. This patient's most likely diagnosis is

   (A) suicide attempt
   (B) salicylate intoxication
   (C) methanol ingestion
   (D) new-onset diabetes mellitus
   (E) viral encephalitis

Answer: (B). Symptoms suggestive of the origin of metabolic acidosis include those associated with the ingestion of acid toxins (e.g., tinnitus of salicylate intoxication, acute loss of visual acuity of methanol ingestion and mental status changes, and flank pain of ethylene glycol ingestion), an infection in a patient with insulin-dependent diabetes mellitus (IDDM), or a history of a prolonged hypotensive episode (e.g., lactic acidosis). (*Chapter 96, Page 837.*)

21.10 Metabolic alkalosis is a primary increase in the plasma concentration of

(A) sodium
(B) potassium
(C) bicarbonate
(D) lactic acid
(E) chloride

Answer: (C). Metabolic alkalosis is a primary increase in plasma bicarbonate concentration (i.e., hyperbicarbonatemia) that causes a compensatory reduction in ventilation and relative hypercapnia (i.e., increased PCO_2). (*Chapter 96, Page 840.*)

21.11 The initial clinical presentation of acute renal failure (ARF) is

(A) increased urine output
(B) decreased urine output
(C) increased urine concentration
(D) dilute urine
(E) increased serum creatinine level

Answer: (B). The initial presentation of ARF is decreased urine output. Clinical manifestations vary, but nausea, weakness, and fatigue are most common. (*Chapter 97, Page 844.*)

21.12 ARF related to renal parenchymal disease most commonly presents in the form of acute tubular necrosis (ATN) and acute interstitial nephritis (AIN). AIN is primarily caused by nephrotoxic drugs. A characteristic finding of AIN is

(A) urinary leukocytosis
(B) increased urinary sodium
(C) increased creatinine clearance
(D) transient urinary eosinophilia
(E) decreased serum protein

Answer: (D). Transient urinary eosinophilia occurs in 80% of AIN. (*Chapter 97, Page 844.*)

21.13 The patient is a 24-year-old white man with ARF. You would consider renal biopsy in which of the following clinical settings?

(A) recent use of high doses of nonsteroidal anti-inflammatory drugs (NSAID)
(B) postrenal failure due to urethral obstruction
(C) sepsis
(D) renal hypoperfusion
(E) urinary casts suggestive of glomerular disease

Answer: (E). Renal biopsy may be indicated in patients with nephrotic syndrome, hematuria, or casts suggestive of glomerular disease, as the biopsy may guide therapy and provide prognostic information. (*Chapter 97, Page 844.*)

21.14 The most common cause of chronic renal failure (CRF) is

(A) diabetes mellitus
(B) congenital renal disease
(C) toxic reaction to medication, especially analgesics
(D) arteriosclerotic vascular disease
(E) none of the above

Answer: (A). Diabetes mellitus is the most common cause of CRF and accounts for more than one-third of all end-stage renal disease (ESRD). Other common causes include hypertension (30%), glomerulonephritis (15%), and polycystic kidney disease (5%). (*Chapter 97, Page 847.*)

21.15 The threshhold for consideration of dialysis or renal transplantation is

(A) a serum creatinine of 3.0 mg/dl
(B) a blood urea nitrogen (BUN) level of 100 mg/dl
(C) weight loss and mental changes
(D) a glomerular filtration rate (GFR) less than 10 ml/min
(E) serum potassium greater than 6.5 mg/dl

Answer: (D). When the GFR becomes less than 10 ml/min, metabolic abnormalities can often no longer be controlled conservatively, and dialysis or renal transplant is considered. (*Chapter 97, Page 847.*)

21.16 The patient is a 10-year-old boy who had hematuria a few weeks ago. Since then, he has developed periorbital edema and some ankle swelling. His blood pressure is 138/86. There are red blood cell (RBC) casts and protein in the urine. This patient's diagnosis appears to be

(A) acute cystitis
(B) glomerulonephritis

(C) chronic renal failure
(D) analgesic-induced nephropathy
(E) Wilms' tumor

Answer: (B). Glomerulonephritis presents with a nephritic syndrome. As the disease progresses, a nephrotic syndrome develops. The nephritic syndrome is characterized by the sudden onset of hematuria often with RBC casts, proteinuria, increasing azotemia, and salt and water retention. This situation causes edema, periorbitally or peripheral (or both), and hypertension. (*Chapter 97, Page 848.*)

21.17 Wilms' tumors account for almost all renal neoplasms during childhood. The tumor is most likely to be discovered by finding

(A) an abdominal mass
(B) hematuria
(C) a UTI
(D) failure to thrive
(E) none of the above

Answer: (A). The median age at diagnosis of a Wilms' tumor is 3 years. The tumor is usually found by discovering an asymptomatic abdominal mass that is generally unilateral. (*Chapter 97, Page 851.*)

21.18 The patient is a 72-year-old man in whom you have just diagnosed cancer of the prostate. He is concerned about prognosis. You can tell him that of men who develop clinically recognized prostate cancer, about how many will die of the disease?

(A) none
(B) 5%
(C) 25%
(D) 50%
(E) 75%

Answer: (C). Only about 25% of men who develop clinically recognized prostate cancer die from it. Additionally, 30 to 40% of men older than age 50 have clinically silent prostate cancer that never results in any health consequences. (*Chapter 98, Page 855.*)

21.19 Advantages of nonscalpel vasectomy over conventional vasectomy include all the following EXCEPT

(A) less bleeding
(B) less chance of injury to tissues surrounding the vas
(C) less discomfort
(D) shorter recovery time
(E) technically easy reversal operation

Answer: (E). This method is safer, with fewer hematomas and infections reported and no skin sutures. It is no more prone to failure than the conventional technique, and the reversal operation is no less difficult with this technique. There is less bleeding, less chance of injury to tissue surrounding the vas, less discomfort, and a shorter recovery time. (*Chapter 99, Page 860.*)

21.20 Which of the following provides curative treatment of human papillomavirus (HPV) infection?

(A) laser
(B) cryotherapy using a nitrous oxide closed probe
(C) trichloracetic acid
(D) 5-fluorouracil (Efudex)
(E) none of the above

Answer: (E). Whether one agrees with the concept of male examinations, there is a basic fact: Today, we cannot cure HPV infection. We can only treat it, reducing the viral load thereby hoping to control it and prevent greater spread of the virus and subsequent dysplastic changes. (*Chapter 99, Page 860.*)

21.21 The most common tumor occurring in men aged 15 to 34 is

(A) lung cancer
(B) adenocarcinoma of the kidney
(C) cancer of the pancreas
(D) testicular cancer
(E) Wilms' tumor

Answer: (D). Testicular cancer is the most common tumor in men aged 15 to 34 and accounts for one of every seven deaths during late adolescence and in young adult men. Case estimates for 1996 were 7,400 cases for all ages, with 370 predicted deaths. (*Chapter 99, Page 861.*)

21.22 The patient is a 10-year-old boy who returned from school 2 hours ago with acute pain in the left testicle. There is no fever, leukocytosis, or pyuria. The immediate management of this patient should be

(A) evaluation for the possibility of testicular torsion
(B) antibiotics to treat probable epididymitis
(C) ice and an athletic supporter to treat a probable contusion of the scrotum
(D) observation for 24 hours
(E) reassurance regarding the psychological aspects of this common problem in prepubertal boys

Answer: (A). Boys with acute testicular pain should be presumed to have testicular torsion until proved otherwise, and it occurs in all age groups with an overall lifetime incidence of about 1.2%. The degree of ischemic injury is in direct proportion to the amount of arterial compression and the interval between onset of symptoms and its correction. (*Chapter 99, Page 862.*)

21.23 The most common type of incontinence in the elderly is

- (A) urge incontinence
- (B) stress incontinence
- (C) overflow incontinence
- (D) functional incontinence
- (E) mixed incontinence

Answer: (A). Urge incontinence is the involuntary loss of urine associated with the abrupt urge to void. Often, the bladder is not completely full. It can result from central neurologic or local loss of control over the bladder. The detrusor muscle is the smooth muscle wall of the bladder, and uninhibited bladder or detrusor contractions overcome urethral resistance. There is usually a warning of an urge to urinate for a few seconds to a few minutes before loss of a significant amount of urine. This is the most common etiology for incontinence in the elderly, causing 50 to 70% of cases in certain populations. (*Chapter 100, Page 866.*)

21.24 The patient is a 46-year-old white gravida 4, para 4 woman with mild hypertension treated with diet and exercise. She has no other significant medical problems. For the past 6 months, she has noticed occasional loss of urine when she laughs or coughs. This patient has

- (A) urge incontinence
- (B) stress incontinence
- (C) overflow incontinence
- (D) functional incontinence
- (E) mixed incontinence

Answer: (B). In ambulatory adult women, stress incontinence is the most common. (*Chapter 100, Page 867.*)

21.25 The patient is a 60-year-old white man with urinary hesitancy, a sense of incomplete voiding, and occasional urinary incontinence. On examination, he has a large symmetrical prostate. This patient appears to have

- (A) urge incontinence
- (B) stress incontinence
- (C) overflow incontinence
- (D) functional incontinence
- (E) mixed incontinence

Answer: (C). Overflow incontinence results when urine is lost from an overdistended, full bladder. This usually occurs in patients with a voiding defect and subsequent urinary retention. Often, they have a history of urinary hesitancy, diminished flow, a need to strain to void, and a sense of incomplete voiding. Drugs or disorders that block urinary outflow or cause bladder outlet obstruction (tumor, prostatic hyperplasia, urethral stricture or spasm) can cause overflow incontinence despite adequate detrusor contractions. (*Chapter 100, Page 867.*)

21.26 Which of the following individuals is at the highest risk for testicular cancer?

- (A) a 16-year-old boy with a 1-hour history of pain in the left testicle
- (B) a 20-year-old man with a history of trauma to the scrotum
- (C) a 60-year-old man with an enlarged scrotum that transilluminates
- (D) a 40-year-old man with a history of mumps orchitis
- (E) a 32-year-old man with an intra-abdominal undescended left testicle

Answer: (E). Intra-abdominal undescended testicles are at highest risk, even after successful corrective surgery; and the malignancy may occur in either testicle. Ten percent of men with a tumor have a history of testicular maldescent. (*Chapter 100, Page 872.*)

21.27 The patient is a 52-year-old white man, here for a small, painless mass, about 1.0 cm in diameter, superior and posterior to the right testis. The mass is easily separable from the testis and is freely mobile. This patient appears to have

- (A) torsion of the appendix testis
- (B) a varicocele
- (C) a hydrocele
- (D) a spermatocele
- (E) a cyst of the vas deferens

Answer: (D). Spermatoceles are small, painless cystic masses that arise from the rete testis, ductuli efferentes, or epididymis. They are common, are often found on routine examination of the scrotum, and are usually superior and posterior to the testis. Easily separable from the testis, most are freely mobile. (*Chapter 100, Page 873.*)

21.28 More than half of all bladder cancers may be related to

(A) exposure to dyes, including arylamine, benzine, and beta-naphthylamine
(B) work with leather
(C) occupational exposure to metal fumes
(D) occupational exposure to rubber
(E) cigarette smoking

Answer: (E). Individuals at increased risk for bladder cancer include those who work with dyes (arylamine, benzine, and beta-naphthylamine), leathers, metals, and rubber. Industrial and occupational carcinogens are thought to be responsible for 21% of bladder cancers. Cigarette smoking increases the risk three- to six-fold and accounts for up to 60% of bladder cancers. (*Chapter 100, Page 874.*)

21.29 The currently effective method of screening mass populations for bladder cancer is

(A) history of UTIs
(B) history of cigarette smoking
(C) urine analysis
(D) urine cytology
(E) none of the above

Answer: (E). At the present time, there is no effective recommended screening method for mass populations. The American Cancer Society recommendations for cancer screening do not include any for the bladder, which was confirmed by the 1996 U.S. Preventive Task Force recommendations. (*Chapter 100, Page 874.*)

21.30 Most bladder cancers are of what histologic type?

(A) transitional cell carcinoma
(B) squamous cell carcinoma
(C) adenocarcinoma
(D) metastatic carcinoma
(E) none of the above

Answer: (A). Transitional cell carcinomas (80 to 90%) predominate, with the remainder being either squamous cell carcinoma or adenocarcinoma of the urinary bladder. Transitional cell carcinoma of the urinary bladder may present as a papillary or solid tumor or a diffusely erythematous neoplastic lesion, carcinoma in situ. (*Chapter 100, Page 875.*)

21.31 The patient is a 58-year-old white man with the acute onset of left flank pain radiating to the perineum,

associated with nausea and vomiting. This patient most likely has

(A) renal trauma
(B) renal colic
(C) a renal tumor
(D) renal infection
(E) infarction of the left renal artery

Answer: (B). Urolithiasis generally presents with renal colic (flank pain, nausea, and vomiting). The pain can be localized in the costovertebral angle or radiate to the perineum. Recurrent emesis may result from acute distension of the renal pelvis or an ileus. The patient is generally afebrile unless a secondary infection is present. (*Chapter 100, Page 875.*)

21.32 The patient is a 57-year-old white man with left flank pain. An intravenous pyelogram reveals a 4-mm stone high in the left ureter. This patient can be counseled that he will probably

(A) develop an infection proximal to the stone
(B) pass the stone spontaneously
(C) require laparascopic surgery for stone removal
(D) require abdominal surgery to remove the stone
(E) require cystoscopy to remove the stone with a "basket"

Answer: (B). The chance of spontaneously passing a stone is 85% for a stone of 4 to 5 mm and 10% for a stone larger than 5 mm. Hydration is emphasized. The patient may require strong analgesics during this time, and all attempts should be made to control the pain. (*Chapter 100, Page 876.*)

DIRECTIONS (Items 21.33 through 21.57): Each of the items in this section is a multiple true–false problem that consists of a stem and four lettered options. Indicate whether each of the four options is TRUE or FALSE.

21.33 Diagnostic imaging should be performed on selected patients with UTIs. Such patients would include which of the following?

(A) a 3-year-old girl with her first episode of a UTI
(B) a 10-year-old boy with cystitis
(C) a 17-year-old sexually active high school girl with her first episode of cystitis
(D) a 12-year-old girl with pyelonephritis

Answer: (A-True, B-True, C-False, D-True). Imaging tests should be conducted after the first episode of UTI in girls younger than 5 years, boys of any age, older sexually inactive girls with recurrent UTI, and any child with pyelonephritis. (*Chapter 95, Page 817.*)

21.34 The patient is a 21-year-old African American primigravida woman at 15 weeks' gestation. You have just diagnosed a UTI. Antibiotics considered reasonably safe for use in this patient would include which of the following?

(A) sulfonamides
(B) cephalosporins
(C) nitrofurantoin
(D) methenamine

Answer: (A-False, B-True, C-False, D-True). The first concern regarding treatment during pregnancy is the safety of antibiotics. Considered reasonably safe are penicillins, cephalosporins, and methenamine. Cautious use can be considered with sulfonamides (allergic reaction, kernicterus, glucose-6-phosphate dehydrogenase [G6PD] deficiency), aminoglycosides (eighth nerve and renal toxicity), nitrofurantoin (neuropathy, G6PD deficiency), clindamycin (allergic reaction, pseudomembranous colitis), and erythromycin estolate (cholestatic hepatitis). (*Chapter 95, Page 818.*)

21.35 The patient is a 22-year-old primigravida woman at 10 weeks' gestation. She has urinary burning and frequency, but no fever is present. This is the first time she has had such symptoms. A urine analysis in your office reveals 10 to 15 white blood cells per high-powered field with a few bacteria present. Your management for this patient might reasonably be which of the following?

(A) oral amoxicillin
(B) norfloxacin
(C) gentamicin
(D) macrocrystalline nitrofurantoin

Answer: (A-True, B-False, C-False, D-True). For cystitis during pregnancy, consider a 7-day regimen that includes oral amoxicillin, macrocrystalline nitrofurantoin, cefpodoxime proxetil, or TMP-SMX. Avoid using fluoroquinolones in pregnant women, and use gentamicin cautiously because of fetal eighth nerve threat. TMP-SMX has not been approved for use during pregnancy but is widely used. (*Chapter 95, Page 819.*)

21.36 True statements regarding UTIs in young men include which of the following?

(A) Homosexuality can be a risk factor.
(B) Circumcision may be a risk factor for UTIs in young men.

(C) UTIs in a young man are more likely to occur if a sex partner is colonized with uropathogens.
(D) Management of symptomatic cystitis in a young man requires a urine culture to establish the pathogen.

Answer: (A-True, B-False, C-True, D-True). Without underlying structural urologic abnormalities, risk factors for UTIs in young men include homosexuality, lack of circumcision, and a sex partner colonized with uropathogens. Management of symptomatic cystitis without obvious complicating factors requires a urine culture to establish the pathogen. (*Chapter 95, Page 820.*)

21.37 An elevated BUN concentration may be found in which of the following clinical settings?

(A) intrinsic renal disease
(B) excessive cellular catabolism
(C) protein deficiency
(D) hemodilution

Answer: (A-True, B-True, C-False, D-False). Elevated BUN concentration (greater than 20 mg/dl) suggests the presence of prerenal azotemia, intrinsic renal disease, postrenal disease, excessive cellular catabolism, or gastrointestinal tract bleeding. Low BUN (less than 10 mg/dl) occurs with protein deficiency and hemodilution. (*Chapter 96, Page 828.*)

21.38 Hypercalcemia in the setting of normal parathyroid hormone (PTH) can be caused by

(A) vitamin D excess
(B) sarcoidosis
(C) hypothyroidism
(D) bony metastasis

Answer: (A-True, B-True, C-False, D-True). Hypercalcemia associated with normal PTH is caused by vitamin D excess, sarcoidosis, hyperthyroidism, increased bone calcium release (e.g., immobilization and bony metastasis), extracellular fluid depletion, thiazides, or milk-alkali syndrome. (*Chapter 96, Page 828.*)

21.39 The patient is a 62-year-old white man with postural hypotension due to hypovolemia. His BUN/creatinine ratio is 10:1. This combination of findings is consistent with which of the following clinical settings?

(A) protein starvation
(B) ARF caused by benign prostatic hypertrophy (BPH)
(C) excessive catabolism
(D) ATN

Answer: (A-True, B-True, C-False, D-True). BUN is retained in volume-depleted states such that the normal 10:1 BUN/creatinine ratio is elevated (e.g., to greater than 20:1) because of renal hypoperfusion resulting in prerenal azotemia and nonintrinsic or functional ARF. Elevation of BUN and maintenance of a BUN/creatinine ratio of 10:1 in the presence of volume depletion may be indicative of protein starvation or ARF caused by postrenal obstruction (e.g., BPH, carcinoma, stones, blood clots, papillary necrosis) or intrinsic renal disease caused by hypotension-induced renal ischemia causing ATN. (*Chapter 96, Page 831.*)

21.40 Causes of volume excess include which of the following?

(A) chronic renal failure
(B) decreased extracellular volume
(C) mineralocorticoid deficiency
(D) infusion of water and sodium at rates exceeding renal excretion

Answer: (A-True, B-True, C-False, D-True). Volume excess, or hypervolemia, can be caused by decreased extracellular volume (ECV), which results in renal sodium and water conservation and edema formation (e.g., hypoalbuminemia and left ventricular dysfunction). Volume excess can also be caused by chronic renal failure, mineralocorticoid excess, and infusion of sodium and water at rates exceeding renal excretion, ultimately resulting in total body hypervolemia and increased ECV. (*Chapter 96, Page 832.*)

21.41 Complications that may be seen with diuretic treatment of volume excess include which of the following?

(A) hypokalemia
(B) hypovolemia
(C) hypermagnesemia
(D) hypoglycemia

Answer: (A-True, B-True, C-False, D-False). Treatment of volume excess with diuretics is associated with many complications, the most significant of which are hypokalemia, hypovolemia, metabolic alkalosis (i.e., thiazides and loop diuretics), metabolic acidosis (carbonic anhydrase inhibitors and the distal tubular diuretics amiloride, triamterene, and spironolactone), hypomagnesemia, and worsening glucose tolerance (especially thiazides). (*Chapter 96, Page 833.*)

21.42 Hypernatremia can be seen in which of the following settings?

(A) prolonged high fever with pure water loss through skin
(B) chronically depressed respirations of a patient in coma
(C) nephrogenic diabetes insipidus
(D) excess addition of sodium salts to body fluid compartments

Answer: (A-True, B-False, C-True, D-True). Hypernatremia can result from pure water loss through skin (e.g., fever), through the respiratory tract (e.g., hyperventilation), and in the presence of nephrogenic and central diabetes insipidus when there is a reduction in secretion or action of antidiuretic hormone. The hypernatremic state can also be caused by excess addition of sodium salts to body fluid compartments. (*Chapter 96, Page 834.*)

21.43 True statements regarding hypokalemia include which of the following?

(A) Hypokalemia is the electrolyte abnormality most commonly seen in family medicine.
(B) The most common cause of hypokalemia is diuretic use.
(C) Hypokalemia usually occurs in the setting of oliguria.
(D) Hypomagnesemia can contribute to hypokalemia.

Answer: (A-True, B-True, C-False, D-True). Hypokalemia, the most frequent electrolyte abnormality seen in family medicine, is usually caused by the use of medullary and cortical loop diuretics (e.g., furosemide and hydrochlorothiazide). Plasma hypokalemia, reflecting potassium loss from all body fluid compartments (i.e., total body potassium depletion), can occur as a result of excessive urinary, gastrointestinal, and skin potassium losses. Renal potassium losses (i.e., $U_K > 25$ mEq/L) leading to total body hypokalemia can result from diuretic use, polyuria, sodium-losing nephropathies, primary mineralocorticoid excess, vomiting, and hypomagnesemia. (*Chapter 96, Page 835.*)

21.44 Some drugs may cause hyperkalemia. These include

(A) furosemide
(B) spironolactone
(C) angiotensin-converting enzyme (ACE) inhibitors
(D) NSAIDs

Answer: (A-False, B-True, C-True, D-True). Drugs capable of causing hypoaldosteronism and hyperkalemia include distal tubular diuretics (e.g., spironolactone, amiloride, and triamterene), ACE inhibitors, and NSAIDs. (*Chapter 96, Page 836.*)

21.45 Respiratory acidosis can be caused by

    (A) excessive stimulation of the central nervous system (CNS) respiratory center
    (B) Guillain-Barré syndrome
    (C) sleep apnea
    (D) hyperventilation

Answer: (A-False, B-True, C-True, D-False). Respiratory acidosis is caused by CNS respiratory center inhibition (e.g., sedatives), disorders of the respiratory and chest wall muscles (e.g., Guillain-Barré syndrome), obstruction to ventilation (e.g., sleep apnea), and pulmonary perfusion and diffusion dysfunction (e.g., severe diffuse pneumonias). (*Chapter 96, Page 841.*)

21.46 In a patient with ARF, dietary restrictions should include reduced intake of

    (A) sodium
    (B) calories
    (C) potassium
    (D) magnesium

Answer: (A-True, B-False, C-True, D-True). Dietary restrictions in ARF include sodium, potassium, phosphorus, protein, and magnesium. Total caloric intake of 35 to 50 kcal/kg/day should be maintained. (*Chapter 97, Page 846.*)

21.47 ACE inhibitors reduce the degree of albuminuria and slow progression of renal disease. ACE inhibitor use is generally recommended in which of the following settings?

    (A) the patient with IDDM with overt albuminuria
    (B) the patient with IDDM with microalbuminuria
    (C) patients with IDDM and hypertension
    (D) Patients with non–insulin-dependent diabetes mellitus (NIDDM) with normal blood pressure and microalbuminuria

Answer: (A-True, B-True, C-True, D-False). ACE inhibitors reduce the degree of albuminuria and slow progression of renal disease. ACE inhibition in IDDM with overt or microalbuminuria regardless of blood pressure slows the progression of the disease. For patients with NIDDM with normal blood pressure and microalbuminuria, the data are insufficient to recommend ACE inhibition. (*Chapter 97, Page 847.*)

21.48 Characteristics of the nephrotic syndrome include which of the following?

    (A) proteinuria
    (B) hyperproteinemia
    (C) peripheral edema
    (D) hypolipidemia

Answer: (A-True, B-False, C-True, D-False). The nephrotic syndrome is characterized by increased proteinuria (greater than 3.5 g/day), hypoproteinemia, peripheral edema, and hyperlipidemia. (*Chapter 97, Page 848.*)

21.49 True statements regarding autosomal dominant polycystic kidney disease (ADPKD) include which of the following?

    (A) The lesions of ADPKD are limited to the kidney.
    (B) ADPKD is present in approximately 10% of patients with end-stage renal disease (ESRD).
    (C) Cystic fibrosis is 15 times more common than ADPKD.
    (D) ADPKD occurs in 1 per 1,000 individuals.

Answer: (A-False, B-True, C-False, D-True). ADPKD occurs in 1 per 1,000 individuals, affecting 500,000 Americans; it is present in approximately 10% of patients with ESRD. It is the most common hereditary disease: 20 times more common than Huntington's chorea, 15 times more common that cystic fibrosis, and 10 times more common than sickle cell disease. ADPKD is a systemic disease. In addition to renal cysts, cysts develop in the liver, pancreas, spleen, seminal vesicles, ovaries, and CNS. (*Chapter 97, Page 850.*)

21.50 Organisms that cause chronic bacterial prostatitis include which of the following?

    (A) *Staphylococcus aureus*
    (B) *Proteus*
    (C) *Pseudomonas*
    (D) *Escherichia coli*

Answer: (A-False, B-True, C-True, D-True). Chronic bacterial prostatitis is a form of prostatitis that should be suspected in any man who has recurrent infection of the urinary tract. The causative bacteria are usually aerobic gram-negative rods including *Escherichia coli, Proteus, Pseudomonas,* and *Klebsiella* or occasionally, the enterococcus. The infection results from urethral colonization and bacteriuria, leading to an ascending infection via the prostatic ducts. (*Chapter 98, Page 852.*)

21.51 The patient is a 73-year-old white male retiree with urinary frequency, urgency, and nocturia. The prostate is enlarged on digital examination. To control this patient's symptoms, you are considering the use of alpha-adrenergic antagonists. True statements regarding this class of medication include which of the following?

(A) These drugs act by increasing smooth muscle tone and augmenting the dynamic component of outflow resistance.
(B) Representative members of this class include terazosin, prazosin, and doxazosin.
(C) The symptomatic benefits of these drugs are generally only of short duration.
(D) The response of alpha-adrenergic antagonists is generally slower than that seen with finasteride.

Answer: (A-False, B-True, C-False, D-False). The alpha-adrenergic antagonist drugs block the receptors of the bladder neck and prostatic urethra, decreasing smooth muscle tone and diminishing the dynamic component of outflow resistance. Representative alpha-blockers used to treat BPH include terazosin (Hytrin), prazosin (Minipress), and doxazosin (Cardura). Alpha-blockers are moderately effective and provide long-term benefit regarding the symptoms of BPH. The response is seen more rapidly than with finasteride. (*Chapter 98, Page 855.*)

21.52 The prostatic specific antigen (PSA) test is sometimes used in screening for cancer of the prostate. In addition to cancer of the prostate, high values may also be seen in which of the following settings?

(A) BPH
(B) prostatitis
(C) following routine digital rectal examination (DRE)
(D) following prostate surgery

Answer: (A-True, B-True, C-False, D-True). The PSA is an enzyme produced by epithelial cells of the prostate that hydrolyzes the ejaculate and has a function in male fertility. The PSA can be elevated in BPH, prostatitis, prostate cancer, prostate trauma, and after prostate surgery. "Routine" DRE does not raise the PSA significantly. (*Chapter 98, Page 856.*)

21.53 True statements regarding vasectomy include which of the following?

(A) Pathologic confirmation of excised tissue is unnecessary because structures are readily visualized during surgery.

(B) Orchitis and epididymitis are uncommon complications of the procedure.
(C) In experienced hands, the failure rate is less than 1%.
(D) The failure rate is stated to be higher with the nonscalpel method than with the conventional method.

Answer: (A-False, B-True, C-True, D-False). Because unforeseen results leading to pregnancy do occur secondary to recanalization or ligation of the wrong structure, pathologic confirmation of the excised tissue is recommended. Orchitis and epididymitis are other uncommon complications. Failure rates for the conventional vasectomy vary from 0.24 to 6.00% (more commonly less than 1% in experienced hands). They are stated to be much lower with the nonscalpel method. (*Chapter 99, Page 859.*)

21.54 Diagnostic tests that may prove useful in the diagnosis of testicular torsion include

(A) determination of serum concentrations of luteinizing hormone and follicle-stimulating hormone
(B) Doppler ultrasound studies
(C) radioactive imaging
(D) dynamic enhanced MRI

Answer: (A-False, B-True, C-True, D-True). Readily available aids in diagnosis include the testicular scan or color Doppler ultrasound studies, with a sensitivity of 80% and a specificity of 100%. Radioactive imaging is considered highly specific in the diagnosis of older children with epididymitis who may have structural or functional urinary tract abnormalities. Dynamic enhanced magnetic resonance imaging (MRI) appears to be helpful for documenting a perfusion deficit due to testicular torsion. (*Chapter 99, Page 863.*)

21.55 The patient is an 82-year-old white woman with involuntary loss of urine associated with the abrupt urge to void. Physical examination is normal, and she has no medical illness. Medications that may be helpful in this setting include which of the following?

(A) propantheline bromide
(B) dicyclomine hydrochloride
(C) spironolactone
(D) imipramine

Answer: (A-True, B-True, C-False, D-True). Anticholinergics, antispasmodics, and tricyclic antidepressants appear to be the most effective drugs for urge incontinence. (*Chapter 100, Page 870.*)

21.56 True statements regarding physical examination of a patient with a varicocele include which of the following?

(A) The Valsalva maneuver may cause a brief decrease in size of the varicocele.
(B) With a patient in the recumbent position and with inspiration, the size of the varicocele may decrease.
(C) If a varicocele is found on the left, causative pathology should be suspected.
(D) Occasionally, the presence of a varix may be associated with a smaller testis on the side of the varicocele.

Answer: (A-False, B-True, C-False, D-True). When the patient performs the Valsalva maneuver, the examiner should feel a brief increase in size and an impulse of blood. With the patient in the recumbent position and with inspiration, this prominence should decrease. If the varicocele does not collapse in the recumbent position, retroperitoneal or renal pathology must be considered. In addition, varicoceles usually occur on the left; if found on the right, secondary pathology is suspected. Occasionally, when there is a discrepancy in testicular size, the smaller testis is associated with the varix. (*Chapter 100, Page 873.*)

21.57 True statements regarding extracorporeal shock wave lithotripsy (ESWL) include

(A) ESWL may be used for calculi within the kidney, ureter, or bladder.
(B) Only about 25% of patients using ESWL are stone-free at the end of 3 months.
(C) The larger the calculus, the greater the probability that a secondary treatment will be required.
(D) Following ESWL, most patients require 5 to 7 days of rest before returning to work.

Answer: (A-True, B-False, C-True, D-False). Most patients return to their normal level of activities within 24 to 48 hours. Previously, ESWL was reserved primarily for renal calculi but now may be used for calculi within the kidney, ureter, or bladder, with a 90% chance of rendering the patient stone-free within 3 months. The larger the calculus, the greater the chance that a secondary treatment will be required. Eighty-seven percent of patients with stones of less than 2 cm are stone-free at 3 months. (*Chapter 100, Page 878.*)

22

The Female Reproductive System

The questions in this chapter constitute a review of the following chapters in *Family Medicine: Principles and Practice, Fifth Edition:*

DIRECTIONS (Items 22.1 through 22.38): Each of the questions or incomplete statements in this section is followed by five suggested answers or completions. Select the ONE that is BEST in each case.

22.1 The patient is a 38-year-old African American woman who reports that yesterday she had an intrauterine device (IUD) inserted at a community clinic. The insertion seemed difficult and painful, and she has continued to have some pelvic discomfort. An ultrasound study reveals the IUD to be outside the uterus. Appropriate management for this patient would be

(A) observation and a repeat examination under sterile conditions in 48 hours
(B) antibiotic therapy to prevent infection
(C) a prescription for oral contraceptives
(D) laparoscopic removal of the IUD
(E) none of the above

Answer: (D). Perforation rates are reported to occur in one per 1,000 IUD insertions and are generally related to the force exerted during insertion. If the IUD cannot be located inside the uterus, an ultrasound study is performed. Any IUD located outside the uterus is electively removed by laparoscopy. Severe peritoneal reactions can occur if an abdominal IUD is not removed. (*Chapter 101, Page 882.*)

22.2 Which *one* of the following types of diaphragm can be worn by most patients?

(A) arcing spring diaphragm
(B) coil spring diaphragm
(C) flat spring diaphragm
(D) wide seal diaphragm
(E) no single diaphragm is appropriate for most patients.

Answer: (A). The arcing spring diaphragm has a strong rim and spring. This diaphragm arcs when folded and makes insertion easy. The arcing diaphragm can be worn by most patients, even those with cystocele, rectocele, or laxity of muscle tone. (*Chapter 101, Page 882.*)

22.3 Which of the following conditions has been reported in patients who wear a diaphragm longer than 36 hours?

(A) toxic shock syndrome (TSS)
(B) pelvic inflammatory disease (PID)
(C) cervical carcinoma in situ
(D) meibomian cysts
(E) actinomycotic pelvic infection

Answer: (A). TSS has been reported when the diaphragm is worn longer than 36 hours, especially in those patients who fail to replenish the spermicide after repeated coitus. (*Chapter 101, Page 882.*)

22.4 The use of spermicides help protect against

(A) pregnancy
(B) gonorrhea
(C) *Chlamydia* infection
(D) human immunodeficiency virus (HIV) infection
(E) all the above

Answer: (E). Clinical studies have indicated that spermicide protects against the gonococcus, *Chlamydia*, and HIV. Laboratory studies have shown that nonoxynol-9 inactivates HIV within 60 seconds of exposure to the spermicide and may be toxic to lymphocytes infected by HIV. (*Chapter 101, Page 883.*)

22.5 There is a higher risk of discontinuing oral contraceptive pill (OCP) use or having a higher failure rate with such use in patients who use which of the following?

(A) alcohol
(B) tobacco
(C) coffee
(D) vitamin C
(E) supplementary calcium tablets

Answer: (B). The proportion of smokers using combination OCPs with 20 to 30 mg of ethinyl estradiol reporting spotting or bleeding is significantly higher than that of nonsmokers. The relative risk of spotting or bleeding for smokers compared with nonsmokers appears to increase with greater levels of smoking, so women smoking 16 or more cigarettes per day have a nearly threefold increased risk of abnormal bleeding while using OCPs. Therefore, smokers may be more likely to discontinue OCPs and so incur higher failure rates. (*Chapter 101, Page 884.*)

22.6 The patient is a 21-year-old college woman who had unprotected sexual intercourse last night. She calls your office today asking for emergency contraception. You may appropriately advise her that the "morning-after pill" is typically administered as follows:

(A) one OCP daily for 5 days
(B) four combination OCPs taken in pairs 12 hours apart within 72 hours of unprotected sexual intercourse
(C) eight OCPs taken as soon as possible after unprotected sexual intercourse
(D) three OCPs taken the morning following intercourse and repeated at 1 week
(E) four progesterone-only pills taken within 24 hours of unprotected intercourse

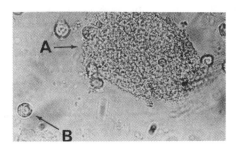

Fig. 22.1. Question 22.8. (From Fischer P. *The Office Laboratory.* Norwalk, CT: Appleton & Lange, 1983. With permission.)

Answer: (B). The emergency contraceptive pill, commonly known as the morning-after pill, is used as a postcoital method of preventing pregnancy. Women who were not able to anticipate and plan contraception might use this method. The regimen is typically administered as four combination OCPs taken in pairs 12 hours apart within 72 hours of unprotected intercourse. Treatment after 72 hours is not likely to be effective. Each OCP usually contains 50 mg ethinyl estradiol and 0.5 mg norgestrel or 1.0 mg levonorgestrel. (*Chapter 101, Pages 886–887.*)

22.7 Emergency contraception can be administered as four combination OCPs taken in pairs 12 hours apart within 72 hours of unprotected intercourse. The primary mode of action of the morning-after pill appears to be

(A) suppression of ovulation
(B) the production a luteolytic effect
(C) tubal transport modification
(D) an embryotoxic effect
(E) the modification of the nidation site

Answer: (E). The primary mode of action of the morning-after pill does not appear to be ovulation suppression, the production of a luteolytic effect, tubal transport modification, or an embryotoxic effect. It appears that the primary mechanism of action is modification of the nidation site, making it unsuitable for implantation. (*Chapter 101, Page 887.*)

22.8 The figure above is a vaginal wet preparation obtained from a 28-year-old single white woman who complains of a 10-day history of vaginal discharge. In this figure, the structure identified by **A** is a

(A) trichomonad
(B) clue cell
(C) lymphocyte
(D) leukocyte
(E) renal epithelial cell

Answer: (B). "Clue cells" are vaginal epithelial cells "studded" with bacteria that adhere for unknown reasons. These epithelial cells look dense and tend to "glitter" when the focus is varied. Although clue cells are present normally in up to 10% of the field, a preponderance of them, especially when combined with a fishy odor on the potassium hydroxide (KOH) preparation, supports the diagnosis of bacterial vaginosis. (*Chapter 102, Page 891.*)

22.9 The most common cause of vaginitis is now

  (A) bacterial vaginosis
  (B) mycotic diseases
  (C) hypersensitivity related to toxic chemicals
  (D) trichomoniasis
  (E) viral infection

Answer: (A). The most common cause of vaginitis is now bacterial vaginosis, followed by mycotic diseases (e.g., *Candida* sp.), with trichomoniasis on the decline. (*Chapter 102, Page 893.*)

22.10 The patient is a 33-year-old white woman who believes that she has a fungal infection of the vagina. Her complaints include vaginal itching and a cheesy discharge. A firm diagnosis of mycotic vaginitis should be based on finding

  (A) vaginal pruritus
  (B) vaginal inflammation with punctate lesions
  (C) a cheesy vaginal exudate
  (D) hyphae present on a KOH preparation
  (E) a positive culture of vaginal secretions

Answer: (D). Although the incidence is rising, contrary to popular belief among patients and physicians, true fungal infections probably account for approximately one-third of all vaginal infections. The textbook presentation is a patient complaining of a vaginal itch and cheesy exudate, with white plaques adherent to the vaginal wall and a KOH preparation showing multiple hyphae. The diagnosis should not be made unless hyphae are seen on the slide. Because as many as 20% of asymptomatic women have positive cultures, it is obvious that culture methods are too sensitive and should be reserved for refractory cases, frequent relapses, or when yeast is suspected clinically but the KOH preparation is negative. (*Chapter 102, Page 894.*)

22.11 The patient is a 29-year-old white female office worker who complains of vaginal itching and urinary frequency. On examination, the vaginal mucosa is inflamed, and there are petechiae on the cervix. The discharge is yellow-green and has a "bubbly" consistency. On the vaginal wet preparation, you are likely to see which organism?

  (A) *Candida albicans*
  (B) *Candida glabrata*
  (C) *Neisseria gonorrhoeae*
  (D) *Gardnerella vaginalis*
  (E) *Trichomonas vaginalis*

Answer: (E). The syndrome caused by *Trichomonas vaginalis* may cause severe itching or pain often accompanied by frequency of urination because of concomitant cystitis from the organism. On examination, the vulva and the vaginal mucosa is fiery red with cervical petechiae ("strawberry cervix"). The typical discharge is yellow-green and bubbly in nature, but any range of color and texture may be seen, making slide examination critical. As noted above, the diagnosis is made by finding motile trichomonads on the saline smear. (*Chapter 102, Page 894.*)

22.12 The patient is a 33-year-old white woman here for a routine examination and Pap smear. She notes a recent increase in the amount of vaginal secretions and an odor that is most noticeable after intercourse. There is a "fishy" odor present following the addition of KOH to a vaginal wet preparation. The cause of this patient's vaginosis is most likely to be

  (A) contact
  (B) mycotic
  (C) trichomoniasis
  (D) bacterial
  (E) atrophic

Answer: (D). Because its course is usually indolent, bacterial vaginosis does not cause an acute change in symptoms. The patient may note only a slight change in normal discharge and an odor that may be more pronounced after intercourse. Patients are frequently inured to the symptoms until treatment is finished and the discharge gone. There may not be an odor immediately on examination, but KOH releases the amines in the epithelial cells and produces the classic fishy odor that is diagnostic when clue cells are present. (*Chapter 102, Page 895.*)

22.13 The patient is a 52-year-old white woman with signs and symptoms of atrophic vaginitis. The treatment of choice for this patient is

  (A) terconazole cream or vaginal suppository
  (B) nystatin applied vaginally and taken as oral tablets

(C) miconazole vaginal cream
(D) estrogen hormone replacement therapy
(E) metronidazole 250 mg t.i.d. for 7 days

Answer: (D). Hormone replacement therapy is the treatment of choice, but vaginal estrogen creams used nightly can provide short-term relief. The patient must be reminded that a vaginal "discharge" may recur as the cells mature back to a premenopausal pattern. (*Chapter 102, Page 895.*)

22.14 The patient is a 52-year-old white woman who complains of vulvar burning and a white vaginal discharge. On examination, you note violaceous papules on the skin with small, lacy, gray, reticular patterns on the inner labia. This patient may have which one of the following diagnoses?

(A) lichen sclerosis
(B) lichen simplex chronicus
(C) lichen planus
(D) vulvar carcinoma
(E) diabetes mellitus

Answer: (C). Lichen planus may involve mucous membranes in other organ systems. There is vulvar burning, leukorrhea, and redness of the inner labia. Patients may have violaceous papules externally and small, lacy, gray, reticular patterns on the inner labia. Without these identifying marks, this lesion may appear similar to that of atrophic vaginitis; it should be entertained as a diagnosis whenever therapy for atrophic vaginitis fails. (*Chapter 102, Page 896.*)

22.15 The definition of *metrorrhagia* is

(A) the loss of more than 90 ml of blood during a menstrual period
(B) menstrual cycles 35 days or more
(C) menstrual periods that occur with a frequency of 20 days or less
(D) bleeding between menstrual cycles
(E) bleeding following sexual intercourse

Answer: (D). Metrorrhagia is bleeding between menstrual cycles. It is associated with ovulatory midcycle spotting or bleeding but may also be a sign of endometrial polyps and uterine malignancy. (*Chapter 103, Page 900.*)

22.16 The most common cause of secondary amenorrhea is

(A) cancer
(B) stress

(C) excessive exercise
(D) eating disorders
(E) pregnancy

Answer: (E). The most common etiology of secondary amenorrhea is pregnancy. (*Chapter 103, Page 900.*)

22.17 The patient is a thin 35-year-old white woman with a 7-month history of amenorrhea. There is no galactorrhea, and her levels of prolactin and thyroid-stimulating hormone (TSH) are normal. Her pregnancy test was negative 2 months ago. Her body hair distribution is normal. This patient's amenorrhea is most likely due to

(A) an eating disorder
(B) anovulation
(C) a functioning pituitary microadenoma
(D) Stein-Levinthal syndrome
(E) a pelvic tumor

Answer: (B). In the presence of normal TSH and the absence of galactorrhea, amenorrhea in women younger than the age of 40 is most likely secondary to anovulation, which results in the production of unopposed estrogen. (*Chapter 103, Page 901.*)

22.18 Postmenopausal osteoporosis is common and can lead to fractures. Of the following fractures, which type accounts for the highest costs and mortality risk?

(A) humerus
(B) vertebral
(C) wrist
(D) tibia
(E) hip

Answer: (E). Up to one-third of women older than age 50 experience a vertebral crush fracture, and more than 250,000 osteoporosis-related hip fractures occur annually. The risk of clinically significant bone loss is related to many genetic and environmental factors. Humerus, vertebral, and wrist fractures are common, but hip fractures account for the highest costs and mortality risk. (*Chapter 103, Page 910.*)

22.19 The patient is a 44-year-old white businesswoman who has had very light and irregular periods for about the past 8 months and no menses for the past three cycles. She has had a few instances of feeling a sensation of warmth. She has a strong desire to know now if this represents the menopause. If you were to do one test to confirm this diagnosis, that test would be to measure the serum level of

(A) luteinizing hormone (LH)
(B) gonadotropin-releasing hormone
(C) follicle-stimulating hormone (FSH)
(D) estradiol
(E) progesterone

Answer: (C). The recognition of menopause is ordinarily not difficult. A woman in her late 40s or early 50s with amenorrhea and classic hot flashes presents little diagnostic uncertainty. Other conditions can mimic hot flashes, however. If doubt exists, serum FSH may be assayed to confirm postmenopausal (high) levels. (*Chapter 104, Page 911.*)

22.20 The patient is a 52-year-old Asian-American woman in the climacteric who reports troublesome hot flashes that are interfering with her work and keeping her awake at night. Hot flashes may respond to all the following medications EXCEPT

(A) estrogens
(B) nicotinic acid
(C) medroxyprogesterone
(D) megestrol
(E) clonidine

Answer: (B). Hot flashes respond reliably to exogenous estrogens. If estrogens are contraindicated, progestins alone can ameliorate hot flashes, although they are not as effective as estrogens. Doses of progestins commonly used are medroxyprogesterone acetate (Cycrin, Provera) 20 mg/day, megestrol acetate (Megace) 40 mg/day, or depot medroxyprogesterone acetate (Depo-Provera) 50 to 150 mg intramuscularly every 1 to 3 months. In women who cannot take estrogens or progestins, several agents may help palliate vasomotor symptoms. Clonidine (Catapres) is somewhat effective, and some women's symptoms are reduced with Bellergal-S (Sandoz), a combination of ergotamine, belladonna alkaloids, and phenobarbital. (*Chapter 104, Page 911.*)

22.21 Estrogens stabilize bone density in postmenopausal women and reduce the risk of hip fracture by 50%. When there are no other risk factors for osteoporosis, estrogen use should begin

(A) with the birth of the first child
(B) 10 years prior to anticipated menopause
(C) early in menopause
(D) 5 to 7 years after the cessation of menses
(E) at the time of vertebral or hip fracture

Answer: (C). Bone loss rapidly escalates at menopause, with substantial loss during the first few years of post-

menopausal estrogen levels. Thus, early institution of hormone prophylaxis is recommended to maximize its effectiveness. (*Chapter 104, Page 913.*)

22.22 The leading cause of death in U.S. women is

(A) domestic violence
(B) coronary heart disease
(C) breast cancer
(D) stroke
(E) lung cancer

Answer: (B). Coronary heart disease is the leading cause of death of U.S. women and a major cause of morbidity. (*Chapter 104, Page 913.*)

22.23 Malignancies known to be estrogen-dependent include all EXCEPT which of the following?

(A) breast cancer
(B) endometrial cancer
(C) thyroid cancer
(D) melanoma
(E) hepatocellular carcinoma

Answer: (C). Malignancies known to be estrogen-dependent include breast cancer, endometrial cancer, melanoma, and hepatocellular carcinoma. (*Chapter 104, Page 914.*)

22.24 A leiomyoma of the uterus is most likely to present with which of the following manifestations?

(A) recurrent vaginal bleeding
(B) amenorrhea
(C) vaginal discharge
(D) a pelvic mass noted at the time of a routine gynecologic examination
(E) pelvic pain

Answer: (D). Most leiomyomas are asymptomatic and noted as a pelvic mass at the time of a routine gynecologic examination. (*Chapter 105, Page 916.*)

22.25 There is an increased incidence of endometrial cancer in patients who have previously had

(A) papillary cancer of the thyroid gland
(B) ovarian cancer
(C) early menopause
(D) multiparity
(E) breast cancer

Answer: (E). Research has identified an association between breast cancer and the risk of developing endometrial carcinoma. This association represents a modest increase in risk, but the increasing number of women presenting with breast cancer represents a potential increase in endometrial cancer. (*Chapter 105, Page 920.*)

22.26 Which of the following cancers causes more deaths than any other cancer of the female reproductive tract?

(A) cervical cancer
(B) ovarian cancer
(C) vulvar cancer
(D) myometrial cancer
(E) endometrial cancer

Answer: (B). Although ovarian cancer ranks second in incidence among gynecologic cancers, it causes more deaths than any other cancer of the female reproductive tract. (*Chapter 105, Page 921.*)

22.27 The patient is a 42-year-old white woman who complains of bilateral breast pain occurring in the upper outer quadrant of the breasts, most commonly occurring just prior to menses and diminishing when menstrual flow begins. This patient's most likely diagnosis is

(A) acute mastitis
(B) fibrocystic changes with mastodynia
(C) mastitis
(D) fibroadenoma
(E) breast cancer

Answer: (B). Mastodynia, the most frequent complaint associated with fibrocystic breasts, is thought to be due to breast swelling. The pain is usually located in the denser upper outer quadrant of the breasts and is bilateral. Onset of pain coincides with the time just prior to menses and diminishes when menses begins. Patients may perceive an enlargement of breast size during this period. A family history of this condition is common. (*Chapter 106, Page 927.*)

22.28 Mastodynia related to fibrocystic changes in the breast may respond to elimination of the use of

(A) alcohol
(B) vitamin C
(C) vitamin E
(D) caffeine
(E) tobacco

Answer: (D). Some patients seem to be sensitive to caffeine, suggesting a trial of caffeine deprivation as a

part of the diagnostic evaluation and management. (*Chapter 106, Page 927.*)

22.29 The patient is a 44-year-old white woman with pain in the upper outer quadrant of the left breast present for about 2 months. Examination reveals a tender cyst 1.5 cm in diameter. Aspiration in the office yields a small amount of bloody fluid; following aspiration, a residual thickening persists. The next step in management of this patient should be

(A) repeat aspiration in 1 month following the next menstrual cycle
(B) serial mammography at quarterly intervals
(C) ultrasonography
(D) excisional biopsy
(E) restriction of dietary caffeine

Answer: (D). Aspiration often provides symptomatic relief in addition to helping establish the diagnosis. If aspiration is performed, clear fluid is obtained, and the mass disappears, follow-up is necessary for at least 3 months to ensure that there is no recurrence. If a residual mass or thickening is present, bloody fluid is obtained, or the mass recurs, an excisional biopsy is performed. (*Chapter 106, Page 927.*)

22.30 The patient is a 26-year-old white woman, 11 days postpartum, who is breast-feeding her infant. She has pain, redness, and swelling in the left breast. This patient's history is most consistent with a diagnosis of

(A) mastodynia
(B) mastitis
(C) fibrocystic breast disease
(D) fibroadenoma
(E) trauma to the breast

Answer: (B). Mastitis presents 1 week or more after delivery. Usually only one breast is affected by moderate-to-severe pain. Typically, only one quadrant or lobule is tender, reddened, swollen, and warm. Axillary adenopathy, purulent drainage fever, and leukocytosis may be present. (*Chapter 106, Page 929.*)

22.31 The patient is a 29-year-old married white woman whose chief complaint is "nipple discharge," which has persisted following pregnancy and breast-feeding 18 months ago. Which of the following symptoms would be considered particularly worrisome?

(A) clear discharge
(B) milky discharge
(C) discharge noted just before the menses

(D) discharge following breast stimulation as part of sexual activity

(E) discharge from a single duct

Answer: (E). Normal, healthy women commonly have some degree of nipple discharge following pregnancy and lactation. This fluid is typically clear or milky and can either spontaneously drain from the breast or be produced by palpation. This discharge may be more frequently noted just before menses. Breast stimulation as part of sexual activity can precipitate nipple discharge. The amount of fluid is small and does not change over time. Nipple discharge from a single duct is ominous. (*Chapter 106, Page 929.*)

22.32 The patient is a 26-year-old white woman currently 5 weeks postpartum who is breast-feeding her infant. For the past 3 weeks, she has had painful nipples. They began with cracking, which she treated with a lanolin ointment. Since that time, the nipples have become increasingly inflamed and painful. She has continued to breast-feed the infant. You suspect that this patient's current problem may be

(A) sensitivity to lanolin

(B) bacterial infection of the skin

(C) fungal infection of the skin

(D) irritation of skin tissue by enzymes in the infant's saliva

(E) Paget's disease of the nipple

Answer: (A). If dried cracked nipples are present, topical vitamin E ointment and USP modified lanolin are commonly recommended "home remedies" for cracked nipples. A word of caution must be issued regarding the use of topical interventions, as they may be associated with sensitivity reactions. This is especially true for lanolin in wool-sensitive individuals. (*Chapter 106, Page 930.*)

22.33 The patient is a 56-year-old white woman with cancer of the right breast. She was found to have a local lesion of 1.5 cm in diameter with no lymph node involvement. Her breast cancer is appropriately categorized as

(A) stage 0

(B) stage I

(C) stage II

(D) stage III

(E) stage IV

Answer: (B). The stages of breast cancer are

Stage 0:   Carcinoma in situ (noninvasive cancer cells in lobule or duct)

Stage I: Local lesion 2 cm or less with no lymph node involvement

Stage II: Lesion with minimal local lymph node involvement or local lesion larger than 2 cm without lymph node involvement

Stage III: Locally advanced lesion with positive axillary nodes and skin or chest wall spread

Stage IV: Metastatic disease (common sites: other breast, liver, lungs, bones, brain) (*Chapter 107, Page 936.*)

22.34 The patient is a 22-year-old African American female restaurant worker with a 2-year history of recurrent pelvic pain. This is her first visit to your office, and you are beginning evaluation of her problem. Given this chief complaint, you might suspect that this patient has a past history of

(A) suicide in a first-degree relative

(B) poor performance in school

(C) imperforate hymen

(D) participation in competitive sports

(E) sexual abuse

Answer: (E). Research has shown a high incidence of sexual abuse associated with chronic pain. Furthermore, current psychiatric diagnoses, especially depression, and substance abuse correlate with pelvic pain. Rates of childhood or adult sexual or physical abuse are as high as 48% in patients presenting with chronic pelvic pain. (*Chapter 108, Page 939.*)

22.35 The patient is a 31-year-old nulliparous white woman with a 9-month history of painful menses and menstrual irregularity. She has noted pelvic pain, especially in the weeks before her periods, and over the past few months there has been dyspareunia. She and her husband have not conceived despite discontinuing contraceptive methods of all types about 7 months ago. Of the following diagnoses, this patient is most likely to have

(A) chronic PID

(B) endometriosis

(C) pelvic congestion syndrome

(D) pelvic adhesions

(E) adenomyosis

Answer: (B). Patients with endometriosis present a wide range of clinical symptoms, and frequently there is poor correlation between these symptoms and the extent of endometrial implants within the pelvis. Dysmenorrhea (50%), infertility (25 to 50%), pelvic pain, and dyspareunia (20%) and menstrual irregularities (12 to 14%) are the most common complaints. Pain can be diffuse or localized to the organs involved. Other less common symptoms include low back pain, dysuria, hematuria, and diarrhea, which classically occur before or during menses. Despite classic descriptions of the disease, endometriosis may present with some, none, or all these symptoms, which may or may not correlate with the menstrual cycle. Textbooks describe the "typical" endometriosis patient as in her late 20 or early 30s, Caucasian, and frequently nulliparous. (*Chapter 108, Page 942.*)

22.36 The diagnosis of endometriosis is based on

(A) historical findings of pelvic pain, dyspareunia, dysmenorrhea, and infertility
(B) classic physical findings
(C) direct visual and histologic confirmation obtained during laparoscopy or laparotomy
(D) serologic testing
(E) biopsy under culposcopic visualization

Answer: (C). The diagnosis of endometriosis requires direct visual and histologic confirmation obtained during laparoscopy or laparotomy. (*Chapter 108, Page 942.*)

22.37 The patient is a 38-year-old white female bus driver who has had recurrent pelvic discomfort over the past year. Laparoscopic examination reveals minimal endometrial disease. The patient does not desire pregnancy. Appropriate management of this patient would be

(A) hysterectomy with bilateral salpingo-oophorectomy
(B) long-term therapy with danazol (Danocrine)
(C) long-term therapy with medroxyprogesterone (Provera)
(D) cyclic therapy with OCPs
(E) laparoscopic aspiration of cysts

Answer: (D). The laparoscopic finding of minimal endometrial disease in women not desiring pregnancy can frequently be managed with cyclic birth control pills to lessen further seeding. More advanced disease usually requires 6 months of danazol or medroxyprogesterone acetate followed by cyclic birth control pills. (*Chapter 108, Page 943.*)

22.38 The diagnosis of TSS requires the presence of specific clinical criteria. These criteria include all EXCEPT which of the following?

(A) hypothermia
(B) scarlatiniform rash

(C) desquamation of palms and soles 1–2 weeks after illness begins
(D) hypotension
(E) exclusion of other causes for these symptoms

Answer: (A). A confirmed diagnosis of TSS requires that all six of the following criteria be met:
1. acute fever
2. scarlatiniform rash
3. desquamation of palms and soles 1 to 2 weeks after illness onset
4. hypotension
5. clinical or laboratory evidence of involvement of at least three organ systems: hematologic, gastrointestinal, neurologic, cardiovascular, hepatic, renal, muscular
6. other causes excluded (e.g., sepsis, measles, drug or toxic ingestion). (*Chapter 108, Page 947.*)

DIRECTIONS (Items 22.39 through 22.66): Each of the items in this section is a multiple true–false problem that consists of a stem and four lettered options. Indicate whether each of the four options is TRUE or FALSE.

22.39 The optimal candidate for an IUD has which of the following characteristics?

(A) is nulliparous
(B) is in a mutually monogamous relationship
(C) has a history of pelvic inflammatory disease
(D) does not desire permanent sterilization

Answer: (A-False, B-True, C-False, D-True). Optimal candidates for IUDs are women who have had at least one child, are in a mutually monogamous relationship, are at low risk for sexually transmitted disease, and do not desire permanent sterilization. Patients who are not candidates for an IUD include those who have an acute pelvic infection or a history of PID, have had previous surgery that might predispose to ectopic pregnancy, have uterine anomalies resulting in distortion of the uterine cavity, or who have known or suspected genital carcinoma. (*Chapter 101, Page 881.*)

22.40 Factors that significantly influence the pregnancy rate associated with the use of a contraceptive cervical cap include which of the following?

(A) length of time the cap is worn
(B) time interval the cap is in place after coitus
(C) use of a spermicide
(D) cap becoming dislodged during coitus

Answer: (A-False, B-False, C-False, D-True). Failure rates of the cervical cap vary from 8.4 to 16.6 pregnancies per 100 woman-years. Neither the length of time the cap is worn nor the time interval the cap is in place after coitus influences the pregnancy rate. The use of spermicide appears to have minimal effect on the women who become pregnant, with 71% reporting that the cap became dislodged during coitus. (*Chapter 101, Page 882.*)

22.41 The patient is a 27-year-old white woman who requests contraception using an injectable progestin. True statements regarding this type of contraceptive include which of the following?

   (A) Following an injection, there is protection for 3 months followed by a 4- to 6-week grace period before the next injection.
   (B) Excessive uterine bleeding may occur.
   (C) The drug may cause irreversible suppression of ovulation.
   (D) Injectable progestin contraception can be safely begun immediately postpartum within 5 days of delivery.

Answer: (A-True, B-True, C-False, D-True). A commonly used injectable progestin, medroxyprogesterone acetate (DMPA; Depo-Provera) has a typical failure rate of 1 per 100 woman-years. One of the reasons for the high efficacy rate is that each 150-mg injection provides 3 months of protection followed by a 4- to 6-week grace period before the next injection. DMPA may cause excessive uterine bleeding, but amenorrhea is to be expected after 12 months of use. Use of DMPA does not result in irreversible suppression of ovulation, but patients must clearly understand that there may be a delay in return to fertility. DMPA can be safely initiated immediately postpartum with the first injection given within 5 days of delivery. (*Chapter 101, Page 886.*)

22.42 Cryptomenorrhea may occur in patients with

   (A) oral contraceptive use
   (B) imperforate hymen
   (C) severe cervical stenosis
   (D) Asherman syndrome

Answer: (A-False, B-True, C-True, D-False). Cryptomenorrhea, or concealed menses, occurs in patients with an imperforate hymen and severe cervical stenosis. Hypomenorrhea refers to unusually light menstrual flow or spotting. It is frequently seen in patients taking oral contraceptives but may also be a sign of Asherman syndrome. (*Chapter 102, Page 899.*)

22.43 Which of the following women satisfy the diagnosis of secondary amenorrhea?

   (A) an 18-year-old woman who has never had a menstrual period
   (B) a 28-year-old woman with previously normal menses who has had no menses for four consecutive cycles
   (C) a 33-year-old woman with a previously normal menstrual history with no menses for eight consecutive cycles
   (D) a 35-year-old woman with a history of previous oligomenorrhea who has had no menses for the past 14 cycles

Answer: (A-False, B-False, C-True, D-True). Secondary amenorrhea is defined as the absence of menses for six consecutive cycles in a previously menstruating woman or for 12 months in a woman with a history of previous oligomenorrhea. (*Chapter 103, Page 900.*)

22.44 The patient is a 34-year-old African-American woman with secondary amenorrhea and an elevated prolactin (PRL) level. As part of your evaluation, you should inquire regarding the possible use of which of the following medications?

   (A) estrogen
   (B) alpha-methyldopa
   (C) tricyclic antidepressants
   (D) none of the above drugs can elevate PRL levels

Answer: (A-True, B-True, C-True, D-False). As many medications elevate PRL levels, a careful drug history is obtained at this point before proceeding further. Medications of special concern include those containing estrogen, alpha-methyldopa, catecholamine-depleting drugs, butyrophenones, dibenzoxzepine, dihydroindolone, diphenylbutylpiperadine, thioxanthenes, and tricyclics. All such drugs may cause elevated PRL levels and concomitantly inhibit estrogen production. (*Chapter 103, Page 901.*)

22.45 Failure to produce uterine bleeding in response to the progesterone challenge test may indicate which of the following?

   (A) inadequate estrogen production
   (B) carcinoma of the endometrium
   (C) a pituitary microadenoma
   (D) an abnormality of the target organ outflow tract

Answer: (A-True, B-False, C-False, D-True). Failure to bleed in response to withdrawal of progesterone almost always indicates inadequate estrogen production or an abnormality of the target organ outflow tract. (*Chapter 103, Page 901.*)

22.46 True statements regarding dysfunctional uterine bleeding (DUB) include which of the following?

(A) DUB tends to be a problem of pubescent and perimenopausal women.
(B) DUB occurs most commonly in women during their child-bearing years.
(C) DUB is a diagnosis of exclusion.
(D) Most DUB is ovulatory.

Answer: (A-True, B-False, C-True, D-False). DUB is without exception a diagnosis of exclusion. It is found most frequently in the pubescent and perimenopausal patient. DUB is classified on the basis of whether the patient is ovulatory (10%) or anovulatory (90%). (*Chapter 103, Page 905.*)

22.47 The patient is a 42-year-old Hispanic woman who complains of excessively heavy menstrual flow in the absence of menstrual cramps. She has read a magazine article about the use of nonsteroidal anti-inflammatory drugs (NSAID) and asks if this medication would be helpful. True statements regarding the use of cyclic NSAID therapy in menorrhagia include which of the following?

(A) These drugs tend to inhibit prostaglandins and increase uterine vasoconstriction.
(B) Although theoretically helpful, in practice, the use of NSAIDs for management of menorrhagia has not proved clinically useful.
(C) The NSAID medication is most successful taken a day or two before the onset of the menses and continued until flow ceases.
(D) Cyclic NSAID therapy should be limited to six cycles of use.

Answer: (A-True, B-False, C-True, D-False). The negative impact of excess prostaglandins on menses can be ameliorated by the administration of NSAIDs, which inhibit prostaglandins, promote platelet degranulation and aggregation, and increase uterine vasoconstriction. The use of NSAIDs for management of menorrhagia has been shown to decrease menstrual blood loss by 30 to 50%. Most of the commonly prescribed NSAIDs have been used to treat menorrhagia, but more data are available on the effectiveness of mefenamic acid and naproxen than others. The management of menorrhagia with NSAIDs is most often successful if the medication is taken 1 to 2 days prior to

the onset of the menstrual cycle and is continued until the flow ceases. Cyclic NSAID therapy may be continued as long as necessary—barring patient intolerance—if it is effective. (*Chapter 103, Page 906.*)

22.48 Danazol, a synthetic androgen with antiestrogen effect, is used primarily to treat endometriosis but has been used for the management of excessive uterine bleeding. True statements regarding this drug include which of the following?

(A) Danazol stimulates release of both FSH and LH.
(B) In the treatment of menorrhagia, danazol compares favorably to both NSAIDs and norethindrone.
(C) Danazol is particularly useful in women who desire conception.
(D) Side effects include acne, hirsutism, weight gain, and decreased libido.

Answer: (A-False, B-True, C-False, D-True). Danazol, a synthetic androgen with antiestrogen effect, inhibits both FSH and LH and suppresses ovulation. It is primarily used to treat endometriosis, but it has also been used for management of excessive uterine bleeding. In the treatment of menorrhagia, danazol has compared favorably with both NSAIDs and norethindrone when results were measured by the decrease in menstrual blood loss. Because it suppresses ovulation, the use of danazol should be restricted to those women who do not desire conception. Unfortunately, the use of danazol is limited by its cost and often unacceptable side effects, which include acne, hirsutism, weight gain, and decreased libido. (*Chapter 103, Page 906.*)

22.49 The patient is a 26-year-old African American woman who has had menorrhagia for the past 8 months. On blood testing, she is likely to have

(A) a normal hemoglobin level
(B) a low hematocrit level
(C) a low serum ferritin level
(D) a low serum vitamin B_{12} level

Answer: (A-False, B-True, C-True, D-False). Iron deficiency anemia secondary to excessive menstrual blood loss is frequent in women with menstrual disorders. As many as two-thirds menorrhagic women have iron deficiency or low serum ferritin. (*Chapter 103, Page 907.*)

22.50 True statements regarding menopause include which of the following?

(A) In the United States, the median age at menopause is 41 years.
(B) Menopause is considered premature if it occurs prior to age 40.
(C) The term *climacteric* refers to the perimenopausal years.
(D) The physiologic transformation of the menopause often extends for years after the last menstrual period.

Answer: (A-False, B-True, C-True, D-True). In the United States, the median age at menopause is approximately 51 years. Menopause is considered premature if it occurs prior to age 40. The changes of the climacteric—also referred to as the perimenopausal years—are a gradual process. Hormone changes may begin as early as age 35, and the physiologic transformation often extends for years after the last menstrual period. (*Chapter 104, Page 909.*)

22.51 The hot flashes of menopause include which of the following characteristics?

(A) intermittent sudden down-regulation in the anterior hypothalamic thermoregulatory centers
(B) abrupt vasoconstriction
(C) bradycardia
(D) increased skin temperature

Answer: (A-True, B-False, C-False, D-True). Hot flashes appear to be due to intermittent sudden down-regulation in the anterior hypothalamic thermoregulatory centers, and they result in abrupt vasodilation, tachycardia, and increased skin temperature, usually lasting 30 seconds to several minutes. Nocturnal hot flashes often interfere with sleep. (*Chapter 104, Page 910.*)

22.52 Irregular bleeding is common in the years prior to the menopause, although other causes of irregular bleeding may occur at this time. Which of the following problems merit investigation in a 46-year-old woman?

(A) menses occurring at 16- to 18-day intervals
(B) absent menses for 3 months accompanied by hot flashes
(C) menses lasting 6 days in duration
(D) resumption of bleeding after 8 months of amenorrhea

Answer: (A-True, B-False, C-False, D-True). Anovulatory cycles occur in most women as ovarian function declines, but many other causes of irregular bleeding may also occur. Investigation should be undertaken for women older than 40 who experience intervals less than 21 days, bleeding longer than 8 days, heavy bleeding, bleeding after 6 months of amenorrhea, or bleeding between periods. (*Chapter 104, Page 912.*)

22.53 Estrogen replacement therapy

(A) increases the risk of coronary heart disease
(B) increases the risk of hypertension
(C) appears unlikely to increase the risk of stroke
(D) increases the risk of venous thromboembolism

Answer: (A-False, B-False, C-True, D-False). Observational studies consistently find a substantial reduction in the risk of coronary heart disease (on the order of 35 to 50%) associated with postmenopausal estrogen use. Estrogen therapy in postmenopausal doses does not increase the risk of hypertension. The effect on the risk of stroke is unclear, but stroke risk appears unlikely to be increased with preventive hormone therapy. There is no evidence that postmenopausal doses of estrogen increase the risk of venous thromboembolism. (*Chapter 104, Page 913.*)

22.54 The patient is a 32-year-old African American woman whose close friend was just diagnosed with cervical carcinoma. She asks about her risk of the disease. Major risk factors for cervical carcinoma include which of the following?

(A) being African American
(B) late age at first intercourse
(C) oral contraceptive use
(D) a sexual partner who has had intercourse with a female who developed cervical cancer

Answer: (A-True, B-False, C-True, D-True). Major risk factors for cervical carcinoma include a present or past history of an abnormal Papanicolaou (Pap) smear; multiple sexual partners; early age at first intercourse; being African American, Hispanic, or Native American; history of genital warts or other sexually transmitted diseases; smoking; oral contraceptives (especially the high-dose estrogen pills used during the 1960s and 1970s); an immunocompromised state; a partner with genital warts; a sexual partner who has had intercourse with a female who developed cervical cancer; and being a woman whose mother had taken diethylstilbestrol during her pregnancy. (*Chapter 105, Page 917.*)

22.55 True statements regarding the Pap smear include which of the following?

(A) The Pap smear is an important diagnostic tool.
(B) False-negative rates are low.
(C) The Pap smear is important in identifying high-risk patients.
(D) Poor patient compliance and inadequate follow-up by the physician remain significant problems.

Answer: (A-False, B-False, C-False, D-True). Not a diagnostic tool but rather a screening method, the Pap smear remains the first step when evaluating for cervical carcinoma. Some of the inadequacies of the screening process are Pap smear false-negatives (5 to 56%), failure to identify high-risk patients, inaccurate or incomplete laboratory reports, poor patient compliance, and inadequate follow-up by the physician. (*Chapter 105, Page 917.*)

22.56 The patient is a 39-year-old Native American woman who is being evaluated for an abnormal Pap test. Biopsy at the time of colposcopy revealed preinvasive disease. Endocervical curettage (ECC) is negative. Appropriate therapy for this patient includes which of the following?

(A) hysterectomy
(B) observation with serial Pap smears at 3-month intervals
(C) large loop electrosurgical excision of the transformation zone
(D) cryotherapy

Answer: (A-False, B-False, C-True, D-True). If the biopsies reveal preinvasive disease and the ECC is negative, cryotherapy, large-loop excision of the transformation zone (LLETZ; British terminology for loop electrosurgical excision procedure [LEEP]), or laser therapy is indicated with a follow-up Pap smear in 3 to 4 months. (*Chapter 105, Page 918.*)

22.57 The patient is a 34-year-old woman whose aunt has recently developed ovarian cancer. She is concerned about risk factors. You may inform her that risk factors for ovarian cancer include

(A) pregnancy
(B) use of oral contraceptives
(C) nulliparity
(D) a positive family history of ovarian cancer

Answer: (A-False, B-False, C-True, D-True). Although a positive family history of ovarian cancer increases a woman's risk 20-fold, 95% of women with ovarian cancer have no family history for it. Pregnancy and the use of oral contraceptives may protect against the development of ovarian cancer. Conversely, nulliparity or low parity and the lack of oral contraceptive use are considered risk factors for ovarian cancer. (*Chapter 105, Page 921.*)

22.58 True statements regarding fibroadenoma of the breast include which of the following?

(A) Fibroadenoma is the most common benign breast tumor.
(B) Fibroadenoma chiefly occurs in middle-aged and older women.
(C) Fibroadenoma occurs more often and at earlier ages in white women than in black women.
(D) Fibroadenomas often calcify and may involute after menopause.

Answer: (A-True, B-False, C-False, D-True). Fibroadenoma is the most common benign breast tumor. It occurs in young women usually within 20 years after the onset of puberty. It is more frequent and occurs at earlier ages in African American than in white women. Multiple lesions may occur and may grow rapidly. Older women characteristically experience a single, solitary, more slowly growing lesion. Fibroadenomas frequently calcify and may involute after menopause. (*Chapter 106, Page 928.*)

22.59 The patient is a 30-year-old Hispanic woman who is 20 days postpartum. She has mastitis of the right breast with mild redness, swelling, and local tenderness but no pitting edema or fluctuation that would suggest abscess development. Appropriate management for this patient might include which of the following?

(A) continuation of breast-feeding including the affected breast
(B) local compresses and oral antibiotics
(C) if the patient wishes to discontinue breast-feeding, breast bindings and ice packs should be used.
(D) medical suppression of lactation

Answer: (A-True, B-True, C-True, D-False). *Staphylococcus aureus* and streptococci are typically the causative organisms. Treatment for mild infections includes local compresses and oral beta-lactamase–resistant antibiotics. If she wishes to continue to nurse, breast-feeding can be continued on the affected breast. The infant is not at risk for developing infection. If the patient wishes to discontinue breast-feeding, breast binding, ice packs, restriction of breast stimulation, and analgesics should be used. Medical suppression of lactation is not justified. (*Chapter 106, Page 929.*)

22.60 Indications for breast biopsy include which of the following?

(A) a cyst that disappears following aspiration
(B) a persistent, dominant mass
(C) breast inflammation that responds to antibiotic therapy
(D) suspicious microcalcifications on mammography

Answer: (A-False, B-True, C-False, D-True). Indications for biopsy include any suspicious lesion, bloody nipple discharge, or bloody fluid following aspiration of a cyst, a mass that persists following cyst aspiration, persistent dominant mass, suspicious skin changes, inflammatory changes unresponsive to antibiotics, suspicious axillary nodes, or suspicious microcalcifications on mammography. (*Chapter 106, Page 932.*)

22.61 Mammography may be of limited value in detection of breast cancer in which of the following women?

(A) women aged 50 to 69
(B) women on hormonal replacement therapy
(C) women with dense fibrotic breasts
(D) women with breast implants

Answer: (A-False, B-True, C-True, D-True). Mammography is of limited value in women on hormonal replacement therapy, younger women, women with dense or fibrotic breasts, and women with breast implants. (*Chapter 107, Page 935.*)

22.62 Tamoxifen is used for women with node-negative breast cancer larger than 1 cm and those with nodal disease. True statements regarding tamoxifen use include which of the following?

(A) Common side effects include hot flashes and menopausal-like symptoms.
(B) Weight loss is often seen.
(C) There is an increased risk of deep venous thrombosis.
(D) Tamoxifen exerts a protective effect against endometrial cancer.

Answer: (A-True, B-False, C-True, D-False). Tamoxifen now has U.S. Food and Drug Administration approval for use in women with node-negative breast cancer larger than 1 cm and those with nodal disease. Com-

mon tamoxifen side effects include hot flashes, weight gain, fluid retention, vaginal dryness, and menopausal-like symptoms. Taking tamoxifen increases the risk of deep venous thrombosis and endometrial cancer by about threefold over that in the general population. (*Chapter 107, Page 936.*)

22.63 The most common causes of chronic pelvic pain in patients younger than age 30 include which of the following?

(A) endometriosis
(B) adenomyosis
(C) chronic PID
(D) leiomyomas

Answer: (A-True, B-False, C-True, D-False). The cause of chronic pain in patients younger than age 30 is most often endometriosis or chronic PID. Older patients are most likely to have adenomyosis, leiomyomas, endometriosis, or symptoms due to pelvic relaxation. (*Chapter 108, Page 940.*)

22.64 In evaluation of the infertile couple, methods of assessing ovulation include which of the following?

(A) basal body temperature
(B) timed serum progesterone levels
(C) urinary screening for gonadotropin-releasing hormone
(D) endometrial biopsy

Answer: (A-True, B-True, C-False, D-True). Assessing ovulation can be accomplished by one or more methods: (1) basal body temperature assessment; (2) timed serum progesterone levels; (3) urinary LH screening; and (4) endometrial biopsy. (*Chapter 108, Page 945.*)

22.65 Hysterosalpingography (HSP) is often useful in the fertility workup. However, this procedure is contraindicated in which of the following settings?

(A) the patient in the early proliferative phase of her cycle
(B) an undiagnosed pelvic mass
(C) presence of PID
(D) allergy to iodine

Answer: (A-False, B-True, C-True, D-True). Hysterosalpingography (HSP) is a safe, high-yield procedure when performed during the early proliferative phase of the cycle. During HSP, a special catheter is passed through the vagina into the endocervical canal through which contrast medium is injected and fluoroscopically followed through the endometrial and fallopian tube lumen. An undiagnosed pelvic mass or PID contraindicates this procedure, as does an iodine or radiocontrast dye allergy. (*Chapter 108, Page 946.*)

22.66 TSS can occur in which of the following patient groups?

   (A) menstruating females using tampons
   (B) nonmenstruating women
   (C) men
   (D) none of the above

Answer: (A-True, B-True, C-True, D-False). Because of the high correlation of TSS with menstruation and tampon use, the perception of TSS as strictly a "tampon disease" persists. More recent data reveal that only half of the reported cases were female, and many of these cases were not associated with menstruation. Most cases of tampon-related TSS occurred during the teenage years; 97% of reported patients were white, and 42% were adolescents. Physicians must recognize that TSS can occur in nonmenstruating women, men, and children of all ages. (*Chapter 108, Page 946.*)

23

The Musculoskeletal System and Connective Tissue

The questions in this chapter constitute a review of the following chapters in *Family Medicine: Principles and Practice, Fifth Edition:*

Disorders of the Back and Neck (Chapter 109)
Disorders of the Upper Extremity (Chapter 110)
Disorders of the Lower Extremity (Chapter 111)
Osteoarthritis (Chapter 112)
Rheumatoid Arthritis and Related Disorders (Chapter 113)
Selected Disorders of the Musculoskeletal System (Chapter 114)

DIRECTIONS (Items 23.1 through 23.45): Each of the questions or incomplete statements in this section is followed by five suggested answers or completions. Select the ONE that is BEST in each case.

23.1 The patient is an 82-year-old white man who reports that for the past 4 months, he has had low back pain associated with numbness, tingling, and pain radiating down both legs. The neurologic symptoms become worse with walking and subside gradually with rest. This patient is most likely to have

(A) a spinal cord tumor
(B) spinal stenosis
(C) an abdominal aortic aneurysm
(D) metastatic cancer of the spine
(E) degenerative joint disease of the spine

Answer: (B). Patients with spinal stenosis report symptoms suggestive of spinal claudication, that is, neurologic symptoms in the legs that worsen with ambulation. Spinal claudication is differentiated from vascular claudication in that the symptoms of spinal claudication have a slower onset and slower resolution. (*Chapter 109, Page 951.*)

23.2 The most common primary malignancy of the vertebral spine is

(A) chordoma
(B) chondrosarcoma
(C) osteogenic carcinoma
(D) multiple myeloma
(E) osteoid osteoma

Answer: (D). Multiple myeloma is the most common primary malignancy of the vertebral spine. Metastatic lesions are the most common cause of cancers of the spine, arising from breast, lung, prostate, thyroid, renal, or gastrointestinal tract primary tumors. (*Chapter 109, Page 954.*)

23.3 Ankylosing spondylitis occurs most commonly in

(A) young women
(B) older women
(C) young men
(D) older men
(E) no age or gender differences

Answer: (C). Ankylosing spondylitis is a spondyloarthropathy most commonly affecting young men. (*Chapter 109, Page 954.*)

23.4 The primary indication for surgery in a patient with low back pain is

(A) the presence of low back pain that is worse with bending or lifting
(B) health insurance coverage
(C) sciatica

(D) abnormal findings on radiographs of the lumbar spine

(E) degenerative disease of the lumbar spine

Answer: (C). The major benefit and primary indication for surgery is relief of sciatica. In well-selected patients, 75% have complete relief of sciatic symptoms after surgery, and an additional 15% have partial relief. (*Chapter 109, Page 957.*)

23.5 The patient is a 36-year-old white woman with a 6-week history of occipital headache radiating to the frontal area, worse on awakening and improving through the day. She has deep aching pain and a burning sensation in both hands, and she perceives a loss of hand dexterity. There is evidence of motor weakness in the hands, and rapid flexion or extension causes a shocklike sensation in the arms. This patient is most likely to have

(A) multiple myeloma

(B) cervical myelopathy

(C) cervical whiplash injury

(D) cervical disc infection

(E) metastatic cancer to the cervical spine

Answer: (B). Unlike cervical radiculopathy, cervical myelopathy rarely presents with neck pain; instead, patients report an occipital headache that radiates anteriorly to the frontal area, is worse on waking, but improves through the day. Patients also report deep aching pain and burning sensations in the hands, loss of hand dexterity, and vertebrobasilar insufficiency, presumably due to osteophytic changes in the cervical spine. On physical examination, patients demonstrate motor weakness and muscle wasting, particularly of the interosseous muscles of the hand. Lhermitte's sign is present in approximately 25% of patients (i.e., rapid flexion or extension of the neck causes a shocklike sensation in the trunk or limbs). (*Chapter 109, Page 959.*)

23.6 Most clavicular fractures involve which area of the clavicle?

(A) proximal third

(B) middle third

(C) distal third

(D) acromioclavicular joint

(E) sternoclavicular joint

Answer: (B). Eighty percent of clavicular fractures occur in the middle third of the clavicle, especially at the junction of the middle and distal thirds. Even when significant displacement or angulation is present, these fractures heal well with minimal intervention. (*Chapter 110, Page 963.*)

23.7 The patient is a 32-year-old white man playing playground basketball when he fell on his left arm and shoulder a short while ago. There is a squaring of the shoulder with a loss of roundness of the deltoid muscle and an apparent anterior mass in the area of the shoulder. The patient holds his arm in slight external rotation and abduction. This patient appears to have

(A) a fracture of the humerus

(B) a fracture of the distal third of the clavicle

(C) an acromioclavicular separation

(D) a posterior dislocation of the shoulder

(E) an anterior dislocation of the shoulder

Answer: (E). The major traumatic injury to the shoulder is dislocation of the humerus from the glenohumeral joint. About 95% of such dislocations are anterior, caused by resisted force to the arm when the shoulder is abducted and externally rotated. Examination of this injury reveals a squaring of the shoulder, loss of the roundness of the deltoid muscle, prominence of the acromial edge, and an anterior mass, which is the humeral head. The arm is held in slight external rotation and abduction. (*Chapter 110, Page 964.*)

23.8 The patient is a 38-year-old African American man whose sport is softball. Following a softball game about 1 week ago, he has noted continuous pain in his right shoulder, especially at night, and radiating down the lateral aspect of the upper arm. On physical examination, the patient has severe pain with attempts to abduct the shoulder beyond 80 degrees. This patient appears to have

(A) a rotator cuff tear

(B) an anterior dislocation of the shoulder

(C) a stress fracture of the humerus

(D) a subacromial bursitis

(E) a bicipital tendonitis

Answer: (A). As a result of chronic impingement, the rotator cuff may tear. Cuff tears are more common in middle-aged or elderly individuals, often due to a hypovascular supply of the supraspinatus tendon as it inserts on the humerus. One hallmark of cuff tears is continuous pain, especially at night, which may radiate down the lateral humerus. Examination of the patient with a rotator cuff injury reveals painful or limited active abduction (between 60 and 120 degrees), where the cuff comes in greatest contact with the overlying acromial arch. (*Chapter 110, Page 965.*)

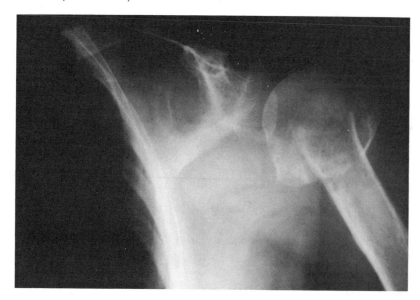

Fig. 23.1. Question 23.10.

23.9 Avascular necrosis of the humeral head may be caused by any of the following EXCEPT

(A) chronic alcoholism
(B) chronic overuse of analgesics
(C) sickle cell disease
(D) systemic lupus erythematosus (SLE)
(E) long-term steroid use

Answer: (B). Although less common than osteonecrosis (avascular necrosis) of the femoral head, osteonecrosis of the humeral head may be caused by a number of illnesses such as alcoholism, sickle cell disease, SLE, and long-term steroid use. Bone scan or magnetic resonance imaging (MRI) may be used for early diagnosis, as radiographs do not show subchondral collapse and humeral head flattening until later in the disorder. Treatment includes rest, analgesics, physical therapy for motion, and in severe cases, joint replacement. (*Chapter 110, Page 966.*)

23.10 The 78-year-old African American woman whose radiograph appears above fell last evening, injuring her shoulder. This radiograph is consistent with

(A) an anterior dislocation of the shoulder
(B) a posterior dislocation of the shoulder
(C) a rupture of the bicipital tendon
(D) an impacted humeral fracture
(E) a fracture of the distal third of the clavicle

Answer: (D). This impacted humeral fracture in an elderly woman is neither displaced nor severely angulated. It was successfully managed with an arm sling for 1 week followed by range-of-motion exercises and a course of physical therapy. (*Chapter 110, Page 966.*)

23.11 The patient is a 3-year-old child whose mother restrained him with a pull on the left arm as he was stepping off a curb into traffic. The child now has a painful left elbow, which he holds in pronation. This child appears to have

(A) a fracture of the radial head
(B) radial head subluxation
(C) lateral epicondylitis
(D) medial epicondylitis
(E) olecranon bursitis

Answer: (B). The most common elbow complaint in children, known as nursemaid's elbow, occurs when sudden longitudinal traction on the wrist or arm causes the annular ligament to become partially entrapped in the radiohumeral joint. The child, younger than 4 years old, presents with a painful elbow held in pronation. (*Chapter 110, Page 967.*)

23.12 The patient is a 54-year-old factory worker with severe heat, redness, tenderness, and swelling over the posterior aspect of his right elbow. You suspect a septic bursitis. The most likely infecting organism is

(A) gonococcus
(B) *Staphylococcus aureus*
(C) Klebsiella
(D) group A *Streptococcus*
(E) none of the above

Answer: (B). When there is marked inflammation, a septic bursitis is suspected. Treatment for a septic bursitis includes surgical drainage of the bursal fluid and intravenous antibiotics. *Staphylococcus aureus* is the most common infecting organism. (*Chapter 110, Page 967.*)

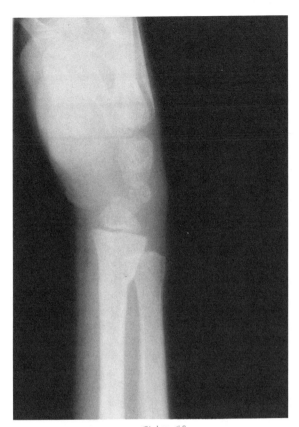

Fig. 23.2. Question 23.13.

23.13 An 8-year-old child, whose wrist radiograph is shown above, fell on his outstretched hand about 90 minutes ago. He complains of pain in the wrist. The radiograph confirms which of the following diagnoses?

(A) Colles' fracture of the wrist
(B) sprained wrist
(C) carpal fracture
(D) torus fracture of the distal radius
(E) fracture of the distal ulna

Answer: (D). The child has buckle (torus) fracture. A small cortical disruption is visible in the metaphysis of the distal radius. (*Chapter 110, Page 968.*)

23.14 The patient is a 35-year-old Asian American male who fell this morning while getting out of his car. The x-ray shows a nondisplaced distal radial fracture that does not involve the joint. This patient should be treated with

(A) percutaneous pinning of the fracture
(B) open reduction of the fracture
(C) cast immobilization for 6 weeks
(D) cast immobilization for 3 months
(E) no therapy is needed

Answer: (C). Nondisplaced distal radial fractures that are nonarticular can usually be treated with cast immobilization for 6 weeks in adults. (*Chapter 110, Page 968.*)

23.15 The most commonly fractured carpal bone is the

(A) capitate
(B) hamate
(C) pisiform
(D) scaphoid (carpal navicular)
(E) trapezium

Answer: (D). Sixty percent of carpal bone fractures involve the scaphoid (or carpal navicular) bone. (*Chapter 110, Page 968.*)

23.16 The patient is a 24-year-old tennis player who fell on her wrist yesterday. She appears to have a wrist sprain, and there is moderately severe tenderness over the scaphoid tubercle (palmar hand surface) and in the anatomic snuffbox. Radiographs of the wrist are normal. Your management for this patient today should be

(A) immobilization in a short arm cast or splint for 7 to 10 days, followed by repeat films
(B) referral for arthroscopy
(C) reassurance that a wrist sprain is a common benign injury of recreational athletes
(D) local injection of corticosteroids
(E) none of the above

Answer: (A). Although a scaphoid fracture is usually identified on a posteroanterior view with the wrist in ulnar deviation, occasionally the fracture is not evident on the initial films. Patients with a "wrist sprain" who have tenderness over the scaphoid tubercle (palmer hand surface) or pain in the anatomic snuffbox, located between the extensor pollicis brevis and extensor pollicis longus tendons, should be immobilized in a short arm cast or splint for 7 to 10 days, at which time repeat films usually demonstrate the fracture. (*Chapter 110, Page 968.*)

23.17 The patient is a 28-year-old white male truck driver involved in a barroom fight last night. He struck his opponent with his right fist and now has a transverse fracture of the distal neck of the fifth metacarpal with 35 degrees of volar angulation. No rotation is present. Appropriate treatment of this fracture is

(A) an ulnar gutter splint with the meta-carpophalangeal (MCP) joint at 90 degrees applied for 3 to 6 weeks
(B) an ulnar gutter splint with the MCP joint at 180 degrees applied for 2 weeks
(C) a splint with the MCP joint in slight hyper-extension applied for 3 to 6 weeks
(D) percutaneous pinning
(E) open reduction followed by a cast for 6 to 8 weeks

Answer: (A). The most common hand fracture is a "boxer's fracture" caused by impaction force and resulting in a fracture of the distal neck of the fifth metacarpal. Because of the mobility of the fourth and fifth metacarpals, volar angulation of the distal fragment of less then 40 degrees is acceptable without the need for bone manipulation. Whereas angulation is acceptable, a rotation injury around the longitudinal axis of any metacarpal necessitates orthopedic referral for surgical pinning. For a boxer's fracture with mild angulation, an ulnar gutter or volar splint with the MCP joint at 90 degrees is applied for 3 to 6 weeks. (*Chapter 110, Page 969.*)

23.18 The patient, whose radiograph is shown here, is a 14-year-old boy who injured his hand playing baseball yesterday. This patient has which of the following?

(A) fracture of the proximal phalanx with normal position and alignment
(B) fracture of the proximal phalanx with mild angulation
(C) fracture of the fourth metacarpal with normal alignment
(D) unicameral bone cyst
(E) volar plate fracture of the middle phalanx

Answer: (B). The radiograph shows a fracture of the proximal phalanx, with only mild angulation. (*Chapter 110, Page 970.*)

23.19 The patient is a 50-year-old white male factory worker who complains of pain at the proximal interphalangeal (PIP) joint of the right second finger. During extension of the finger, there is a catching of the PIP joint. This patient's problem is called a

(A) mallet finger
(B) trigger finger
(C) gamekeeper's finger
(D) PIP joint dislocation
(E) de Quervain's disease

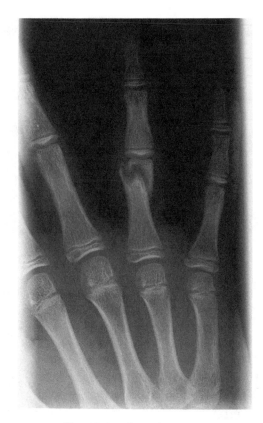

Fig. 23.3. Question 23.18.

Answer: (B). As the flexor tendon courses through the hand, a nodular thickening at the MCP level may prevent free passage of the tendon. The cause is inflammation of the A_1 pulley, the first of five pulleys that guide the flexor tendon into the finger. Although the problem is located at the MCP level, the patient frequently complains of more distal pain at the interphalangeal joint of the thumb or PIP joint of the finger. During extension of the finger, there is a catching or locking of the PIP joint as the stenosed tendon becomes trapped in the pulley. (*Chapter 110, Page 971.*)

23.20 The injury currently called a skier's (or gamekeeper's) thumb is caused by sudden hyperabduction that damages the

(A) radial collateral ligament
(B) ulnar collateral ligament
(C) carpal navicular bone
(D) flexor tendons of the thumb
(E) extensor tendons of the thumb

Answer: (B). Damage to the ulnar collateral ligament that occurs with sudden hyperabduction is termed a *gamekeeper's* or *skier's thumb*. This ligament is vital for open grasp and pinch action of the hand. Swelling and

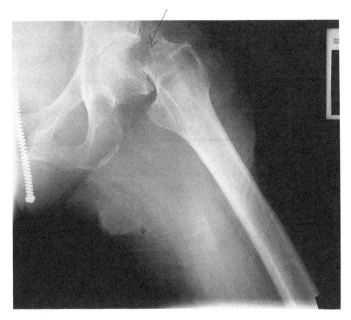

Fig. 23.4. Question 23.21. (Courtesy of A. Allen, M.D., Department of Radiology, University of Tennessee Medical Center.)

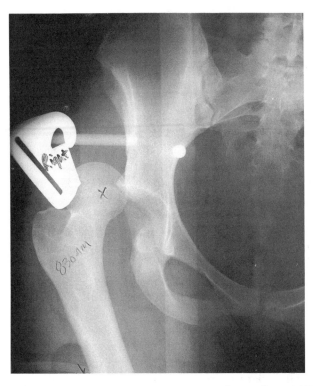

Fig. 23.5. Question 23.23. (Courtesy of A. Allen, M.D., Department of Radiology, University of Tennessee Medical Center.)

tenderness of the ulnar side of the MCP joint suggest this injury. (*Chapter 110, Pages 971–972.*)

23.21 The 84-year-old patient whose radiograph of the hip is shown above fell at the nursing home a few hours ago and has pain in the left hip. The radiograph shows a

(A) osteoid osteoma of the femur
(B) unicameral bone cyst of the hip
(C) dislocation of the hip
(D) femoral neck fracture with displacement
(E) femoral neck fracture without displacement

Answer: (D). The radiograph shows a femoral neck fracture (intracapsular) with displacement. (*Chapter 111, Page 975.*)

23.22 Most hip dislocations occur

(A) anteriorly
(B) posteriorly
(C) centrally
(D) laterally
(E) none of the above

Answer: (B). Dislocations occur most commonly in the posterior direction (85 to 90%) but can also occur in an anterior or central direction. (*Chapter 111, Page 975.*)

23.23 The patient whose radiograph of the right hip is shown here is a 22-year-old African American woman

involved in an automobile crash about 3 hours ago. She has severe pain in her right hip. The radiograph shows a

(A) femoral neck fracture without displacement
(B) femoral neck fracture with displacement
(C) osteoid osteoma of the right hip
(D) posterior dislocation of the right hip
(E) avulsion of the anterior superior iliac spine

Answer: (D). The patient has a posterior dislocation of the right hip. Note the internal rotation and adduction of the hip with subsequent loss of the lesser trochanter silhouette. (*Chapter 111, Page 976.*)

23.24 The patient is a 17-year-old soccer player who "caught his foot" while attempting to kick a ball. There is pain in the lower anterior thigh that is worse on active contraction and passive stretching. Ely's test is positive. This young athlete appears to have an acute injury to which muscle?

(A) gracilis
(B) sartorius
(C) rectus femoris
(D) hamstring
(E) gastrocnemius

Answer: (C). The most common thigh injury is to the rectus femoris muscle and commonly occurs at the distal muscle-tendon unit. The rectus femoris is the most central and superficial of the quadriceps muscles of the anterior thigh, and the distal portion is the leading edge in the flexed knee. Injury to the quadriceps muscles may show a visibly swollen, tender area at the site of the muscle tear. Pain is felt on active contraction and passive stretching. Isolation of this muscle is best done in the prone position with a mild passive stretch to flexion. In the prone position, Ely's test is performed by passive flexion of the knee to 90 degrees while observing the involved hip. Spontaneous hip flexion on the involved side with this maneuver is a positive test, which shows a tight rectus femoris due to spasm. (*Chapter 111, Page 977.*)

23.25 Myositis ossificans is a complication of

(A) fracture of the femur
(B) thigh contusion and hematoma
(C) chronic strain of the hamstring muscles
(D) lack of proper warm-up before exercise
(E) increasing running distance too rapidly

Answer: (B). Myositis ossificans is a complication of significant thigh contusion and hematoma. (*Chapter 111, Page 977.*)

23.26 The patient is a 28-year-old white woman who runs about 15 miles weekly. For the past month, she has had pain in the right knee. On examination, there is tenderness and swelling at the site of the insertion of the tendons onto the medial tibia. This patient appears to have

(A) pes anserine bursitis
(B) a quadriceps tendon rupture
(C) an injury to the medial meniscus of the knee
(D) a medial collateral ligament (MCL) strain
(E) osteochondritis dissecans of the medial tibial plateau

Answer: (A). Clinical diagnosis of pes anserine bursitis is based on tenderness over the insertion of the tendons onto the medial tibia (gracilis, sartorius, semitendinosus aponeurosis) along with swelling. Questionable cases ought to have MRI to rule out other internal derangements of the knee. MRI typically shows fluid underneath the tendons of the pes anserinus at the medial aspect of the tibia near the joint line. (*Chapter 111, Page 978.*)

23.27 In the examination of a patient with a knee injury, one maneuver is performed with the patient in the supine position and the knee in full flexion. The tibia is internally and externally rotated while placing a mild varus and valgus stress on the knee. This maneuver can help identify meniscal damage. This maneuver is called

(A) Lockman's test
(B) McMurray's test
(C) anterior drawer maneuver
(D) posterior drawer maneuver
(E) Ely's test

Answer: (B). McMurray's test is performed with the patient in the supine position and the knee in full flexion. The tibia is internally and externally rotated while placing a mild varus and valgus stress on the knee to induce entrapment of an injured meniscus, resulting in either a snap or pain. (*Chapter 111, Page 978.*)

23.28 The most common injury of the major knee stabilizers involves the

(A) anterior cruciate ligament (ACL)
(B) MCL
(C) lateral collateral ligament (LCL)
(D) posterior cruciate ligament
(E) patellar tendon

Answer: (B). The MCL is the weakest and therefore the most commonly injured of the three major knee stabilizers (ACL, MCL, LCL). (*Chapter 111, Page 980.*)

23.29 The patient whose radiographs are shown on the next page is a 26-year-old tennis player with chronic pain in the right knee. The pain is aching and poorly localized. It is aggravated by activity and twisting motions. Physical examination shows mild swelling of the knee and some atrophy of the quadriceps muscle. This patient appears to have

(A) a chondral fracture of the right knee
(B) patellar dislocation
(C) an ACL tear
(D) osteochondritis dissecans
(E) an injury to the medial meniscus of the knee

Answer: (D). The films show osteochondritis dissecans of the medial femoral condyle of the right knee. Anteroposterior (**A**) and lateral (**B**) views. There is an articular defect of the medial femoral condyle that is best appreciated on the lateral view. (*Chapter 111, Pages 980–981.*)

23.30 The patient is a 28-year-old white male recreational athlete who has an acute painful sprain of the left

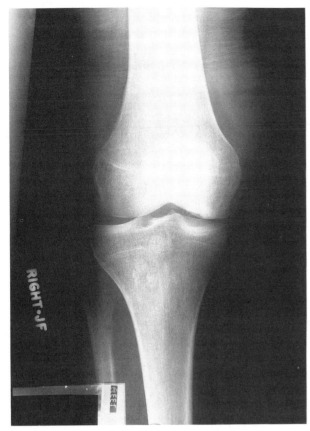
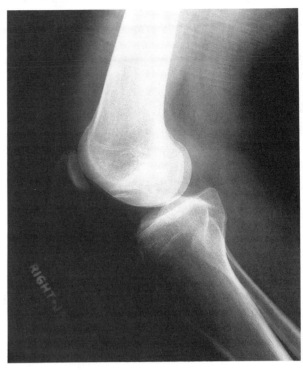

A   B

Fig. 23.6. Question 23.29. (Courtesy of A. Allen, M.D., Department of Radiology, University of Tennessee Medical Center.)

ankle. Radiographs show lateral swelling but no fracture. The optimum treatment for this patient will be

(A) local injection of lidocaine
(B) bracing to limit lateral motion
(C) casting for 3 weeks
(D) internal fixation
(E) bed rest and wheelchair use for 7 to 10 days

Answer: (B). When treating the acute ankle sprain, it is important to note that patients treated with "dynamic" bracing (protection of lateral motion while allowing full planter and dorsiflexion) versus those with static bracing (i.e., immobilization, casting) have earlier, more comprehensive functional recovery. Early mobilization also allows earlier return to functional capacity and may be more comfortable for the patient. (*Chapter 111, Page 982.*)

23.31 In examination of a 42-year-old white man with a suspected Achilles tendon rupture, the patient is placed in a prone position, and the relaxed calf muscles are squeezed forcefully. Absence of foot plantarflexion describes a positive

(A) Lachman's test
(B) McMurray's test
(C) Ely's test
(D) Thompson's test
(E) Hadlund's test

Answer: (D). By squeezing the relaxed prone calf, there should be movement of the foot into plantarflexion. Absence of this motion describes a positive Thompson's test. (*Chapter 111, Page 982.*)

23.32 An osteoid osteoma is a benign bone lesion that is characterized by

(A) chronic pain
(B) local deformity
(C) edema
(D) redness and heat
(E) atrophy of overlying muscles

Answer: (A). An osteoid osteoma is a benign bone lesion that can occur on any bone of the foot but is seen most often on the tarsal bones. It causes chronic pain, and one-third of patients describe nocturnal pain. (*Chapter 111, Page 985.*)

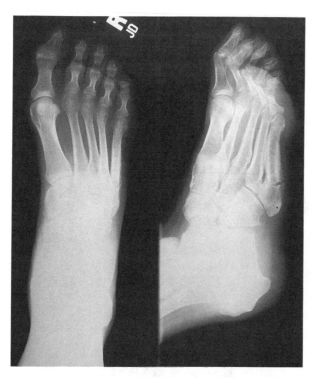

Fig. 23.7. Question 23.33. (Courtesy of M. Holt, M.D., Department of Orthopedics, University of Tennessee Medical Center.)

23.33 The patient whose radiographs are shown here is a 36-year-old white female runner who twisted her right ankle a few days ago. She has pain in the lateral right foot. Her radiographs reveal which of the following?

(A) a Lisfranc injury
(B) an acute ankle sprain
(C) a recurrent ankle sprain
(D) a Jones fracture
(E) an avulsion of the peroneus tendon insertion

Answer: (D). The patient has a transverse fracture at the base of the fifth metatarsal (Jones fracture). These fractures may be associated with complications resulting from nonunion or delayed union. It is managed closely with immobilization. A bone graft is considered if nonunion is suspected. (*Chapter 111, Page 986.*)

23.34 The patient is a 62-year-old white woman with pain in a number of joints including her hands. There is cartilaginous and bony enlargement of the PIP. Such joint enlargement is called

(A) Heberden's nodes
(B) Bouchard's nodes
(C) Roth's nodes
(D) tophi
(E) rheumatoid nodules

Answer: (B). Physical findings associated with hand osteoarthritis include Heberden's nodes of the distal interphalangeal joints, representing cartilaginous and bony enlargement of the dorsolateral and dorsomedial aspects. Bouchard's nodes are similar findings at the PIP joints. (*Chapter 112, Page 989.*)

23.35 Osteoarthritis (OA) can be diagnosed based on which of the following laboratory test results?

(A) erythrocyte sedimentation rate (ESR)
(B) autoantibodies
(C) rheumatoid factor
(D) joint fluid analysis
(E) none of the above

Answer: (E). There are no specific laboratory tests for OA. Unlike with the inflammatory arthritides (e.g., rheumatoid arthritis [RA]), the ESR and hemogram are normal, and autoantibodies are not present. If there is joint effusion, the synovial fluid is noninflammatory, with fewer than 2,000 white blood cells (WBC), a predominance of mononuclear WBCs, and a good mucin clot. (*Chapter 112, Page 989.*)

23.36 The patient is a 32-year-old white woman who has been diagnosed with RA. In an attempt to avoid joint destruction and disability, you have decided to use a disease-modifying antirheumatic drug (DMARD) early in the course of her disease. Your best choice among the DMARDs is probably

(A) parenteral gold
(B) methotrexate
(C) chloroquine
(D) azathioprine
(E) cyclosporine

Answer: (B). Parenteral gold was accepted for many years as the most effective of the DMARDs, but weekly low-dose methotrexate has emerged as the most frequently used DMARD in the United States and is considered by many rheumatologists as the DMARD of choice. (*Chapter 113, Page 998.*)

23.37 The most common complaint of patients with SLE is

(A) malar rash
(B) pain related to pericarditis
(C) joint pain
(D) cough
(E) seizures

Answer: (C). Arthralgias are the most common complaint of SLE patients and are often present at the time of initial diagnosis. Up to 76% of patients develop arthritis associated with disease activity. The classic malar butterfly rash is present in only one-third of patients. (*Chapter 113, Page 1000.*)

23.38 The patient is a 48-year-old white man with a long history of low back pain and stiffness that is becoming worse. Radiographs of the back are read as showing "bamboo spine." This clinical picture is most consistent with

(A) ankylosing spondylitis
(B) RA
(C) polymyalgia rheumatica
(D) SLE
(E) degenerative arthritis of the spine

Answer: (A). The diagnosis of ankylosing spondylitis can be confirmed radiographically if there is evidence of sacroiliitis. If the disease has progressed, patients have the "bamboo spine" seen on radiographs. (*Chapter 113, Page 1003.*)

23.39 The most characteristic finding in polymyalgia rheumatica is

(A) elevated creatine phosphokinase (CPK) levels
(B) elevated ESR
(C) occurrence in patients aged 30 to 50 years
(D) distal joint pain
(E) coexistence of temporal arteritis in almost all patients

Answer: (B). Polymyalgia rheumatica has a prevalence of approximately 1 in 150 persons older than age 50. On clinical examination, patients are tender to palpation, but their strength is intact and CPK levels are normal, ruling out muscle destruction. The most characteristic finding in polymyalgia rheumatics is an elevated ESR. In fact, many patients have ESRs in excess of 100 mm/hour. It is estimated that one-fourth to one-half of patients with polymyalgia rheumatica also have temporal arteritis. (*Chapter 113, Page 1003.*)

23.40 The patient is a 36-year-old white woman who strained her right shoulder while lifting a heavy package into the trunk of her car. The strain occurred about 2 weeks ago. She continues to have pain in the right upper back and shoulder. Examination reveals a "trigger point" in the right upper trapezius muscle. The trigger point is tender and palpation of this point elicits a twitch response with pain referred to the right

shoulder and upper arm. The patient has no fatigue or other generalized symptoms. This patient's problem is most accurately described as

(A) muscle strain
(B) myositis
(C) reflex sympathetic dystrophy (RSD)
(D) fibromyalgia
(E) myofascial pain syndrome (MPS)

Answer: (E). MPS is the name given to the common clinical syndrome of persistent regional or local pain in muscle(s) accompanied by "trigger points" on palpation of the involved muscles. The trigger point has local tenderness, the presence of a "taut band," and a twitch response. Palpation of the trigger point characteristically produces pain referred beyond it. The syndrome may be acute and is often seen after strain or trauma to a muscle. Nonmusculoskeletal symptoms, such as fatigue, are unusual. (*Chapter 114, Page 1007.*)

23.41 The patient is a 34-year-old white woman who injured her right hand when it was accidentally shut in a car door. This occurred about 3 months ago. An initial increase in skin temperature and edema progressed to a burning pain in the involved extremity, cool skin, decreased hair growth, localized sweating, and decreased range of motion with some muscle atrophy. This patient might benefit from referral for which one of the following treatment modalities?

(A) stellate ganglion blockade
(B) cervical laminectomy
(C) cervical sympathectomy
(D) intrathecal injection of corticosteroids
(E) none of the above

Answer: (A). Chemical blockade, such as a stellate ganglion blockade or a regional Bier block, is often helpful early in the course of reflex sympathetic dystrophy. Multiple blocks may be required. Surgical sympathectomies may be required in persistent cases. (*Chapter 114, Page 1008.*)

23.42 Morton's neuroma (MN) is an entrapment neuropathy of the interdigital nerve. It is a common cause of forefoot pain, especially in women. Which of the following is the most noteworthy risk factor for MN?

(A) family history
(B) RA
(C) improper shoe selection
(D) pes planus
(E) diabetes mellitus

Answer: (C). The factor most conducive to prevention of MN is shoe selection. People should be encouraged to use a shoe wide enough to accommodate the foot comfortably and to avoid high-heeled shoes. (*Chapter 114, Pages 1009–1010.*)

23.43 The pathognomonic sign of Dupuytren's contracture (DC) is

(A) anesthesia of the fourth and fifth fingers
(B) motor weakness of the fourth and fifth fingers
(C) atrophy of muscles of the forearm
(D) a nodule in the palm of the hand
(E) ulnar deviation at the MCP joints

Answer: (D). The pathognomonic sign of DC is a nodule in the palm, usually located at the base of the ring finger. The other fingers or thumb may also be involved but less commonly than the ring finger. This nodule may be painful or pruritic. (*Chapter 114, Page 1010.*)

23.44 The patient is a 14-year-old white male football player. Although he can recall no injury, he has noted a 2-month history of progressive pain and swelling involving the right knee. Examination of the right knee reveals tenderness and swelling involving the metaphysis of the right tibia. Your leading concern is that this patient may have which of the following?

(A) osteochondroma
(B) osteosarcoma
(C) chondroma
(D) osteoid osteoma
(E) metastatic tumor to the bone

Answer: (B). Primary osteosarcomas occur most commonly in children and young adults and are most common in males. There appears to be a genetic predisposition. The secondary osteosarcomas generally develop in adults in areas of abnormal bone (e.g., Paget's disease) or in response to some sort of carcinogen exposure (most commonly irradiation). The most common presenting complaints of patients with osteosarcoma are local pain, tenderness, and swelling. It most often occurs in the medullary cavity of the metaphyseal end of the long bones of the extremities. (*Chapter 114, Pages 1011–1012.*)

23.45 The patient whose bone scan and plain film are shown on the next page is a 75-year-old white man with a 6-month history of pain in the lower back and pelvis. He has also noted a decrease in his hearing acuity. The pain is worse at night. Laboratory analysis shows an elevated serum alkaline phosphatase level.

Serum calcium and phosphorus levels are normal. This patient's diagnosis appears to be

(A) metastatic cancer to the bones of the left pelvis
(B) Paget's disease of bone
(C) osteogenic sarcoma of the left hip
(D) Ewing's sarcoma of the left pelvis
(E) osteoid osteoma

Answer: (B). The bone scan shows extensive uptake in half of the pelvis in this patient with nocturnal pelvic pain. The plain film shows coarse trabeculae over the acetabulum (*black arrow*) and a thickening of the iliopectineal line (*white arrow*), findings seen with Paget's disease. Paget's disease is often asymptomatic and discovered incidentally by radiography. When symptomatic, night-time bone pain is usually the first symptom. Because of bone softening, bowing of the tibias, pathologic fractures, and increased kyphosis are commonly seen. An increasing head circumference, deafness, and a waddling gait are other relatively common symptoms. A markedly elevated serum alkaline phosphatase level and normal calcium and phosphorus are the usual laboratory pattern. An elevated 24-hour urinary hydroxyproline level, indicative of rapid bone turnover, is also seen. Radiographic findings include expanded bone with increased density. Early on, radiolucent lesions are common, especially in the skull and pelvis. Later mixed, then sclerotic lesions are seen. (*Chapter 114, Page 1014.*)

DIRECTIONS (Items 23.46 through 23.61): Each of the items in this section is a multiple true–false problem that consists of a stem and four lettered options. Indicate whether each of the four options is TRUE or FALSE.

23.46 True statements regarding sciatica include which of the following?

(A) Of patients with acute low back pain, approximately one-fourth develop sciatica.
(B) There is an increased risk of sciatica with long-distance driving, especially truck driving.
(C) The incidence of sciatica peaks during the fourth and fifth decades of life.
(D) Most patients with persistent sciatica require surgery.

Answer: (A-False, B-True, C-True, D-False). Of patients with acute low back pain, only 1.5% develop sciatica (i.e., painful paresthesias or motor weakness in the distribution of a nerve root). The lifetime prevalence of sciatica is 40%, and sciatica afflicts 11% of patients with

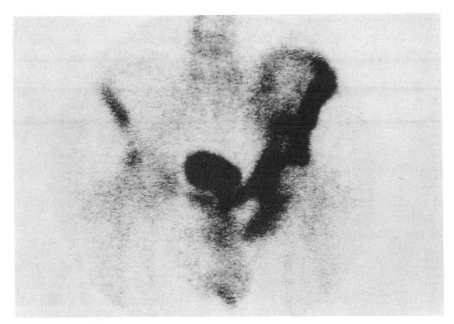

A

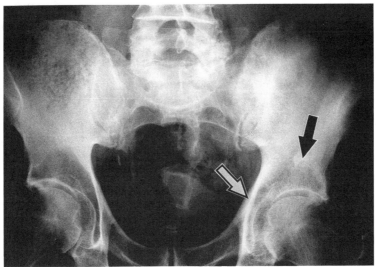

B

Fig. 23.8. Question 23.45.

low back pain that lasts more than 2 weeks. Sciatica is associated with long-distance driving, truck driving, cigarette smoking, and repeated lifting in a twisted posture. It is most common during the fourth and fifth decades of life, peaking during the fourth decade. Most patients with sciatica, even those with significant neurologic abnormalities, recover without surgery. Only 5 to 10% of patients with persistent sciatica require surgery. (*Chapter 109, Page 950.*)

23.47 Aerobic fitness training is an effective means of preventing low back injury and rehabilitating patients in whom low back pain has developed. Useful exercises for this purpose include which of the following?

(A) jogging
(B) swimming
(C) cycling
(D) jumping rope

Answer: (A-True, B-True, C-False, D-False). Typical exercises include walking, jogging, or aerobics; swimming is a useful alternative when weight-bearing exercise is painful. Cycling is not recommended because the sitting position increases the biomechanical workload on the lumbar spine. Jumping rope should be avoided because it places a high compression load on the spine and requires a high level of intensity before aerobic benefit is achieved. (*Chapter 109, Page 956.*)

23.48 The patient is a 28-year-old white man who was driving a car that was struck from behind by a pickup truck. The accident occurred yesterday, and now the patient complains of severe pain in the neck. True statements regarding cervical whiplash injury include which of the following?

(A) In cervical whiplash, the initial injury is hyperflexion.
(B) The cervical spine injury centers on the C5–6 interspace.
(C) There is often an injury to the anterior longitudinal ligament of the cervical spine.
(D) Complaints of visual disturbance are not part of the cervical whiplash syndrome and indicate malingering.

Answer: (A-False, B-True, C-True, D-False). After a rear-end impact in a motor vehicle accident, the patient is accelerated forward and the neck is thrown into hyperextension, which centers on the C5–6 interspace, followed by flexion of the neck, which is limited by the chin striking the chest. Hyperextension commonly causes an injury to the anterior longitudinal ligament of the cervical spine and other soft tissue injuries of the anterior neck, including muscle tears, muscle hemorrhage, esophageal hemorrhage, or disc disruption. Muscles most commonly injured include the sternocleidomastoid, scalenus, and longus colli muscles. Patients may also develop visual disturbances, possibly due to vertebral, basilar, or other vascular injury or injury to the cervical sympathetic chain. (*Chapter 109, Page 960.*)

23.49 De Quervain's tenosynovitis includes which of the following tendons?

(A) extensor carpi ulnaris
(B) abductor pollicis longus
(C) flexor pollicis longus
(D) extensor pollicis brevis

Answer: (A-False, B-True, C-False, D-True). A stenosing tendonitis, de Quervain's tenosynovitis, occurs in the first extensor compartment of the wrist, comprising the abductor pollicis longus and extensor pollicis brevis. (*Chapter 110, Page 969.*)

23.50 Characteristics of DC include which of the following?

(A) There is a familial tendency.
(B) The problem is more common in middle-aged persons.
(C) The problem is more common in women than in men.
(D) The cause is vascular injury to the tendon sheath.

Answer: (A-True, B-True, C-False, D-False). Although the etiology is unknown, there is a familial tendency with DC occurring more frequently in middle-aged men of northern European descent. (*Chapter 110, Pages 969–970.*)

23.51 True statements regarding fractures of the neck of the femur include which of the following?

(A) Fractures of the neck of the femur may be painless.
(B) Fractures of the neck of the femur may be associated with little bruising or swelling.
(C) It is sometimes possible for a patient to ambulate with a nondisplaced fracture of the femur.
(D) A displaced fracture of the femoral neck causes internal rotation of the lower extremity.

Answer: (A-False, B-True, C-True, D-False). Fractures of the neck of the femur are painful and can be associated with little bruising or swelling. It is important to note that a nondisplaced fracture can be ambulated on, albeit with some degree of pain. A displaced fracture of the hip causes shortening and external rotation. (*Chapter 111, Page 975.*)

23.52 True statements regarding RA include which of the following?

(A) The disease occurs in all racial and ethnic groups.
(B) RA occurs more commonly in men than in women.
(C) The estimated worldwide prevalence of RA is about 1%.
(D) The peak age of RA occurrence is between the second and third decades of life.

Answer: (A-True, B-False, C-True, D-False). RA occurs in all racial and ethnic groups. It is seen more commonly in women by a 3:1 ratio. One U.S. study found RA in 6% of women and 2% of men, although estimates of its worldwide prevalence generally are about 1%. RA occurs in all age groups but is more common with increasing age, peaking between the fourth and sixth decades of life. (*Chapter 113, Page 992.*)

23.53 The early manifestations of RA include which of the following?

(A) pain in the small joints of the hands and feet
(B) morning stiffness
(C) fatigue and malaise
(D) large joint pain and swelling

Answer: (A-True, B-True, C-True, D-False). Patients usually first experience small joint involvement in the hands and feet, particularly the PIPs and MCPs. Morning stiffness lasting more than 1 hour in these joints is suggestive of RA. Edema and inflammatory products are absorbed by lymphatics and venules with motion. Patients often have constitutional symptoms as well, such as fatigue, malaise, low-grade fever, anorexia, weight loss, and anemia. Large joints become symptomatic later in the course of the disease. (*Chapter 113, Page 993.*)

23.54 ANA titers may be useful in the diagnosis of RA. True statements about the use of ANA titers include which of the following?

(A) ANA titers should be ordered early in the evaluation of patients with joint pain and stiffness.
(B) ANA titers are elevated in almost all patients with RA.
(C) ANA titers are highly specific for RA.
(D) An elevated ANA titer may be seen in a patient with Sjögren syndrome.

Answer: (A-False, B-False, C-False, D-True). ANA titers are ordered only in patients with systemic symptoms. ANA titers may be elevated in up to 30% of patients with RA; if abnormal, the physician should entertain the diagnoses of SLE, Sjögren syndrome, and scleroderma as well. (*Chapter 113, Page 994.*)

23.55 True statements regarding the use of aspirin in treating RA include which of the following?

(A) Aspirin, even at high doses, is less effective than nonsteroidal anti-inflammatory drugs (NSAID).
(B) Compliance with aspirin use can be monitored by using serum salicylate levels.
(C) High-dose aspirin is often less well tolerated than other NSAIDs.
(D) The maximum daily dose of aspirin is 2.4 g divided four times daily.

Answer: (A-False, B-True, C-True, D-False). Aspirin at high-doses is as effective in RA patients as other, much more expensive NSAIDs, and compliance can be monitored via serum salicylate levels. However, high dose aspirin is often less well tolerated than other NSAIDs.

Patients should be started on 3.6 g divided four times daily. If this dosage is tolerated but not optimally effective, it can be increased to 4.2 g daily. (*Chapter 113, Page 995.*)

23.56 The characteristics of Reiter syndrome include which of the following?

(A) arthritis
(B) cerebritis
(C) conjunctivitis
(D) colitis

Answer: (A-True, B-False, C-True, D-False). The hallmark signs of Reiter syndrome is the triad of arthritis, conjunctivitis, and urethritis. (*Chapter 113, Page 1001.*)

23.57 Your patient is a 52-year-old Hispanic woman with blanching and numbness of the fingertips that occurs in cold exposure. Subsequently, there is cyanosis and then erythema on rewarming. This patient may benefit from which of the following measures?

(A) prophylactic use of dextroamphetamine
(B) pseudoephedrine to abort an attack
(C) nifedipine
(D) relaxation and stress managements strategies

Answer: (A-False, B-False, C-True, D-True). Conservative approaches to treatment of Raynaud's disease include the obvious, such as warm socks or mittens and cold avoidance. Patients are encouraged to stop smoking and to avoid vasoconstrictive drugs such as amphetamines, cocaine, and over-the-counter decongestants. Caffeine may also exacerbate symptoms by causing a rebound vasoconstriction after an initial vasodilation. In patients with vasospasm associated with emotional stress, relaxation and stress management strategies have also been helpful. When conservative strategies fail, patients may respond to calcium channel blockers. Nifedipine has been the most widely studied at doses of 10 mg sublingually for immediate treatment of acute vasospasm or 30 to 60 mg of nifedipine taken daily on a chronic basis. (*Chapter 113, Page 1002.*)

23.58 True statements regarding psoriatic arthritis include which of the following?

(A) The disease usually involves proximal joints.
(B) Tenosynovitis may occur.
(C) A flare-up of the skin disease may precede an exacerbation of joint symptoms.
(D) The arthritis is generally treated with (NSAIDs) or antimalarials.

Answer: (A-False, B-True, C-True, D-True). Psoriatic arthritis is found in patients with psoriasis, distal joint involvement, tenosynovitis, and enthesopathy. Psoriatic arthritis is generally treated with NSAIDs or antimalarials. In up to one-third of patients, a flare-up in the skin disease may precede a flare of joint symptoms. (*Chapter 113, Page 1003.*)

23.59 True statements regarding fibromyalgia (FM) include which of the following?

(A) FM patients have a higher incidence of migraine headaches than the general population.
(B) Common complaints of FM patients generally do not include sensory symptoms such as numbness or tingling.
(C) The incidence of mitral valve prolapse in FM patients is about the same as in the general population.
(D) FM patients have a higher incidence of depression than the normal population.

Answer: (A-True, B-False, C-False, D-True). FM patients also have a higher incidence of migraine and tension headaches than the general population. Approximately 84% of people with FM complain of numbness or tingling somewhere in the body. Echocardiographic evidence of mitral valve prolapse is seen in up to 75% of FM patients. Patients with FM have a higher incidence of depression, and controversy remains as to whether FM symptoms are a manifestation of a psychosomatic syndrome, or, conversely, depression results from chronic pain. (*Chapter 114, Page 1005.*)

23.60 True statements regarding RSD include which of the following?

(A) RSD is a pain syndrome associated with loss of function.
(B) The most common cause is coronary artery disease.
(C) There is evidence of autonomic dysfunction.
(D) RSD often follows trauma that may seem relatively minor.

Answer: (A-True, B-False, C-True, D-True). RSD is a pain syndrome in which the pain is accompanied by loss of function and evidence of autonomic dysfunction. RSD usually occurs after trauma, although the trauma may be relatively minor. (*Chapter 114, Page 1007.*)

23.61 True statements regarding Ewing's sarcoma include which of the following?

(A) Ewing's sarcoma occurs most commonly in older adults and the elderly.
(B) The disease occurs more commonly in whites than in blacks.
(C) The tumors are found chiefly in the skull and vertebrae.
(D) "Onion-skin" appearance of the periosteum is a late radiographic finding.

Answer: (A-False, B-True, C-False, D-True). Ewing's sarcoma is a tumor of uncertain origin. It is most common in children and young adults. It is more common in whites than blacks. The tumor may occur in any bone but has some predilection for long tubular bones and the pelvis. The presenting complaints include pain, swelling, tenderness, and erythema, which makes it resemble osteomyelitis. Early, there may be no radiographic abnormalities, but later a typical lytic lesion with an "onion-skin" appearance of the periosteum is seen. (*Chapter 114, Page 1011.*)

24

The Skin and Subcutaneous Tissue

The questions in this chapter constitute a review of the following *chapters in Family Medicine: Principles and Practice, Fifth Edition:*

    Common Dermatoses (Chapter 115)
    Skin Infections and Infestations (Chapter 116)
    Skin Tumors (Chapter 117)
    Selected Disorders of the Skin (Chapter 118)

DIRECTIONS (Items 24.1 through 24.24): Each of the questions or incomplete statements in this section is followed by five suggested answers or completions. Select the ONE that is BEST in each case.

24.1 The patient is a 23-year-old married white female nurse with severe nodulocystic acne. Initial therapy has not brought relief, and you are considering the use of oral isotretinoin (Accutane). For this patient, the most significant risk of oral isotretinoin is

    (A) xerosis
    (B) cheilitis
    (C) arthralgia
    (D) teratogenicity
    (E) elevated liver enzymes

Answer: (D). Although this medicine can be profoundly effective, it has "black box" warnings about its teratogenicity and its association with pseudotumor cerebri. There are also numerous less severe side effects, including xerosis, cheilitis, epistaxis, myalgias, arthralgias, and elevated liver enzymes. Liver function tests, triglyceride levels, and complete blood counts should be frequently monitored. The highly teratogenic potential must be made clear to all female patients, and this medicine must be used with extreme caution in all women with childbearing potential. (*Chapter 114, Page 1017.*)

24.2 The photograph on the next page is of a 22-year-old white male mechanic with pruritic lesions, including excoriations and lichenification, on the flexor surfaces of the upper extremities. This patient appears to have

    (A) pityriasis rosea
    (B) atopic dermatitis
    (C) miliaria
    (D) psoriasis
    (E) seborrheic dermatitis

Answer: (B). The patient has atopic dermatitis in the popliteal fossae. (*Chapter 115, Page 1018.*)

24.3 Miliaria is caused by

    (A) allergies
    (B) an immunoglobulin deficiency
    (C) emotional stress
    (D) blockage of eccrine sweat glands
    (E) superficial fungal infection of the skin

Answer: (D). Miliaria (heat rash) is a common condition resulting from the blockage of eccrine sweat glands. There is an inflammatory response to the sweat that leaks through the ruptured duct, and papular or vesicular lesions result. It usually occurs after repeated exposure to hot and humid environments. (*Chapter 115, Page 1019.*)

24.4 The patient whose photograph is shown on the next page is a 30-year-old white male furniture mover with a 2-week history of salmon-pink patches on the chest and upper arms. This patient appears to have

    (A) pityriasis rosea
    (B) miliaria

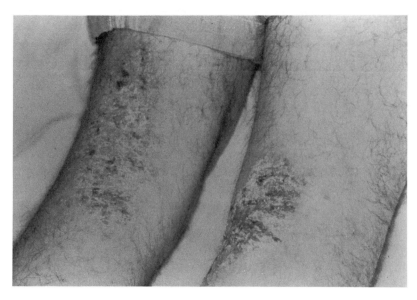

Fig. 24.1. Question 24.2.

(C) psoriasis
(D) atopic dermatitis
(E) seborrheic dermatitis

Answer: (A). Pityriasis rosea often starts with a single, 2- to 10-cm, oval, papulosquamous, salmon-pink patch (or plaque) on the trunk or proximal upper extremity. This "herald patch" is followed by a generalized eruption of discrete, small, oval plaques on the trunk and proximal extremities, sparing the palms and soles and oral cavity. These plaques align their long axis with the skin lines, thus giving the rash a characteristic "Christmas tree" appearance. (*Chapter 115, Page 1019.*)

24.5 The lesions of psoriasis often show pinpoint bleeding if a scale is removed. This phenomenon is called

(A) Roth's sign
(B) Janeway's sign
(C) Auspitz's sign
(D) Goeckerman's sign
(E) Wood's sign

Answer: (C). Psoriasis is a chronic recurrent disorder characterized by an inflammatory, scaling, hyperproliferative papulosquamous eruption. Lesions are well-defined plaques with a thick, adherent, silvery-white scale. If the scale is removed, pinpoint bleeding can be seen (Auspitz's sign). (*Chapter 115, Page 1020.*)

24.6 The patient whose knee is shown in the photograph on the next page has a 1- to 2-year history of erythematous plaques with thick silvery scales, especially on the elbows and knees. This patient has

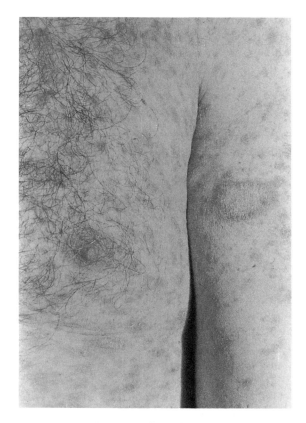

Fig. 24.2. Question 24.4.

(A) dyshidrotic excema
(B) seborrheic dermatitis
(C) pityriasis rosea
(D) psoriasis
(E) miliaria

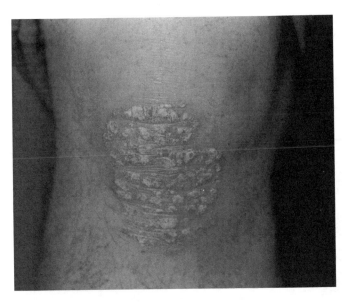

Fig. 24.3. Question 24.6.

Answer: (D). The classic presentation of psoriasis with its erythematous plaques and thick silvery scales on elbows or knees is usually easy to diagnose, but there are numerous morphologic variants. (*Chapter 115, Page 1020.*)

24.7 There is an increased incidence of seborrheic dermatitis in patients who have

(A) rheumatoid arthritis
(B) acquired immunodeficiency syndrome (AIDS)
(C) cancer of the lung
(D) diabetes mellitus
(E) depression

Answer: (B). An increased incidence (up to 80%) has been described in patients with AIDS, and these patients often present with a severe persistent eruption. (*Chapter 115, Page 1022.*)

24.8 The patient is a 35-year-old white male construction worker who has a red-brown macular skin rash in the genital area that has been present for 6 weeks. The rash glows a coral-pink color on Wood's lamp examination. This patient appears to have

(A) tinea cruris
(B) erythrasma
(C) erysipelas
(D) impetigo
(E) ecthyma

Answer: (B). Erythrasma is a superficial, often asymptomatic infection that causes red-brown macular skin dis-

coloration, generally in the genital area. The infection, easily confused with tinea cruris, may also affect the axillae and intertriginous skinfolds, particularly in obese individuals. Erythrasma is more common in males. Individuals affected notice skin color changes and present with this complaint. Wood's light examination is helpful, as the infected area glows a coral-pink color. The causative agent of infection is *Corynebacterium minutissimum,* a porphyrin-producing bacterium, and this porphyrin production accounts for the fluorescence under Wood's light illuminations. (*Chapter 116, Page 1027.*)

24.9 The patient is a 32-year-old white female flight attendant who recently visited friends in Arizona, where she spent some time in their hot-tub. She now has widespread folliculitis. The causative organism is likely to be

(A) *Staphylococcus aureus*
(B) *Corynebacterium minutissimum*
(C) *Pseudomonas aeruginosa*
(D) *Candida albicans*
(E) *Trichomycosis axillaris*

Answer: (C). Hot-tub folliculitis, a special type of folliculitis, bears mention. Following exposure to a poorly maintained hot-tub or Jacuzzi, a folliculitis may occur. The causative agent for the folliculitis is *Pseudomonas aeruginosa*. The illness is self-limited in most patients, and resulting serious illness is rare. (*Chapter 116, Page 1029.*)

24.10 When an abscess is present, the site of the abscess may have significant implications. A cervical or facial abscess is especially significant as it may lead to

(A) acute parotitis
(B) airway compromise
(C) acute necrotizing gingivitis
(D) oral thrush
(E) cervical lymphadenopathy

Answer: (B). Cervical and facial abscesses are particularly worrisome and may herald airway compromise. (*Chapter 116, Page 1030.*)

24.11 The patient whose photograph is shown on the next page has a painful vesicular rash of the chest wall. This rash is caused by

(A) *Staphylococcus aureus*
(B) reactivation of varicella-zoster virus (VZV)
(C) herpes simplex virus

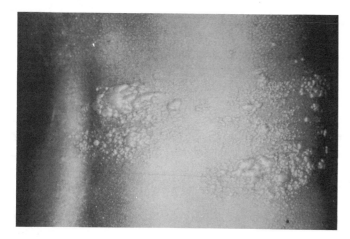

Fig. 24.4. Question 24.11.

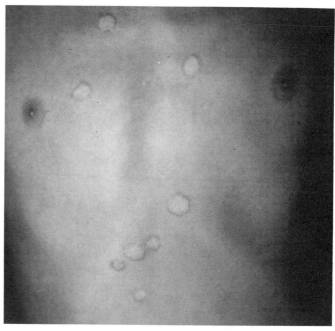

Fig. 24.5. Question 24.14.

(D) necrotizing fasciitis
(E) *Pseudomonas aeruginosa*

Answer: (B). Zoster is the result of reactivation of VZV residing in the dorsal nerve root ganglia. (*Chapter 116, Page 1032.*)

24.12 The primary infection of oral herpes is an episode of

(A) childhood varicella infection
(B) gingivostomatitis
(C) a vesicular genital lesion
(D) an infection of the vermillion border of the lip
(E) none of the above

Answer: (B). The primary infection of oral herpes (herpes labialis) is an episode of gingivostomatitis accompanied by systemic symptoms of headache, fever, and upper respiratory symptoms. (*Chapter 116, Page 1033.*)

24.13 Hand, foot, and mouth disease is caused by

(A) a Coxsackie virus
(B) VZV
(C) anaerobic bacteria
(D) *Haemophilus influenzae*
(E) herpes simplex virus type II

Answer: (A). Hand, foot, and mouth disease is a curious illness affecting the body parts noted in its name. The incubation period for the illness is not known, although it is known to be caused by Coxsackie A16 virus. (*Chapter 116, Page 1034.*)

24.14 The patient whose photograph is shown above is a 16-year-old white boy with a 1-week history of rash on the anterior chest. This patient appears to have

(A) tinea versicolor
(B) pityriasis rosea
(C) erythrasma
(D) tinea corporis
(E) impetigo

Answer: (D). Tinea corporis and tinea faciei are most commonly seen in children. Lesions with reddish, scaling, raised borders surround a central zone that is faded but often scaling. (*Chapter 116, Page 1036.*)

24.15 The patient is a 43-year-old white female factory worker. Over the past 3 to 4 months, she has noticed a small brown nodule of the anterior lower leg. The nodule has a firm consistency and attempts to elevate the nodule between the thumb and forefinger cause a retraction "dimpling" underneath the skin surface. This patient is most likely to have which of the following?

(A) malignant melanoma
(B) dermatofibroma
(C) hemangioma
(D) Kaposi's sarcoma (KS)
(E) lipoma

Answer: (B). Dermatofibromas are small, pink to brown, sometimes scaly, 3- to 7-mm hard nodules; they are commonly located on the anterior surface of the leg. Dermatofibromas are a localized nodular/fibrous tissue response to what may be an insignificant skin injury or inflammation. They are distinguished clinically by the "dimple sign" (retraction underneath the skin surface with attempts to elevate between the thumb and forefinger). (*Chapter 117, Page 1041.*)

24.16 The patient is a newborn girl with two small, raised, bright-red lesions, one on the chest and one on the shoulder, that were present at birth. You should advise the parents that

(A) the lesions should be surgically excised at 3 months of age
(B) the best treatment is cryotherapy at 2 months of age
(C) the lesions are best treated with intralesional steroid injections
(D) the lesions indicate a high risk of angiomatous polyps in the gastrointestinal tract
(E) the lesions will probably disappear spontaneously in time

Answer: (E). Strawberry nevi represent a collection of dilated vessels located in the dermis. They manifest as raised bright red lesions, usually present at birth or evolving in the first few months of life. Complete involution, commencing by age 3 years, occurs with more than 90% of these lesions. Because spontaneous involution is the norm, observation and parental reassurance are the cornerstones of management. (*Chapter 117, Page 1041.*)

24.17 The most commonly occurring type of skin cancer is

(A) basal cell carcinoma
(B) lentigo maligna
(C) malignant melanoma
(D) metastatic cancer to the skin
(E) squamous cell carcinoma (SSC)

Answer: (A). Basal cell carcinoma accounts for nearly 75% of all skin cancers; 400,000 new patients are diagnosed each year. Ninety percent of lesions occur on sun-exposed areas of the head and neck and one-third on the nose. (*Chapter 117, Page 1045.*)

24.18 Malignant melanoma occurs most commonly

(A) in the genital area
(B) on sun-exposed areas

(C) on the torso
(D) on the face
(E) as malignant transformation of actinic keratoses (AK)

Answer: (B). Although melanoma may occur on any body surface, most occur on sun-exposed areas. (*Chapter 117, Page 1046.*)

24.19 The patient is a 32-year-old white male waiter whom you have followed for the past 2 years because he has human immunodeficiency virus (HIV) infection. For the past 2 months, he has noted a 2-cm lesion on the right forearm that appears as a violaceous macule with some associated edema of the skin. The biopsy of this lesion is likely to be reported as

(A) AK
(B) keratoacanthoma
(C) KS
(D) basal cell carcinoma
(E) lentigo maligna

Answer: (C). A tumor of the vascular endothelium, KS can occur on any body surface including the palms, soles, and mucous membranes. KS has also been reported in all organs of the body except the brain. The lesions typically appear as violaceous or erythematous macules with associated cutaneous edema and can be easily confused with other pigmented skin lesions. Biopsy is essential during the initial evaluation of such lesions. (*Chapter 117, Page 1046.*)

24.20 In considering the best technique to remove skin lesions, the shave biopsy is most appropriately used with lesions that are known to be

(A) metastatic
(B) premalignant
(C) malignant
(D) nonmalignant
(E) none of the above

Answer: (D). The shave biopsy is best adapted to lesions known to be nonmalignant. (*Chapter 117, Page 1048.*)

24.21 The patient is a 42-year-old white woman. For the past year, she has noted several hypopigmented areas of the face and neck. In evaluation of this patient, it might be reasonable to order which of the following studies?

(A) estrogen levels
(B) thyroid studies

(C) carcinoembryonic antigen
(D) genetic screening
(E) pregnancy test

Answer: (B). Vitiligo is associated with thyroid disorders in up to 30% of cases, and there are reported associations with alopecia areata, pernicious anemia, other autoimmune and endocrine disorders, and melanoma. (*Chapter 118, Page 1050.*)

24.22 The patient is a 7-year-old girl whom you have treated from time to time for mild atopic dermatitis. For the past 3 to 4 months, she has had several lesions on the cheeks and arms that began with light redness and progressed to hypopigmentation. The next step in the management of this child should be

(A) incisional biopsy for diagnosis
(B) injection of intralesional steroids
(C) reassurance
(D) application of topical antifungal cream
(E) application of topical antibiotic ointment

Answer: (C). Pityriasis alba is a common skin disorder in prepubertal children with a history of atopic dermatitis. The lesions begin with erythema and progress to hypopigmentation and are located primarily on the cheeks and lateral arms. It is more common in dark-skinned individuals in sunny climates. The condition is transient and nonscarring, gradually fading after puberty. Treatment is not mandatory, but when inflammation appears, topical steroids are helpful. (*Chapter 118, Page 1050.*)

24.23 The first step in the management of corns and calluses is

(A) surgical excision
(B) trimming the lesion with a sharp blade
(C) use of a keratinolytic medication
(D) filing with an emery board or pumice stone
(E) removal of pressure

Answer: (E). Removal of pressure is the first step in the conservative management of these lesions. (*Chapter 118, Page 1052.*)

24.24 The patient is a 26-year-old white woman who is 9 weeks postpartum. She has noted significant hair loss, with decreased hair density, but there are no patches of complete baldness. This patient's condition is called

(A) anagen defluvium
(B) telogen effluvium
(C) tinea capitus

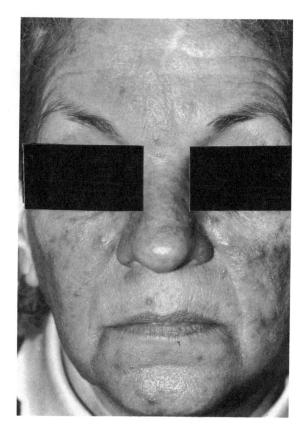

Fig. 24.6. Question 24.25.

(D) trichotillomania
(E) alopecia areata

Answer: (B). Telogen effluvium is the most common form of pathologic hair loss. It is a process that leads to decreased hair density but not usually to complete baldness. (*Chapter 118, Page 1054.*)

DIRECTIONS (Items 24.25 through 21.36): Each of the items in this section is a multiple true–false problem that consists of a stem and four lettered options. Indicate whether each of the options is TRUE or FALSE.

24.25 The patient pictured is a 52-year-old white female receptionist with a chronic facial rash including flushing, papules, and pustules. True statements regarding this patient's problem include which of the following?

(A) The rash is most common between the ages of 30 and 60.
(B) Although there is significant involvement of facial skin, the eyes and surrounding tissues are spared.
(C) Severe involvement can lead to rhinophyma.

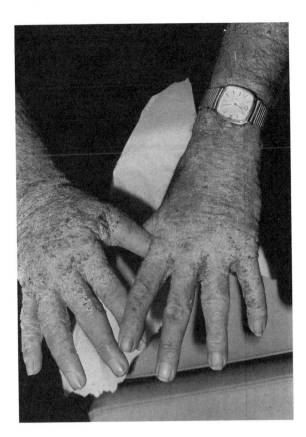

Fig. 24.7. Question 24.26.

(D) The most severe lesions are found on the neck and upper back.

Answer: (A-True, B-False, C-True, D-False). A chronic facial dermatosis, acne rosacea typically appears in patients between the ages of 30 and 60. It is characterized by acneiform lesions such as papules, pustules, and occasionally nodules. Most lesions are on the forehead, cheeks, and nose. Patients also have facial flushing, generalized erythema, and telangiectasias; they may have moderate-to-severe sebaceous gland hyperplasia. Ocular manifestations such as conjunctivitis, blepharitis, and episcleritis can be found in about half of the patients. Severe involvement of the nose can lead to soft tissue hypertrophy and rhinophyma. (*Chapter 115, Pages 1022–1023.*)

24.26 The photograph shown is of the hands of a 48-year-old restaurant dishwasher who has had a pruritic rash of the hands and wrists for 2 to 3 months. True statements regarding the management of this patient's condition include which of the following?

(A) The first step will be removal of the irritant or allergy.
(B) Cool compresses may help relieve pruritus.

(C) In the acute phase, creams or lotions are recommended as they are less irritating than most ointments.
(D) Topical lidocaine may be used at bedtime to relieve pruritus.

Answer: (A-True, B-True, C-False, D-False). This patient has contact dermatitis, irritant type. Treatment is symptomatic after removal of the irritant or allergen. Cool compresses can provide relief from the pruritus, particularly if there is any weeping. Oral antihistamines may be needed along with topical steroids. Ointment compounds are recommended, as they are less irritating and sensitizing than most creams or lotions. The patient should avoid any topical preparations with benzocaine or other "-caines," as they may aggravate the condition. (*Chapter 115, Page 1025.*)

24.27 True statements regarding the rash of rubella include which of the following?

(A) The rash may be the first manifestation of the disease.
(B) The rash begins on the torso and spreads to the face and other areas.
(C) The rash of rubella often affects the perioral area.
(D) Lymphadenopathy often accompanies the rash.

Answer: (A-True, B-False, C-True, D-True). The illness of rubella generally begins as a rash, and unlike measles, there is virtually no prodrome. The rash is similar to that of measles; it begins on the face and exhibits a butterfly pattern. The rash of rubella often affects the perioral area, and this distinction is useful if a concern about scarlet fever also exists. Lymphadenopathy may become prominent during the illness. (*Chapter 116, Page 1031.*)

24.28 The patient pictured on the next page is a 17-year-old black male high school student with a long-standing rash of the face and upper chest. The lesions are confluent and slightly scaly and appear lighter during the summer months. True statements regarding this person's skin rash include which of the following?

(A) The rash is properly called pityriasis versicolor.
(B) The illness is common in prepubertal children.
(C) The rash occurs more commonly in dry cool environments.
(D) The lesions interfere with tanning of the affected skin.

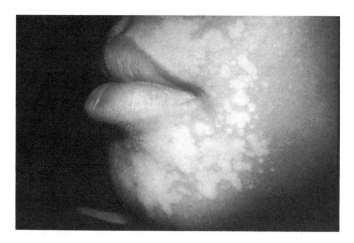

Fig. 24.8. Question 24.28.

Answer: (A-True, B-False, C-False, D-True). *Tinea versicolor* is a common infection that is more properly referred to as *pityriasis versicolor*. *Tinea* is incorrectly used, as the rash is not one caused by a dermatophyte. Rather, it is due to infection by the yeast *Pityrosporum* (*Malassezia*) *furfur*. The illness is rare before puberty. It is more common in humid warm environments, and the causative organism requires an environment rich in lipids. Thus the rash of the illness is found on the chest and back and may spread to the lateral buttocks. The skin lesions are generally coffee-colored and are up to 1 cm in size. As the rash spreads, the lesions become confluent and slightly scaly. The skin lesions themselves show little change in color seasonally, although the pigmentation of surrounding skin makes the lesions appear lighter during months when skin becomes tan and darker during nontanning months. (*Chapter 116, Pages 1037–1038.*)

24.29 The patient is a 46-year-old homeless man, and you have diagnosed body lice. True statements regarding this patient's problem include which of the following?

(A) Body lice burrow 3 to 5 mm into the skin, and finding such a burrow is important in making the diagnosis.
(B) Body lice attach to clothing, particularly the seams.
(C) Pruritus from body lice occurs from a reaction to the body protein of the louse in its skin burrow.
(D) The body louse can transmit rickettsial disease, including Rocky Mountain spotted fever.

Answer: (A-False, B-True, C-False, D-True). Body lice are most common among the homeless. These lice do not actually attach to the body but to clothing, particularly the seams. Intense pruritus from exposure to the louse saliva during blood meals results in widespread excoriations arranged in a linear fashion. *Pediculosis humanus corporis* is capable of transmitting various rickettsial diseases, including spotted fever and trench fevers. (*Chapter 116, Page 1039.*)

24.30 Keratoacanthomas are rapidly growing, round, flesh-colored lesions with a typical central crater. Characteristics of the keratoacanthoma include which of the following?

(A) These lesions occur most commonly in young African American women.
(B) A keratoacanthoma may be mistaken for squamous cell carcinoma.
(C) The keratoacanthoma usually does not exceed 3 cm in greatest dimension.
(D) Keratoacanthomas rarely undergo spontaneous regression.

Answer: (A-False, B-True, C-True, D-False). They occur most commonly in Caucasian men older than 50 years of age. Clinically and histologically, keratoacanthomas may be mistaken for SCC. In contrast to SCCs, which have unlimited growth potential, most keratoacanthomas usually do not exceed 3 cm in greatest dimension. In addition, unlike SCCs, keratoacanthomas spontaneously regress within 2 to 6 months. (*Chapter 116, Page 1042.*)

24.31 The patient is a 72-year-old white man who has several AKs of the forehead and scalp. He asks about the possibility of change to a skin cancer. True statements that you might use in your reply include which of the following?

(A) Approximately 15 to 20% of people with AK develop cutaneous SCC during their lifetime.
(B) SCC almost always arises from an AK.
(C) Infiltration and elevation of an AK suggests malignant change.
(D) Tenderness of an AK suggests malignant change.

Answer: (A-True, B-False, C-True, D-True). Although the risk of malignant transformation is unknown, it is estimated that 15 to 20% of people with AKs eventually develop cutaneous SCC during their lifetime. AKs are not the sole precursors of SCC. Studies have shown that 40% may arise de novo in normal skin.

Infiltration, elevation, or tenderness of an AK suggests malignant change. (*Chapter 117, Page 1043.*)

24.32 The patient is a 32-year-old white man who lives in a "single room occupancy" hotel when he can find work; sometimes he is homeless. On examining the patient because of a cough and fever, you notice a painless white wrinkled lesion affecting the lateral aspects of the tongue. The lesion does not "wipe off" with an applicator. This patient

(A) should be suspected of having a HIV infection
(B) appears to have lichen planus
(C) should be treated with nystatin oral suspension
(D) should have a definitive diagnosis established by biopsy

Answer: (A-True, B-False, C-False, D-True). Because of its association with AIDS, hairy leukoplakia is an important oral lesion. It is now recognized as one of the early dermatologic "warning signs" of HIV infection, as 75% of individuals in whom hairy leukoplakia is diagnosed manifest AIDS within 3 years. Hairy leukoplakia may appear clinically similar to idiopathic leukoplakia or leukoplakia associated with tobacco use. It most often presents as an asymptomatic, whitish, wrinkled lesion affecting the lateral aspects of the tongue. However, as with other leukoplakic lesions, it may also involve the buccal mucosa, floor of the mouth, or palate. Differential diagnosis includes candidiasis, other leukoplakias, lichen planus, and traumatic hyperplasia. As with other leukoplakic oral lesions, definitive diagnosis is established by biopsy. (*Chapter 117, Page 1043.*)

24.33 The patient is a 76-year-old white man who is uncircumcised. For the past 2 months, he has noted a velvety reddish plaque on the glans penis. This patient appears to have

(A) lentigo maligna
(B) a type of Bowen's disease
(C) erythroplasia of Queyrat
(D) a keratoacanthoma

Answer: (A-False, B-True, C-True, D-False). When Bowen's disease affects the glans penis, it is referred to as erythroplasia of Queyrat. These lesions typically present as bright, erythematous, velvety, nonscaly plaques in elderly uncircumcised men. (*Chapter 117, Page 1044.*)

24.34 Medications that can cause a photosensitivity reaction include which of the following?

(A) furosemide
(B) sulfonamides
(C) tetracyclines
(D) thiazides

Answer: (A-True, B-True, C-True, D-True). Some of the more common medications that cause a photosensitivity reaction are furosemide, nonsteroidal anti-inflammatory drugs sulfonamides, tetracyclines, and thiazides. (*Chapter 118, Page 1051.*)

24.35 True statements regarding cutaneous lupus erythematosus (LE) include which of the following?

(A) Chronic cutaneous LE is associated with a high incidence of systemic disease.
(B) The disease is more common in females.
(C) Chronic cutaneous LE is more common in Caucasian than in African American patients.
(D) In chronic cutaneous LE, the antinuclear antibody (ANA) and erythrocyte sedimentation rate (ESR) are usually both elevated.

Answer: (A-False, B-True, C-False, D-False). Chronic cutaneous LE (discoid LE) carries a low incidence of systemic diseases. It is more common in females and has a peak incidence during the fourth decade of life. The incidence of chronic cutaneous LE is 3 per 100,000 among white females and 8 per 100,000 in black females. The ANA, anti-dsDNA, and ESR are all usually within normal limits. (*Chapter 118, Page 1051.*)

24.36 The patient is a 34-year-old white man who is having bitemporal hair loss. He reports that his father had male pattern baldness. True statements regarding androgenic alopecia (male pattern baldness) include which of the following?

(A) This type of baldness does not occur in women.
(B) Male pattern baldness can begin as early as the adolescent years.
(C) Less than 20% of Caucasian men have noticeable hair loss by age 50.
(D) The condition follows an autosomal dominant pattern of inheritance with incomplete penetrance.

Answer: (A-False, B-True, C-False, D-True). Androgenic alopecia, or male pattern baldness, is exceedingly common and manifests as bitemporal thinning of the hair followed by loss of hair over the crown. This type of thinning can occur in women as well as men, although the hair loss is generally less severe in women. Male pattern baldness can begin as early as the adolescent years, with more than 50% of Caucasian men having noticeable hair loss by age 50. The condition follows an autosomal dominant pattern of inheritance with incomplete penetrance. Certain ethnic groups, including Japanese, Chinese, and American Indians, are relatively immune to the condition. (*Chapter 118, Page 1054.*)

25

The Endocrine and Metabolic System

The questions in this chapter constitute a review of the following chapters in *Family Medicine: Principles and Practice, Fifth Edition*:

Dyslipidemias (Chapter 119)
Diabetes Mellitus (Chapter 120)
Thyroid Disease (Chapter 121)
Osteoporosis (Chapter 122)
Gout (Chapter 123)
Selected Disorders of the Endocrine and Metabolic System (Chapter 124)

DIRECTIONS (Items 25.1 through 25.29): Each of the questions or incomplete statements in this section is followed by five suggested answers or completions. Select the ONE that is BEST in each case.

25.1 The possibility that a patient might have hypertriglyceridemia should be considered whenever an individual has which of the following diagnoses?

(A) urolithiasis
(B) chronic obstructive lung disease
(C) noncalculous cholecystitis
(D) splenomegaly
(E) pancreatitis

Answer: (E). Hypertriglyceridemias are considered in any patient with pancreatitis. Dyslipidemias with triglyceride (TG) levels greater than 1,000 mg/dl have a high risk of associated pancreatitis most likely due to microvascular obstruction; but TG levels drop precipitously during acute attacks, which may mask the etiology of this life-threatening condition. A careful family history, family lipid screening, and remeasurement of TG levels after recovery can identify hypertriglyceridemia as the cause of pancreatitis. (*Chapter 119, Page 1058.*)

25.2 Consumption of which of the following may be associated with an elevation of high-density lipoprotein (HDL) levels?

(A) fiber
(B) ethanol
(C) fish oil
(D) vitamin E
(E) folic acid

Answer: (B). No specific foods or nutrients cause an increase in HDL levels, with the exception of ethanol. Whereas moderate alcohol intake has been associated with elevations in HDL, ethanol may contribute to obesity and elevated TG and blood pressure. In addition, ethanol is toxic to heart muscle, raises blood pressure and TG levels, is addictive, and has variable effects on subspecies of HDL. Therefore, alcohol should not generally be recommended as a treatment for low HDL. (*Chapter 119, Page 1060.*)

25.3 In the treatment of dyslipidemias, which one of the following is limited to use for high-risk hypertriglyceridemias?

(A) niacin
(B) clofibrate
(C) gemfibrozil
(D) lovastatin
(E) cholestyramine

Answer: (B). Clofibrate (Atromid-S), a fibric acid similar to gemfibrozil, is limited to use for high-risk hypertriglyceridemias owing to safety concerns raised in clinical trials. (*Chapter 119, Page 1061.*)

25.4 The patient is a 40-year-old white male executive with a family history of coronary artery disease and whose lipid profile is normal, with the exception of a HDL level of 22 mg/dl (normal range, 30 to 80 mg/dl). The only medication likely to be effective is

(A) niacin
(B) clofibrate
(C) gemfibrozil
(D) lovastatin
(E) cholestyramine

Answer: (A). The only medication shown to date to be effective in patients with isolated low HDL (less than 35 mg/dl) is niacin. Isolated HDL deficiencies are slow to respond to treatment if they respond at all. (*Chapter 119, Page 1064.*)

25.5 The patient is a 55-year-old businessman with a history of coronary artery disease. His serum TG level is 620 mg/dl (normal range, 40 to 150 mg/dl). The patient also has peptic ulcer disease and diabetes mellitus (DM). The treatment of choice for this patient is

(A) niacin
(B) clofibrate
(C) gemfibrozil
(D) lovastatin
(E) cholestyramine

Answer: (C). Gemfibrozil is the treatment of choice for hypertriglyceridemia associated with diabetes, gout, gastritis, or ulcer disease due to the potential for niacin to exacerbate these conditions. (*Chapter 119, Page 1064.*)

25.6 The *earliest* marker of diabetic nephropathy is

(A) elevated blood urea nitrogen level
(B) elevated serum creatinine level
(C) urinary casts
(D) microalbuminuria
(E) elevated diastolic blood pressure

Answer: (D). Markers of nephropathy are also important to measure. The earliest marker, microalbuminuria, is not only a forerunner of overt clinical nephropathy but also a marker for greatly increased cardiovascular risk in both type I and type II patients. Microalbuminuria can be conveniently measured in spot urine specimens or by overnight albumin excretion rates. (*Chapter 119, Page 1068.*)

25.7 The current dietary recommendation for an individual with diabetes is

(A) at least 50% carbohydrate, less than 30% fat, and 20% or less protein
(B) at least 65% carbohydrate, less than 20% fat, and 15% or less protein
(C) at least 40% carbohydrate, less than 40% fat, and 20% or less protein
(D) use of sugar-free foods only
(E) none of the above

Answer: (A). For individuals with diabetes, the current dietary recommendations are a diet containing at least 50% carbohydrate, less than 30% fat, and 20% or less protein. (*Chapter 119, Pages 1068–1069.*)

25.8 The patient is a 52-year-old white woman. She is a newly diagnosed diabetic with fasting blood sugars in the range of 150 to 170 mg/dl. You have elected to begin treatment with acarbose. She inquires about the most common side effect that she might encounter. The appropriate answer to her question would be

(A) increased intestinal gas formation
(B) hypoglycemia, especially during nocturnal hours
(C) cutaneous flushing
(D) elevated liver enzymes
(E) urinary retention

Answer: (A). Monotherapy with acarbose is indicated in the newly diagnosed, mildly hyperglycemic patient. Increased intestinal gas formation is the most common adverse effect and does improve with time. (*Chapter 120, Pages 1073–1074.*)

25.9 Diabetic ketoacidosis (DKA) should be treated with

(A) metformin
(B) intravenous insulin therapy
(C) subcutaneous insulin with dosage adjustments four times daily on a sliding scale
(D) troglitazone
(E) glucagon

Answer: (B). In a patient with DKA, intravenous insulin therapy is initiated at a dose of 0.1 U/kg/hour. With rapid titration every 1 to 2 hours, a 75- to 100-mg/dl/hour decrease in glucose should be achieved. Insulin therapy at this relatively high dose is needed to combat the insulin resistance of the hormonal milieu of DKA (i.e., high levels of glucagon, cortisol, growth hormone, and catecholamines). (*Chapter 120, Page 1075.*)

25.10 The patient is a 32-year-old white type I diabetic woman who currently has poor glycemic control. She desires contraception. The most effective form of contraception for this patient is

(A) intrauterine contraceptive device
(B) cervical cap
(C) condom
(D) vaginal contraceptive jelly
(E) oral contraceptives (OC)

Answer: (E). The use of OCs in women with type I or type II DM has been an area of controversy, with many believing that significant elevations occur in blood glucose along with an increased risk of vascular complications. However, the incidence of such problems is minimal given a woman who is normotensive and has an absence of vascular disease; therefore in such a patient OCs can be safely used. Even for a woman in poor glycemic control, OCs are still the most effective form of contraception. (*Chapter 120, Page 1075.*)

25.11 The most *frequent* physical sign seen in patients with thyrotoxicosis is

(A) tachycardia
(B) goiter
(C) atrial fibrillation
(D) brisk deep tendon reflexes
(E) tremor

Answer: (B). Goiter is the most frequent sign, but the enlargement may be only mild or difficult to appreciate, especially when it occupies a substernal location. (*Chapter 121, Page 1078.*)

25.12 The cause of Graves' disease is

(A) infectious
(B) malignancy
(C) ischemic
(D) autoimmune
(E) none of the above

Answer: (D). The disease, described by Robert Graves in 1835, is the most common cause of hyperthyroidism. Its etiology is an autoimmune process, closely related to chronic lymphocytic (Hashimoto's) thyroiditis. (*Chapter 121, Page 1079.*)

25.13 The patient is a 32-year-old white woman with a heart rate of 110, a fine tremor of the hands, and a history of a 15-lb weight loss over the past 4 months. Lid lag and exophthalmos are prominent. Which one

of the following drugs is likely to be effective in controlling the tachycardia and tremor?

(A) beta-blockers
(B) alpha-blockers
(C) alpha-agonists
(D) phenytoin
(E) digitalis

Answer: (A). Therapy of Graves' disease is directed toward controlling the effects of excess thyroid hormone and reducing the production of additional hormone. Beta-blockers are especially effective in controlling the tachycardia, tremor, and other symptoms related to excess hormone. (*Chapter 121, Page 1080.*)

25.14 The patient is a 30-year-old white woman with a 1.5-cm nodule in her thyroid gland. There has been a 3-lb weight loss, and there is a mild tremor to the hands. Her diagnostic studies include an elevated free T4, a low thyroid-stimulating hormone (TSH), and a hot nodule on radioiodine scan. The patient is most likely to have

(A) Hashimoto's thyroiditis
(B) goiter
(C) an autonomously functioning thyroid nodule
(D) Grave's disease
(E) carcinoma of the thyroid

Answer: (C). An autonomously functioning thyroid nodule may cause thyrotoxicosis with typical hyperthyroid symptoms. Physical examination reveals a thyroid nodule, and findings specific to Grave's disease are absent. The diagnosis is confirmed with elevated free thyroxine index (FTI) (or free T4), low TSH, and a hot nodule on radioiodine scan. (*Chapter 121, Page 1081.*)

25.15 The patient is a 46-year-old white woman who has been found to have a normal FTI and a high level of TSH. Based on these laboratory findings, the most appropriate diagnosis for this patient is which of the following?

(A) acute thyroiditis
(B) Hashimoto's thyroiditis
(C) congenital hypothyroidism
(D) subclinical hypothyroidism
(E) euthyroid sick syndrome

Answer: (D). Hypothyroidism is diagnosed by finding an elevated TSH and a low serum FTI or free T_4. Patients with an FTI in the normal range and a high

TSH are functionally hypothyroid relative to their own bodily requirements (subclinical hypothyroidism). (*Chapter 121, Page 1083.*)

25.16 The patient is a 54-year-old African American woman with hyperthyroidism for whom you are beginning therapy with L-thyroxine. The use of this medication should be monitored by periodic assessment of

(A) TSH levels
(B) triiodothyronine levels
(C) thyroid scan
(D) free T$_4$ levels
(E) FTI

Answer: (A). Oral synthetic L-thyroxine (Synthroid) is the treatment of choice for hypothyroidism. The usual starting dosage is approximately 75 µg/day, but elderly patients and patients with heart disease are usually started much lower and slowly titrated upward. The goal of therapy is to restore the euthyroid state. Administration of excess thyroxine is avoided, and the dosage is adjusted by using a sensitive assay to maintain TSH within the normal range. (*Chapter 121, Page 1083.*)

25.17 The most common type of thyroid cancer is

(A) papillary carcinoma
(B) follicular carcinoma
(C) medullary carcinoma
(D) anaplastic carcinoma
(E) metastatic carcinoma

Answer: (A). Papillary carcinoma comprises 60 to 80% of all thyroid cancer. The tumor is slow-growing, and there is good long-term survival if surgical removal is performed while the cancer is still confined to the thyroid gland. (*Chapter 121, Page 1085.*)

25.18 The most important risk factor for osteoporosis is

(A) female gender
(B) northern European ancestry
(C) family history
(D) low calcium intake
(E) age

Answer: (E). Age is the most important risk factor for osteoporosis. After age 50, the risk of hip fracture doubles every 5 to 10 years. (*Chapter 122, Page 1088.*)

25.19 In a patient with early osteoporosis, the best method for assessing the risk of fracture of the femur and spine is which of the following?

(A) serial serum calcium levels
(B) plain radiographs
(C) single-photon absorptiometry (SPA)
(D) dual x-ray absorptiometry (DXA)
(E) dual photon absorptiometry (DPA)

Answer: (D). Plain radiography is insensitive to early osteoporosis and to small changes in bone mass. Several noninvasive techniques have been developed to quantitate bone mineral content and density and have been found to predict fracture risk during relatively short follow-up periods. SPA, DPA, QCT, and DXA are the main methods available for clinical use. Ultrasound measurements are investigational. The least expensive method, SPA, can accurately measure bone mineral density only in the extremities, whereas DPA can assess the hip and spine, correcting for soft tissue density, but with an inconveniently long scan time. DXA of the femur and spine is more precise and rapid than DPA, and it is becoming accepted as the best method for assessing fracture risk. (*Chapter 122, Page 1089.*)

25.20 The definitive diagnosis of acute gout is made by

(A) typical history and physical examination
(B) a uric acid level greater than 10 mg/dl
(C) an elevated erythrocyte sedimentation rate
(D) joint aspiration and examination of synovial fluid under polarized light
(E) a prompt response to colchicine therapy

Answer: (D). Acute gout can be diagnosed on clinical grounds, especially in a patient with a history of gout; examination of synovial fluid under polarized light provides the only definitive diagnosis. Acute synovitis due to deposition of pyrophosphate crystals (pseudogout) becomes more common after age 65, so joint aspiration is particularly important for this age group. (*Chapter 123, Page 1095.*)

25.21 The patient is a 32-year-old white woman with galactorrhea, oligomenorrhea, and vaginal dryness. A serum prolactin level is elevated. Further studies, including magnetic resonance imaging (MRI) of the skull, will be indicated if the serum prolactin level exceeds what level?

(A) 10 ng/ml
(B) 20 ng/ml
(C) 50 ng/ml
(D) 100 ng/ml
(E) 200 ng/ml

Answer: (E). Serum prolactin levels greater than 200 ng/ml are usually due to pituitary adenomas, which are best visualized by MRI with gadolinium enhancement. (*Chapter 124, Page 1099.*)

25.22 The best method to distinguish diabetes insipidus (DI) from other causes of polyuria is the use of

(A) serum insulin levels
(B) the glycohemoglobin level
(C) serial serum sodium determinations
(D) water deprivation test
(E) dexamethasone challenge

Answer: (D). A water deprivation test is used to distinguish DI from other causes of polyuria. In a controlled setting, water intake is restricted, and the weight and the sodium and osmolarity of the plasma and urine are measured hourly. The patient should not be allowed to lose more than 5% of body weight. Dilute urine in the face of concentrated serum suggests DI. Then, vasopressin (5 units sc) is administered to differentiate central DI from nephrogenic DI. (*Chapter 124, Page 1101.*)

25.23 In girls, the first event of puberty is which of the following?

(A) breast development and skeletal growth
(B) appearance of pubic hair
(C) appearance of axillary hair
(D) menarche
(E) change in pitch of the voice

Answer: (A). In girls, puberty is heralded by breast development and skeletal growth, followed by the appearance of pubic and axillary hair and then menarche. (*Chapter 124, Page 1101.*)

25.24 In boys the first change noted in puberty is

(A) appearance of pubic hair
(B) testicular enlargement
(C) enlargement of the penis
(D) increase in length of the femur and tibia
(E) skeletal growth of the spine

Answer: (B). In boys puberty is announced by testicular enlargement and is followed by the appearance of pubic hair and enlargement of the penis. Skeletal growth is a late event of male puberty. (*Chapter 124, Page 1101.*)

25.25 The most common cause of hyperparathyroidism is

(A) a functioning benign adenoma
(B) metastatic cancer
(C) functioning carcinoma of the parathyroid gland
(D) an autoimmune disease
(E) Paget's disease

Answer: (A). Hyperparathyroidism produces hypercalcemia, a frequent medical problem, through increased bone resorption; it is due to an autonomously functioning benign adenoma 80% of the time. Idiopathic or familial parathyroid hyperplasia accounts for most of the rest. (*Chapter 124, Page 1104.*)

25.26 The level of serum calcium reported may be influenced by the serum level of

(A) sodium
(B) protein
(C) glucose
(D) TGs
(E) bilirubin

Answer: (B). A serum calcium level greater than 10.5 mg/dl is considered elevated in most laboratories. But because almost half of the total serum calcium is protein-bound, an adjustment may be required if a variation in the serum protein level also exists. An increase of protein by 1 g/dl raises the measured total serum calcium by about 0.8 mg/dl. (*Chapter 124, Page 1104.*)

25.27 Addison's disease is best diagnosed by

(A) a typical history and physical examination
(B) the adrenocorticotropic hormone (ACTH) stimulation test
(C) low serum sodium and high serum potassium levels
(D) a positive response to glucocorticoid hormone replacement
(E) low serum cortisol levels

Answer: (B). Addison's disease is diagnosed by demonstrating the inability of the adrenal cortex to increase cortisol production during an ACTH stimulation test. Low serum cortisol levels alone are not diagnostic of Addison's disease unless accompanied by persistently elevated levels of ACTH. (*Chapter 124, Page 1105.*)

25.28 The most common cause of Cushing's syndrome is

(A) a carcinoma of the adrenal cortex
(B) carcinoma of the lung
(C) an adenoma of the adrenal gland

(D)   long-term use of exogenous glucocorticoids
(E)   a functioning adenoma of the pituitary gland

Answer: (D). Cushing's syndrome commonly results from the long-term use of exogenous glucocorticoids. On rare occasions, it may be caused by a glucocorticoid-producing adrenal adenoma or carcinoma, an ACTH-secreting pituitary adenoma (Cushing's disease), or another ACTH-producing neoplasm (usually lung). (*Chapter 124, Page 1105.*)

25.29 The patient is a 45-year-old white man who has a 4- to 6-month history of paresthesias and occasional tetanic spasms of the wrist. He lately has had some confusion, and he suffered a seizure during his sleep last night. Physical examination in the office reveals a positive Chvostek's sign. There is a prolonged QT interval on the electrocardiogram (ECG). You suspect that this patient has which one of the following diagnoses?

(A)   DM with early ketoacidosis
(B)   hypoparathyroidism
(C)   a series of transient ischemic attacks
(D)   acute adrenal insufficiency
(E)   hypothyroidism

Answer: (B). The symptoms and signs of hypoparathyroidism are related to the degree of hypocalcemia and are primarily neurologic: paresthesias, Chvostek's sign, carpopedal spasms, tetany, delirium, seizures. Patients with mild symptoms might mimic patients with dementia, depression, or psychosis. A prolonged QT interval may be noted on ECG. (*Chapter 124, Page 1105.*)

DIRECTIONS (Items 25.30 through 25.47): Each of the items in this section is a multiple true–false problem that consists of a stem and four lettered options. Indicate whether each of the four options is TRUE or FALSE.

25.30 Secondary causes of dyslipidemias include which of the following?

(A)   hypothyroidism
(B)   nephrosis
(C)   noncalculous cholecystitis
(D)   obesity

Answer: (A-True, B-True, C-False, D-True). The following secondary causes of dyslipidemias should be ruled out prior to extensive testing or treatment: diabetes; hypothyroidism; nephrosis; obstructive liver disease; myeloma; obesity; excess dietary alcohol, fat, or calories; and medications (steroids, beta-blockers, diuretics, or *cis*-retinoic acid). (*Chapter 119, Page 1057.*)

25.31 Vitamins that may reduce lipoprotein atherogenicity include which of the following?

(A)   vitamin A
(B)   vitamin C
(C)   vitamin D
(D)   vitamin E

Answer: (A-False, B-True, C-False, D-True). Research suggests that antioxidant nutrients (vitamin C, beta-carotene, and vitamin E) can reduce lipoprotein atherogenicity by providing protection from oxidation. (*Chapter 119, Page 1059.*)

25.32 True statements regarding the use of glycohemoglobin testing in the management of DM include which of the following?

(A)   Glycohemoglobins reflect average blood glucose levels over the previous 60 to 90 days.
(B)   Glycohemoglobin levels are useful for confirming the degree of glycemic control.
(C)   Glycohemoglobins have not proved useful for identifying errors in home blood glucose monitoring (HBGM) results.
(D)   Glycohemoglobin levels should not be reported to patients because such knowledge can cause undue concern.

Answer: (A-True, B-True, C-False, D-False). Glycohemoglobins reflect the average blood glucose over the previous 60 to 90 days. They are useful not only for confirming the degree of glycemic control but also for identifying possible falsification or errors in HBGM results. Glycohemoglobins are useful motivating tools for the patient; it often becomes a perceived challenge to reduce the result within the constraints of hypoglycemia. (*Chapter 119, Page 1068.*)

25.33 Hypertension in the diabetic patient exacerbates retinopathy, nephropathy, and macrovascular disease. In addition, when lifestyle modifications fail to control the blood pressure, pharmacologic therapy is needed. True statements regarding antihypertensive therapy in the diabetic patient include which of the following?

(A)   Beta-blockers and diuretics are excellent choices in the diabetic patient, because they stabilize glycemic control.
(B)   Angiotensin-converting enzyme (ACE) inhibitors are a good choice in diabetic patients with proteinuria.

(C) Calcium channel blockers should be avoided in patients with coronary artery disease.
(D) Monotherapy is frequently unsuccessful, especially in the setting of diabetic nephropathy.

Answer: (A-False, B-True, C-False, D-True). In treating hypertension in the diabetic patient, beta-blockers and diuretics should be avoided whenever possible, as they worsen insulin resistance. ACE inhibitors are a good choice in the proteinuric patient; calcium channel blockers are a good choice for the angina patient; and alpha-blockers are a good choice in the patient with benign prostatic hyperplasia. Monotherapy is frequently unsuccessful, especially in the setting of nephropathy, such that combination therapy is frequently needed with special attention to underlying concomitant medical problems. (*Chapter 119, Page 1070.*)

25.34 Appropriate early treatment of type II diabetes mellitus (DM) includes which of the following?

(A) diet
(B) weight control
(C) exercise
(D) early insulin therapy

Answer: (A-True, B-True, C-True, D-False). In most instances, type II DM is a syndrome of insulin resistance coupled with variable secretory defects, both of which can be compounded by glucotoxicity. Insulin resistance is related to genetic factors, obesity, and sedentary life style. The mainstay of treatment for the type II diabetic patient is correction of insulin resistance through diet and exercise and reversal of glucotoxicity acutely through reestablishment of euglycemia. It is important to avoid premature and unnecessary insulin therapy in these individuals and to stress to them the importance of diet and exercise as the most physiologic approach to controlling their metabolic disorder. (*Chapter 120, Page 1072.*)

25.35 The patient is a 28-year-old white type I diabetic man. He plans to play in a basketball league this winter and asks about adjusting his diet and insulin dosage. Appropriate options include which of the following?

(A) a reduction in insulin dosage prior to the activity
(B) an increase in insulin dosage prior to the activity
(C) increased carbohydrate intake prior to the physical activity
(D) decreased carbohydrate activity prior to the physical activity

Answer: (A-True, B-False, C-True, D-False). Many episodes of severe hypoglycemia occur in the context of unplanned physical activity and dietary errors; likewise, many episodes of ketoacidosis occur during episodes of intercurrent illness. For physical activity, a reduction in insulin dosage of 1 to 2 units per 20 to 30 minutes of activity generally suffices, pending the intensity of the activity. The other option is to augment carbohydrate intake (i.e., 15 g carbohydrate prior to every 20 to 30 minutes of activity). (*Chapter 120, Page 1071.*)

25.36 Metformin is useful in the treatment of type II DM. True statements regarding this medication include which of the following?

(A) The drug directly increases insulin secretion from the pancreas.
(B) Metformin improves insulin sensitivity.
(C) When metformin is used as monotherapy, the physician and patient must remain alert for hypoglycemia.
(D) The drug would be appropriate for an obese type II diabetic patient.

Answer: (A-False, B-True, C-False, D-True). Metformin hydrochloride (Glucophage) improves insulin sensitivity, enhancing peripheral glucose uptake and utilization, and decreases hepatic glucose production. As it has no effect on insulin secretion, when used as monotherapy it cannot induce hypoglycemia. Ideal candidates for treatment are overweight or obese type II diabetic patients. (*Chapter 120, Page 1072.*)

25.37 The patient is a 26-year-old white woman with gestational diabetes mellitus (GDM). Following delivery, you should anticipate that

(A) she will become hypoglycemic
(B) she will become euglycemic
(C) she will require insulin therapy
(D) she has a long-term risk of developing overt type II DM

Answer: (A-False, B-True, C-False, D-True). Most women with GDM have reestablishment of euglycemia immediately postpartum. These individuals, however, should be counseled on the long-term risks of prior GDM for developing overt type II DM, which may occur in as many as 70% of these individuals. (*Chapter 120, Page 1074.*)

25.38 Severe DKA is characterized by

(A) consumption of large amounts of fluids
(B) urinary retention

(C) edema with weight gain
(D) Kussmaul's respirations

Answer: (A-True, B-False, C-False, D-True). Diagnosis of DKA is fairly characteristic in the newly presenting or established type I diabetic patient. The history of polydipsia, polyuria, weight loss, and Kussmaul's respirations are virtually pathognomonic. (*Chapter 120, Page 1075.*)

25.39 Common physical findings in patients with thyrotoxicosis include

(A) smooth moist skin
(B) lid lag
(C) exophthalmos
(D) fine tremor of the outstretched hands

Answer: (A-True, B-True, C-False, D-True). In the patient with thyrotoxicosis, the skin tends to be warm, moist, and velvety smooth. A fine tremor of outstretched hands is usually present, and deep tendon reflexes are often brisk with a rapid relaxation phase. Lid lag may be present with any cause of thyrotoxicosis; exophthalmos is specific to Graves' disease. (*Chapter 121, Page 1078.*)

25.40 A 48-year-old black woman taking estrogen replacement therapy is likely to have which of the following?

(A) high levels of thyroid-binding proteins
(B) elevated serum total T_4 levels
(C) elevated TSH
(D) none of the above

Answer: (A-True, B-True, C-False, D-False). Euthyroid patients may have an elevated total T_4 due to excess thyroid-binding proteins, such as during pregnancy, with use of estrogens, or with some inherited disorders. (*Chapter 121, Page 1078.*)

25.41 The patient is a 50-year-old postmenopausal Asian American female who has always had a low intake of milk and dairy products because such foods tend to cause abdominal cramps and gas. She is not taking estrogen supplementation. You and she decide to begin calcium supplementation to prevent osteoporosis. Appropriate choices would include which of the following?

(A) calcium carbonate tablets
(B) calcium citrate tablets
(C) calcium lactate tablets
(D) calcium from dolomite or bone meal

Answer: (A-True, B-True, C-False, D-False). Chewable calcium carbonate tablets (Tums, Os-Cal 500 Chewable), calcium citrate tablets (Citracal) or liquid (calcium-fortified orange juice), or other tablets meeting U.S.P. standards for dissolution are recommended for calcium supplementation. Calcium carbonate requires acid for absorption and may be ineffective in the elderly or those taking drugs to inhibit acid secretion. Calcium lactate is contraindicated in persons with lactose intolerance. Calcium from dolomite or bone meal should be avoided because it is poorly absorbed and may contain lead. (*Chapter 122, Page 1090.*)

25.42 True statements regarding the medication alendronate (Fosamax) include which of the following?

(A) The drug inhibits bone resorption.
(B) Osteomalacia is a common long-term side effect.
(C) Use of alendronate can help reduce both vertebral and appendicular fracture incidence.
(D) One side effect of alendronate therapy can be esophagitis.

Answer: (A-True, B-False, C-True, D-True). The second-generation bisphosphonate alendronate (Fosamax) more potently inhibits bone resorption without causing osteomalacia and therefore can be given continuously. A dose of 10 mg/day on an empty stomach is approved by the U.S. Food and Drug Administration for treatment of osteoporosis. In 3-year controlled trials, this regimen increased bone mineral density by 8% and decreased both vertebral and appendicular fracture incidence. The long-term safety of bisphosphonates has not been established. Concern has arisen about esophagitis as a side effect of alendronate. (*Chapter 122, Page 1092.*)

25.43 The patient is a 62-year-old man with an acute attack of gout. Appropriate treatment options at this time include which of the following?

(A) allopurinol
(B) probenecid
(C) indomethacin
(D) colchicine

Answer: (A-False, B-False, C-True, D-True). Attacks of acute gout are most commonly managed by nonsteroidal anti-inflammatory agents (NSAID). High doses are needed. Although all NSAIDs are probably effective for acute gout, indomethacin (Indocin) is commonly used. Acute gout can also be treated with colchicine in a dose of 0.6 mg/hour by mouth up to a total of 5 or 6 mg until relief or severe gastrointestinal side effects occur. Hypouricemic agents (e.g., allopurinol or probenecid) worsen an acute gouty attack and are never used during one. (*Chapter 123, Page 1096.*)

25.44 The medical treatment of hyperuricemia includes the use of two agents with different modes of action: uricosuric agents or allopurinol (Zyloprim). True statements regarding the choice among these two medications include which of the following?

(A) Allopurinol is preferred in patients with nephrolithiasis.
(B) Uricosuric agents are preferred in patients with tophi.
(C) Uricosuric agents are preferred in patients with renal disease.
(D) Allopurinol is indicated in patients with congenital overproduction of uric acid.

Answer: (A-True, B-False, C-False, D-True). Medical treatment of hyperuricemia involves use of either uricosuric agents or allopurinol (Zyloprim), an agent that interferes with uric acid metabolism. The choice of agent depends on patient characteristics. Allopurinol is indicated in patients with nephrolithiasis, tophi, or renal disease. It is also indicated in patients with congenital overproduction of uric acid. (*Chapter 123, Page 1096.*)

25.45 Clinical features of hyperprolactinemia include which of the following?

(A) galactorrhea
(B) hypermenorrhea
(C) excessive vaginal secretions
(D) dyspareunia

Answer: (A-True, B-False, C-False, D-True). The principal clinical features of hyperprolactinemia are stimulation of milk production and suppression of gonadal function through processes that are not well understood. Women present with galactorrhea, amenorrhea or oligomenorrhea, infertility, vaginal dryness, and dyspareunia. (*Chapter 124, Page 1098.*)

25.46 The patient is a 13-year-old boy playing on a middle school football team. He has recently experienced a significant increase in muscle mass, and you wonder if he is taking androgens. True statements regarding the use of exogenous androgens include which of the following?

(A) Exogenous androgens cause physical development including increased muscle mass.
(B) Exogenous androgens cause sexual development without testicular enlargement.
(C) Exogenous androgens cause bilateral testicular enlargement.
(D) Exogenous androgens cause unilateral testicular enlargement.

Answer: (A-True, B-True, C-False, D-False). Participation in sports may lead to a desire to "bulk up." Androgens of exogenous or adrenal origin cause physical and sexual development without testicular enlargement. Unilateral testicular enlargement suggests neoplasia. (*Chapter 124, Page 1103.*)

25.47 True statements regarding pheochromocytoma include which of the following?

(A) These tumors cause symptoms related to their secretion of mineralocorticoids.
(B) Most pheochromocytomas are found in the adrenal medulla.
(C) The typical patient is age 65 to 85 years of age.
(D) The characteristic sign of pheochromocytoma is hypertension.

Answer: (A-False, B-True, C-False, D-True). Pheochromocytomas are rare chromaffin cell tumors that secrete catecholamines. Most pheochromocytomas are found in the adrenal medulla, but approximately 20% originate from extra-adrenal neural crest tissue. These tumors can be found in association with neurofibromatosis (von Recklinghausen's disease). Patients are typically middle-aged on presentation. Hypertension is the hallmark sign of these tumors and is persistent in about half of the patients. (*Chapter 124, Page 1106.*)

26
The Blood and Hematopoietic System

The questions in this chapter constitute a review of the following chapters in *Family Medicine: Principles and Practice*, Fifth Edition:

> Anemia (Chapter 125)
> Selected Disorders of the Blood and Hematopoietic System (Chapter 126)

DIRECTIONS (Items 26.1 through 26.14): Each of the questions or incomplete statements in this section is followed by five suggested answers or completions. Select the ONE that is BEST in each case.

26.1 The patient is a 42-year-old attorney with symptoms of fatigue, weakness, and decreased exercise tolerance. Examination reveals a mild anemia with a hemoglobin of 11.2 g/dl. The most likely cause of his anemia is

(A) dietary deficiency of iron
(B) gastrointestinal (GI) bleeding
(C) renal disease
(D) hemolysis
(E) cancer

Answer: (B). GI blood loss is probably the most frequent cause of anemia in adults and is an important area to investigate. In women, it is important to inquire about the potential increase in blood loss through menstruation. Chronic medical conditions such as hepatic, renal, endocrine, and inflammatory diseases can lead to anemia, as can malignancies and infections. (*Chapter 125, Page 1108.*)

26.2 The normal reticulocyte count, reported as reticulocytes/100 red blood cells (RBC) is about

(A) 1%
(B) 5%
(C) 10%
(D) 15%
(E) 20%

Answer: (A). Reticulocytes are newly formed RBCs. A new RBC remains a reticulocyte for 1.0 to 1.5 days, after which the RBC circulates for about 120 days. Thus, the blood normally contains about 1 reticulocyte/100 RBCs. The reticulocyte count is usually reported as reticulocytes per 100 RBCs (a percentage). (*Chapter 125, Page 1109.*)

26.3 For women, the recommended dietary allowance (RDA) for iron is

(A) 1 mg/day
(B) 15 mg/day
(C) 100 mg/day
(D) 300 mg/day
(E) 1,000 mg/day

Answer: (B). Iron deficiency anemia (IDA) is probably the most common cause of anemia in the United States. The RDA for iron is 10 mg/day for men and 15 mg/day for women. Meats, eggs, vegetables, legumes, and cereals are principal sources of iron in the American diet. (*Chapter 125, Page 1109.*)

26.4 Beta-thalassemia trait can be diagnosed by

(A) examination of radiographs of the wrists
(B) hemoglobin electrophoresis
(C) detection of elliptocytes on the peripheral blood smear
(D) detection of Howell-Jolly bodies on the peripheral blood smear
(E) careful history and physical examination

Answer: (B). Beta-thalassemia trait can be diagnosed by hemoglobin electrophoresis with elevated levels of hemoglobins A_2 and occasionally F. With alpha-thalassemia trait, the hemoglobin electrophoresis is normal, and diagnosis is usually made by exclusion, although precise molecular analysis is available. (*Chapter 125, Pages 1110–1111.*)

26.5 Which of the following is a sensitive and specific sign of megaloblastic anemia?

(A) spherocytes
(B) neutrophil hypersegmentation
(C) target cells
(D) burr cells
(E) Heinz bodies

Answer: (B). A sensitive specific sign of megaloblastic anemia is neutrophil hypersegmentation, which represents a disorder of DNA synthesis of erythrocyte precursors. (*Chapter 125, Page 1114.*)

26.6 Classic pernicious anemia is caused by

(A) hypervitaminosis
(B) inadequate dietary intake of vitamin B_{12}
(C) gastric mucosal atrophy
(D) interference of vitamin B_{12} absorption caused by excessive use of antacids
(E) peptic ulcer disease

Answer: (C). Pernicious anemia results from atrophy of the gastric mucosa leading to cessation of intrinsic factor secretion. Others at risk for vitamin B_{12} deficiency anemia include patients who have gastric and ileal surgeries and those with ileal absorption disorders, such as Crohn's disease, sprue, or tapeworm infection. (*Chapter 125, Page 1114.*)

26.7 Hemophilia A is an autosomal recessive X-linked deficiency of

(A) factor III
(B) factor IV
(C) factor V
(D) factor VIII
(E) thromboplastin

Answer: (D). Hemophilia A is an autosomal recessive X-linked deficiency of factor VIII. (*Chapter 126, Page 1116.*)

26.8 von Willebrand's disease (vWD) is inherited in which of the following patterns?

(A) an X-linked recessive
(B) an autosomal dominant
(C) an X-linked dominant pattern with females as asymptomatic carriers
(D) an autosomal recessive with incomplete penetrance
(E) a genetic mutation with sporadic expression

Answer: (B). vWD is an inherited hemorrhagic disorder characterized by deficiency of von Willebrand factor (vWF). vWF is necessary for normal interaction of platelets with vessel walls. vWD is inherited in an autosomal dominant pattern, with males and females equally affected. (*Chapter 126, Page 1117.*)

26.9 The patient is a 6-year-old boy who had scattered petechiae which led to a diagnosis of idiopathic thrombocytopenia purpura (ITP). The petechiae have now subsided, and his platelet count is 50,000/mm³. Which of the following is the appropriate treatment for this patient?

(A) immunosuppressive agents
(B) gamma-globulin
(C) splenectomy
(D) corticosteroids
(E) observation

Answer: (E). Treatment is unnecessary in patients with mild thrombocytopenia and is reserved for the patient who is bleeding because of thrombocytopenia or whose platelet count is less than 20,000/mm³. The goal of therapy is to stop the bleeding and return the platelet count to more than 20,000/mm³. (*Chapter 126, Page 1118.*)

26.10 The patient is an 8-year-old white boy recently treated in the emergency department for otitis media with a sulfonamide preparation. Now, 1 week later, the patient has a macular rash on the arms, legs, and buttocks, with a few areas of purpura. Urine analysis shows some blood cells and protein in the urine. This patient appears to have

(A) vWD
(B) hemophilia B
(C) folate deficiency
(D) ITP
(E) Henoch-Schönlein purpura (HSP)

Answer: (E). HSP (allergic purpura) primarily affects the kidneys, GI tract, and joints. The etiology is unknown. HSP has been seen after viral and streptococcal infections. Drugs (sulfonamides and penicillin) have been implicated as causative agents, and there are data to support an immune mechanism as a cause. HSP is most often seen in children aged 2 to 10 years (male/female ratio 2:1) but can occur at any age. There is an increased incidence during early spring and early autumn.

HSP presents with fever followed by a macular or urticarial rash on the buttocks, legs, and arms that becomes purpuric. Lesions can occur in crops. Other findings include edema (legs, hands, scalp, eyes), abdominal pain, vomiting, diarrhea, intussusception, arthritis, and hypertension. Kidney involvement is manifested by proteinuria, hematuria, renal failure, or nephrotic syndrome. Iritis, pericarditis, pleurisy, and neurologic disorders are seen less frequently. (*Chapter 126, Pages 1119–1120.*)

26.11 The patient is a 61-year-old white male immigrant from Denmark. He has type I diabetes. For the past 6 to 8 months, he has noted aching joints, loss of libido, and a brown skin discoloration. On physical examination, both the liver and spleen appear enlarged. This patient's most likely diagnosis is

(A) polycythemia
(B) multiple myeloma
(C) alcoholic cirrhosis
(D) idiopathic splenomegaly
(E) hemochromatosis

Answer: (E). The clinical manifestations of hemochromatosis include brown or gray skin discoloration, hepatosplenomegaly, carcinoma of the liver, hepatic cirrhosis, abdominal pain, congestive cardiomyopathy, insulin-dependent diabetes mellitus, arthralgias, loss of libido, and hypogonadism. (*Chapter 126, Page 1129.*)

26.12 Persons with sickle cell anemia often suffer splenic infarctions, which put them at increased risk for

(A) cirrhosis of the liver
(B) pulmonary embolism
(C) autoimmune disease
(D) carcinoma of the spleen
(E) pneumococcal infections

Answer: (E). Patients with sickle cell anemia are at increased risk of pneumococcal infections due to splenic infarctions. (*Chapter 126, Page 1123.*)

26.13 Sickle cell anemia can be prevented by

(A) gene therapy
(B) monoclonal antibody therapy

(C) immunization
(D) immunosuppression
(E) none of the above

Answer: (E). Sickle cell anemia cannot be prevented, but it can be detected in utero. Genetic counseling should be offered to the parents of a child with sickle cell anemia. (*Chapter 126, Page 1124.*)

26.14 Multiple myeloma is a malignancy of which of the following cells?

(A) megakaryocytes
(B) plasma cells
(C) reticulocytes
(D) stem cells
(E) mast cells

Answer: (B). Multiple myeloma is a plasma cell (beta-lymphoid) malignancy. Expansion of the plasma cell mass and the secreted products of the cells cause the symptoms associated with multiple myeloma. (*Chapter 126, Page 1124.*)

DIRECTIONS (Items 26.15 through 26.23): Each of the items in this section is a multiple true–false problem that consists of a stem and four lettered options. Indicate whether each of the four options is TRUE or FALSE.

26.15 The patient is a 79-year-old white man with IDA related to an inadequate diet. You are beginning iron replacement therapy. The patient asks if there are any foods or medicines that might interfere with the iron therapy. Substances that can reduce iron absorption include

(A) coffee
(B) vitamin C
(C) meats
(D) calcium-rich antacids

Answer: (A-True, B-False, C-False, D-True). Substances that can reduce absorption include bran, eggs, milk, tea, coffee, calcium-rich antacids, and drugs such as cimetidine. However, taking the ferrous sulfate with vitamin C-containing products and meats can improve absorption. (*Chapter 125, Page 1110.*)

26.16 Laboratory testing can be very helpful in the diagnosis of a hemolytic anemia. Laboratory features indicating hemolysis include

(A) elevated serum lactate dehydrogenase (LDH) levels

(B) low levels of indirect bilirubin
(C) elevated levels of plasma haptoglobin
(D) a positive direct Coombs' test in patients with autoimmune hemolytic anemia

Answer: (A-True, B-False, C-False, D-True). Laboratory features that may be indicative of hemolysis include elevated serum LDH and indirect bilirubin levels. Haptoglobin, a plasma protein that binds and clears hemoglobin released into the plasma, is often decreased with hemolysis. A direct Coombs' test is frequently positive with autoimmune hemolytic anemia. (*Chapter 125, Page 1112.*)

26.17 Characteristics of the anemia of chronic disease (ACD) include which of the following?

(A) The anemia is usually normocytic.
(B) Hemoglobin levels are usually less than 7 g/dl.
(C) The serum iron and transferrin saturation are typically low.
(D) The ferritin level is typically low.

Answer: (A-True, B-False, C-True, D-False). The pathogenesis of ACD is multifactorial and not fully understood. Some of the mechanisms include a reduction in RBC lifespan, defects in iron transfer to the developing erythroid cells, and a relative erythropoietin deficiency. Although the anemia is customarily normocytic, it can be microcytic. The Hgb levels usually are between 7 and 11 g/dl. The serum iron and transferrin saturation are typically low, which may confuse ACD with IDA. However, ACD can be distinguished from IDA because the ferritin is commonly normal or elevated and the total iron binding capacity is normal or low. (*Chapter 125, Page 1112.*)

26.18 Impaired absorption of folate may occur in patients taking which of the following?

(A) vitamin B$_{12}$ injections
(B) multiple vitamin supplements
(C) oral contraceptives
(D) phenytoin

Answer: (A-False, B-False C-True, D-True). Impaired absorption of folate may occur in patients taking oral contraceptives or anticonvulsants, such as phenobarbital and phenytoin. Patients who have liver cirrhosis may develop folate deficiency owing to the decreased storage and metabolism capabilities of the liver. Patients with uremia can lose folate during dialysis. (*Chapter 125, Page 1114.*)

26.19 True statements regarding hemophilia A include which of the following?

(A) Males have hemophilia A and females are usually asymptomatic carriers of the hemophilia A gene.
(B) All daughters of a hemophiliac father are carriers of the gene.
(C) All sons of a hemophiliac father are carriers of the hemophilia A gene.
(D) The male children of a female hemophilia A carrier have a 50% chance of being affected by the gene.

Answer: (A-True, B-True, C-False, D-True). Because of the mode of transmission and gene expression, males have hemophilia A, and females are usually asymptomatic carriers of the hemophilia A gene. All daughters of a hemophiliac father are carriers of the hemophilia A gene; all his sons are normal. The male children of a female hemophilia A carrier have a 50% chance of being affected by the gene. (*Chapter 126, Page 1116.*)

26.20 Laboratory findings characteristic of vWD include which of the following?

(A) prolonged bleeding time
(B) prolonged prothrombin time (PT)
(C) normal activated partial thromboplastin time (APTT)
(D) a decreased platelet count

Answer: (A-True, B-False, C-True, D-False). The diagnosis of vWD is confirmed by laboratory findings of prolonged bleeding time, decreased factor VIII levels, decreased vWF activity, and decreased vWF antigen. The PT, APTT, and platelet count are usually normal. (*Chapter 126, Page 1117.*)

26.21 Vitamin K is a fat-soluble compound essential to the synthesis of factors II, VII, IX, and X. Deficiency states of vitamin K can occur in which of the following settings?

(A) a vegetarian diet
(B) the newborn
(C) patients undergoing heparin anticoagulation
(D) with long-term antibiotic use

Answer: (A-False, B-True, C-False, D-True). The sources of vitamin K are dietary (especially green leafy vegetables) and synthesis of vitamin K by intestinal bacteria. The daily adult requirement of vitamin K is 100 to 200 mg/day. Deficiency states of vitamin K can be seen in the newborn (hemorrhagic disease), the elderly, patients with liver disease, after ingestion of vitamin K antagonists (i.e., warfarin), or with long-term antibiotic use (elimination of gastrointestinal flora). (*Chapter 126, Pages 1117–1118.*)

26.22 True statements regarding ITP include which of the following?

(A) The fundamental pathology is decreased platelet production.
(B) ITP can be associated with a collagen vascular disease.
(C) ITP can occur in the setting of a viral illness.
(D) Acute ITP occurs chiefly between the ages of 20 and 50 years.

Answer: (A-False, B-True, C-True, D-False). ITP is caused by interaction of immunoglobulin G and other antibodies with megakaryocytes or platelets, resulting in increased platelet destruction. ITP can present as a primary problem or be associated with such conditions as malignancies, collagen vascular disease, or viral illnesses. Acute ITP is most common in children, and chronic ITP is more common in adults, with a male/female ratio of 1:3. Acute ITP occurs most commonly between the ages of 2 and 9 years; chronic ITP occurs chiefly between the ages of 20 and 50 years. (*Chapter 126, Page 1118.*)

26.23 Disseminated intravascular coagulation (DIC) is a syndrome of accelerated fibrin deposition in blood vessels and lysis of RBCs. The bleeding in DIC is caused by the consumption of fibrin and its procoagulants. The diagnosis is suspected clinically and confirmed by laboratory findings of

(A) prolonged PT
(B) normal partial thromboplastin time
(C) increased fibrin levels
(D) thrombocytopenia

Answer: (A-True, B-False, C-False, D-True). The diagnosis is suspected clinically and confirmed by laboratory findings of elevated fibrin degradation products, prolonged PT and partial thromboplastin time, decreased fibrin levels, and thrombocytopenia. (*Chapter 126, Page 1120.*)

27

Principles and Applications

The questions in this chapter constitute a review of the following chapters in *Family Medicine: Principles and Practice, Fifth Edition:*

Family Medicine: Current Issues and Future
  Practice (Chapter 1)
Human Development and Aging (Chapter 2)
Approach to the Patient (Chapter 3)
Sociocultural Issues in Health Care (Chapter 4)
Families and Health (Chapter 5)
Population-Based Health Care (Chapter 6)
Clinical Guidelines (Chapter 127)
Information Management (Chapter 128)
Managed Care (Chapter 129)
Profile of Family Physicians in the United States (Chapter 130)

DIRECTIONS (Items 27.1 through 27.13): Each of the questions or incomplete statements in this section is followed by five suggested answers or completions. Select the ONE that is BEST in each case.

27.1 When the specialty of family practice was established in 1969, all except which of the following were critical innovations?

(A) 3 year residency training
(B) certifying board for Family Practice
(C) mandatory recertification
(D) mandatory continuing medical education
(E) practicing physicians "grandfathered" as board-certified

Answer: (E). Four critical innovations formed the basis of the new specialty in the United States. Three-year *residency training* positions were established, in contrast to a single year of internship, perhaps supple-

mented by a 2-year general practice residency, which was the prior norm for general practitioners. A *certifying board*—the American Board of Family Practice—was established; until 1979, a physician could qualify to sit for the certifying examination based on practice eligibility, but since then, all candidates for specialty certification must be graduates of approved 3-year family practice residency programs. *Mandatory recertification* was pioneered by the American Board of Family Practice, and all U.S. board-certified family physicians must take a recertification examination every 7 years; several other specialties have since followed this lead. Finally, *mandatory continuing medical education* was required by the American Academy of Family Physicians (AAFP) and the American Board of Family Practice. The latter organization requires 300 approved hours of approved continuing medical education every 6 years as one component of the recertification process. (*Chapter 1, Page 1.*)

27.2 What percentage of graduating medical students in U.S. medical schools currently choose careers in family practice?

(A) 4%
(B) 8%
(C) 12%
(D) 16%
(E) 20%

Answer: (D). There are 670,000 physicians (FP) in the United States today. Of this number, 52,000 are family physicians and 20,000 general practitioners. There are 452 family practice residency training programs in community hospitals and academic medical centers; and in 1997 in the United States, 16% of graduating medical students chose careers in family practice. (*Chapter 1, Page 2.*)

27.3 The most important characteristic of infancy and childhood is the need for

- (A) nurturance
- (B) immunizations
- (C) vitamin supplementation
- (D) car seat use
- (E) fluoridated drinking water

Answer: (A). Perhaps the most important characteristic of this stage is the need for nurturance. Even prior to birth, the fetus must be nutritionally nurtured and protected from harm. The adverse effects of smoking and drugs on fetal development are well established, but the real "work" of parenting begins with the birth of the child. Almost from the moment of birth, mother–child bonding begins to take place. This process has been shown to have significant effects on the child, affecting emotional, social, and intellectual development. The role of the father in the bonding process is also critical to the child's well-being but has been less studied than the role of the mother. (*Chapter 2, Pages 6–7.*)

27.4 The health status of Native Americans is affected by a number of factors. These include all the following EXCEPT

- (A) geographic isolation in villages, communities, and large reservations
- (B) poor transportation
- (C) travel often requiring long distances on dirt roads or by air
- (D) low levels of sexually transmitted disease and drug use owing to high levels of family support
- (E) lack of efficient communication systems

Answer: (D). Native Americans suffer some of the worst health in the nation and the lowest social status even among minorities and underserved people. Access to health care for Native Americans is more difficult than for the rest of the U.S. population because of their geographic isolation in villages and communities in states that are large in area and have large reservations, poor transportation, lack of efficient communications systems, and lack of running water and sewage disposal. Travel may require long distances on dirt roads or by air. Native Americans are younger, less educated, less likely to be employed, and poorer than the general population. These factors, combined with high rates of sexually transmitted disease and drug

use, favor the spread of human immunodeficiency virus. Alcoholism exacts a terrible toll among many Native Americans. Tribal, cultural, educational, economic, and geographic diversity exist among Native Americans and affect their health care. (*Chapter 4, Page 21.*)

27.5 The ability of a family to adapt to change

- (A) is tested throughout the life cycle from birth to aging of the parents, through advanced age and death
- (B) is not an important factor in serious or chronic illness
- (C) can undermine the solidarity that a family needs in times of stress
- (D) requires strong leadership by a dominant family member
- (E) will place the family at an ecologic disadvantage during times of rapid economic and social change

Answer: (A). The hallmark of a healthy family is the ability to adapt to change. The universal challenges of the family life cycle tests every family with some or all of the classic themes: births, young children, adolescence, young adults establishing new relationships beyond the family, emancipation of young adults to form their own families, maturing and aging of the parents, and finally truly advanced age and death. These life-cycle challenges are compounded by the adaptation to serious or chronic illness. For example, insulin-dependent diabetes mellitus often has its onset at the peak of adolescent rebellion from parental values and behavior—not an ideal time to have an illness that is best treated with carefully patterned diet, exercise, and precise compliance with medical treatment. In addition, successful coping with illness frequently requires a family to be extremely flexible about all manner of powerful issues: who stays at home, who goes to work, who helps with the children, who takes care of aging grandparents, where families live, what a family does for fun, and who will be available to lead the family emotionally. (*Chapter 5, Page 27.*)

27.6 The current transformation of our health care system is being driven by

- (A) the administrative branch of the federal government
- (B) boards of directors of health maintenance organizations (HMOs)
- (C) problems in the domains of cost, quality, and access

(D) medical school graduates' career choices and international medical graduates entering the workforce

(E) a long-range planning committee reporting to the U.S. Senate

Answer: (C). The current transformation of our health care system has been driven by problems in three domains: cost, quality, and access. The cost of providing medical care has risen at a dramatic rate, and an ever-increasing portion of our gross domestic product is being devoted to health. As a result, we have seen a variety of complex changes in the organization, financing, and delivery of health care. Since the mid-1980s, there has been a marked alteration in community-based medical practices. Free-standing individual and small group practices are vanishing across the United States as we see a dramatic horizontal and vertical consolidation within the health delivery system. Care is increasingly organized and delivered by large health care systems, not individual practices or hospitals. (*Chapter 6, Page 33.*)

27.7 Community-oriented primary care (COPC) is a systematic strategy to address the health care of the community and individuals in an integrated fashion. The COPC process requires all the following elements EXCEPT which of the following?

(A) defining and characterizing the community or denominator population

(B) identifying health and health care problems

(C) organizing primary care providers and others into a vertically integrated provider group

(D) the intervention or modification of practice patterns

(E) monitoring the impact of the intervention

Answer: (C). The COPC paradigm can easily be used within a primary care practice. Such a practice must be comprehensive and able to provide the array of services necessary to meet the needs of the population it serves. Care must be accessible and continuous over time. Furthermore, the primary care provider must act as the coordinator of care when multiple individuals are involved in delivering services and information. The COPC process provides a methodology for identifying and addressing the major health problems of a population. It applies the principles of management to the planning and implementation of health care. In fact, its structure is remarkably similar to that used by quality assurance and continuous quality improvement programs. The COPC process requires four elements:

1. defining and characterizing the community or denominator population
2. identifying health and health care problems
3. intervention or modification of practice patterns
4. monitoring the impact of the intervention (*Chapter 6, Page 35.*)

27.8 Reimbursement for FPs in managed care organizations (MCOs) may include which of the following?

(A) discounted fee for service

(B) accepting limited risk for the utilization of services

(C) capitation rates paid for enrolled patients

(D) full-risk contracting

(E) all of the above

Answer: (E). Reimbursement to FPs in MCOs can take several forms. During the early stages of managed care, the FP usually receives a discounted fee for service. When FPs get accustomed to managed care and realize that they may do better financially by accepting some risk for the utilization of services, they accept a capitated rate for each enrolled patient. This capitation rate may be specifically for primary care services, or it may be for all physician services, with the FP paying the specialist. Full-risk contracting refers to a physician network or integrated delivery system receiving the entire capitated amount for health care and then paying for all services, usually at predetermined rates that may be fee-for-service or subcapitation. (*Chapter 129, Pages 1140–1141.*)

27.9 The first MCOs in the United States were

(A) staff model HMOs

(B) independent practice organizations

(C) preferred provider organizations

(D) physician networks

(E) physician-hospital organizations

Answer: (A). The original MCOs were staff model HMOs. Physicians worked as staff employees for an organization for health care to a defined population. (*Chapter 129, Page 1140.*)

27.10 When compared with those in independent practice, the income for FPs in MCOs is generally

(A) higher

(B) the same

(C) lower

(D) much lower

(E) unknown

Answer: (A). Income for FPs in MCOs is generally higher than in independent practice, with the income going to specialists generally reduced. (*Chapter 129, Page 1141.*)

27.11 According to National Ambulatory Medical Care Survey (NAMCS) data regarding office visits to physicians, the greatest proportion of all physician visits in the United States are made to

   (A) general physicians and FPs
   (B) pediatricians
   (C) general internists
   (D) obstetrician-gynecologists
   (E) pediatricians and general internists combined

Answer: (A). The greatest proportion of all physician visits in the United States are made to general physicians and FPs. In 1993 there were 197.6 million estimated visits to these specialists, whereas the estimated number of office visits to pediatricians and general internists was 179.4 million. There were 10% more office visits to general physicians and FPs than to pediatricians and general internists combined. (*Chapter 130, Page 1146.*)

27.12 In the NAMCS, the average duration of an office visit during which there is contact between the patient and the FP was

   (A) 6.7 minutes
   (B) 9.3 minutes
   (C) 12.1 minutes
   (D) 15.9 minutes
   (E) 20.3 minutes

Answer: (D). The average duration of an office visit during which there was contact between the patient and the physician was 18.4 minutes for all specialties, 15.9 minutes for FPs, 14.4 minutes for pediatricians, 20.3 minutes for general internists, and 17.9 minutes for obstetricians. (*Chapter 130, Page 1150.*)

27.13 In the NAMCS, the rate at which the FP referred the patient to another physician was approximately

   (A) 5%
   (B) 10%
   (C) 15%
   (D) 20%
   (E) 25%

Answer: (A). Data from the NAMCS are available related to the disposition and follow-up required by the attending physician. In this survey, the FP referred the patient to another physician during approximately 5% of visits. (*Chapter 130, Page 1150.*)

DIRECTIONS (Items 27.14 through 27.32): Each of the items in this section is a multiple true–false problem that consists of a stem and four lettered options. Indicate whether each of the four options is TRUE or FALSE.

27.14 Family practice care in the United States has been characterized by

   (A) aggressive action
   (B) a longitudinal approach to health care
   (C) a humanistic approach
   (D) an emphasis on victory over disease

Answer: (A-False, B-True, C-True, D-False). Throughout its history, family practice has served a counterculture role. Medical care in the United States has been described as characterized by aggressive action, a mechanistic approach, problem orientation, and an emphasis on victory over disease. Into this setting came family practice. In contrast to an aggressive assault on disease, family physicians championed longitudinal health care, which allowed both patient and physician to understand the nature of illness and to share decisions over time. A humanistic approach integrated with the evolving new technology was advocated. The emphasis of family practice was on the broad-based care of the person and family, rather than a narrow focus on the disease problem. Finally, family physicians advocated improving the quality of life, particularly important when patients suffer chronic or terminal illness. (*Chapter 1, Page 2.*)

27.15 Certificates of added qualifications are available to FP with appropriate training in which of the following areas?

   (A) school health
   (B) geriatric care
   (C) primary care neurology
   (D) sports medicine

Answer: (A-False, B-True, C-False, D-True). In addition to a full-scope office-based practice, many FPs develop special interests. Geriatric care and sports medicine are two favorites of FPs, and there are certificates of added qualifications available for both of these areas. Others have developed expertise in adolescent medicine, administrative medicine, or occupational medicine. (*Chapter 1, Page 2.*)

27.16 In the twenty-first century, FPs will need to have new areas of competence. These include the ability to

(A) anticipate and meet community needs
(B) understand the economics of health care
(C) use research to advance the knowledge base of the discipline
(D) find new ways to deal with community-wide health problems

Answer: (A-True, B-True, C-True, D-True). As we look ahead to the twenty-first century, it is apparent that FPs must develop new areas of competence while maintaining roots as personal physicians and patient advocates. Thus, FPs must anticipate community needs such as terminal care outside the hospital and home care for the acquired immunodeficiency syndrome patient, as well as population-based problems such as tobacco use and teen pregnancy. Integrationist activities must be expanded, serving the coordinating role for patients with multiple problems including those needing the services of various subspecialists. The economics of medicine must be understood; some FPs who have failed to learn how payments flow in capitated care have suffered badly. FPs must continue to enhance their clinical skills as new developments occur; and as a specialty, FPs must use research to advance the knowledge base of the discipline. New ways must be found to deal with community-wide health problems such as domestic violence. Finally, FPs and, in fact, all physicians must learn how to influence legislative action as health care becomes increasingly politicized. (*Chapter 1, Page 4.*)

27.17 True statements concerning gender socialization during childhood include which of the following?

(A) Children begin to express gender-specific behaviors at an early age.
(B) It is possible to shield children from most gender-identified materials until puberty.
(C) A child may exhibit gender-specific behaviors even when parents have tried to raise their child in a manner that avoids such behaviors at an early age.
(D) The FP should encourage parents to reinforce gender-specific behavior as soon as it is clear that the child has developed his or her gender identity.

Answer: (A-True, B-False, C-True, D-False). The concept of gender socialization is interesting to consider. It appears that at an early age children begin to express gender-specific behaviors. Little girls may make their own dolls, and boys may fashion guns out of sticks. It is virtually impossible to not expose children to gender-identified material. Some parents are upset that they have tried to raise their child with a sensitivity toward preventing stereotyped behaviors, yet the child exhibits them. A child should be given a wide range of opportunities for expression and exploration based on interest and aptitude, rather than gender. (*Chapter 2, Pages 7–8.*)

27.18 The psychosocial tasks of adolescence are

(A) beginning separation from the family
(B) developing a self-identity
(C) developing a sexual identity
(D) depending less on one's peers for support than during earlier childhood stages of development

Answer: (A-True, B-True, C-True, D-False). The adolescent stage of human development has been called the second stage of individuation and is perhaps the most turbulent. The body at puberty is going through marked change, a true metamorphosis. Rapid growth and hormonal changes affect the young person on a daily, often variable, basis. In a way, it is a misnomer to term this period a "stage." So much change is occurring that it is more appropriately conceived of as an explosion! Psychosocially, the tasks of this stage are clear: begin separation from the family, develop a self-identity, develop a sexual identity, begin to depend on one's peers (rather than the family) for support, and start formulating plans for a means of supporting one's self. How these tasks are accomplished defines transition to a healthy adulthood. (*Chapter 2, Page 8.*)

27.19 Visits by a young adult woman to the FP might reasonably involve

(A) assessment of the woman's stress level
(B) discussion of concerns about child-rearing
(C) discussion of her relationship with her partner
(D) career concerns

Answer: (A-True, B-True, C-True, D-True). Contacts with the physician during this stage are often by women and are related to birth control, pregnancy, or well-child visits. Many opportunities are available for anticipatory guidance and counseling. The physician should assess the stress level of the woman and facilitate discussing her concerns about child-rearing, her relationship with her partner, and career concerns. (*Chapter 2, Page 9.*)

27.20 Middle age

   (A) may be described as a conflict between generativity and stagnation

   (B) may involve a consolidation of social and occupational roles

   (C) occurs at a time when children are growing up and leaving home

   (D) is a time when individuals should avoid new challenges

Answer: (A-True, B-True, C-True, D-False). Erikson spoke of middle age as characterized by a conflict between generativity and stagnation. This stage is often attended by consolidation of one's social and occupational roles. The uncertainty and testing of the young adult stage has passed. Many are firmly fixed in their careers, sometimes disproportionately so. Children are growing up and leaving home. For many, it is a time of relative economic stability and intellectual accomplishments. The question often arises concerning the appropriate goals in life, often termed the *mid-life-crisis.*

An important adaptational response to this stage is the development of new challenges to replace those already met. For some, it means changing jobs or duties within a job. Some take on added responsibilities or managerial roles. Others increase their involvement in church and community affairs or exercise programs. Whatever the method, such endeavors are probably preferable to gaining all of one's sense of accomplishment through other individuals' activities, such as from one's spouse or children. (*Chapter 1, Page 9.*)

27.21 True statements regarding retirement include which of the following?

   (A) Through many generations of human experience, social scientists know a great deal about the human experience of retirement.

   (B) Retirement, even when freely chosen, is a risk factor for development or exacerbation of health problems.

   (C) Many elders become involved in educational pursuits during retirement.

   (D) For most retirees, income is insufficient for their needs.

Answer: (A-False, B-True, C-True, D-False). Retirement, as a social phenomenon, is a relatively recent human experience. Much is still being learned about the positive and negative effects of retirement. In general, retirement that is freely chosen and well planned is strongly correlated with positive health out-

comes. Time for exercise, both physical and psychosocial, may increase. Many elders become involved in educational pursuits or advocacy programs. For most, retirement income is sufficient for their needs. Opportunities for contacts with grandchildren usually increase. For some, the chance to travel is gratifying. (*Chapter 2, Page 10.*)

27.22 True statements regarding old age as a stage of life include which of the following?

   (A) Most older persons perceive themselves as in good health.

   (B) Older people are typically unadaptable and tend to view disability in a negative light.

   (C) More than half of all persons older than age 75 are unable to perform at least one activity of daily living such as bathing or dressing.

   (D) Sickness should be considered a normal part of this stage of life.

Answer: (A-True, B-False, C-True, D-False). Regardless of income, most older persons perceive themselves as being in good health. This viewpoint is interesting considering that more than 50% of those older than 75 are unable to perform at least one activity of daily living (e.g., bathing, dressing). This dichotomy probably can be explained by two perceptions: (1) older people are remarkably adaptable and learn to view disability in a positive light; and (2) some older people are accepting of medically related changes that could potentially be reversed by better care. Older individuals are able to view changes in physical function with more equanimity than younger persons faced with the same degree of impairment. However, there is also a prevalent myth in our society that "old equals sick." Sickness is common, but it should not be considered normal. (*Chapter 2, Page 11.*)

27.23 Which of the following statements is/are true regarding hospice care?

   (A) Hospice care helps dying people maintain a higher quality of life.

   (B) The majority of hospice patients are older than age 65.

   (C) Persons in hospice care find the end of their lives satisfying only when there is some prospect for medical improvement.

   (D) Medicare does not fund hospice care.

Answer: (A-True, B-True, C-False, D-False). Since the early 1980s, the hospice movement has helped persons who are dying maintain a higher quality of life. Almost two-thirds of hospice patients are older than age 65. By emphasizing patient-directed approaches to symptom control, even in those with no prospect for medical improvement, individuals can live more satisfying lives. The major objectives of care are pain control; prevention of constipation, depression, or other symptoms; involvement of families; and care at home. Medicare has recognized the benefits of this approach by funding hospice care since 1992. (*Chapter 2, Page 11.*)

27.24 A patient-centered approach to health care

(A) improves psychosocial outcomes but has not been shown to improve biomedical results
(B) requires understanding the physician–patient relationship, including both the patients' and physicians' perspectives
(C) requires communication skills, organization of the interaction, patient education, and appropriately structured medical records
(D) is undermined if the physician attempts negotiation and consensus formation with the patient and family

Answer: (A-False, B-True, C-True, D-False). Research has shown that a patient-centered approach improves biomedical and psychosocial outcomes. For instance, patients whose physicians are patient-centered not only are more likely to receive education and preventive care, they also experience improvement in their psychosocial, medical, and surgical outcomes in ways that are not clearly explained through the biomedical model. Mastery of the patient-centered model requires understanding the physician–patient relationship including both the patient's and the physician's perspectives. Communication skills, organization of the interaction, patient education, medical records, and negotiation and consensus formation are needed for this approach. (*Chapter 3, Page 13.*)

27.25 True statements regarding the physician–patient interaction include which of the following?

(A) Only open-ended questions should be used, and an attempt to maintain a focus during the interaction will deny the patient the opportunity to tell the story in his or her own words.
(B) When the patient presents with a long list of questions, the physician should allow a full discussion of all topics on the list.
(C) The passage of time can be a useful diagnostic or therapeutic tool.

(D) Even when the patient has a number of complicated medical or psychosocial issues, it is important that all be addressed at the time of the initial visit.

Answer: (A-False, B-False, C-True, D-False). It is important to elicit the patient's story with open-ended questions, but it is also important to maintain a focus during the interaction. If the patient presents with a long list of questions, a quick review of this list, with input from the patient about which items are of most concern to them, can help the physician budget time and prioritize the topics of discussion.

Because the FP provides continuing care, he or she may choose to use time as a diagnostic or therapeutic tool. For instance, for the active child with a fever but no localizing signs, the physician may choose to wait a day or two and then reevaluate the child before performing any diagnostic tests. For the patient with ongoing or complicated medical or psychosocial issues, some problems may need to wait until the more major problems are stabilized. The physician must remember to note these less pressing issues, though, to not omit discussion of them at a later time. (*Chapter 3, Page 16.*)

27.26 Patient noncompliance may be caused by

(A) misinformation
(B) fear
(C) lack of consensus between patient and the physician about a plan of action
(D) a nonjudgmental inquiring attitude on the part of the physician that often communicates uncertainty

Answer: (A-True, B-True, C-True, D-False). Patient noncompliance may result from an informed reconsideration of the treatment plan by the patient, misinformation, fear of the diagnostic procedure or treatment, or a lack of consensus between the physician and patient about the importance of the proposed diagnostic or treatment plans. In many of these cases, the patient's noncompliant behavior is a reasonable response and can be easily addressed by considering the underlying reasons. It takes some patients a significant amount of time to comply with physician recommendations, especially if they involve significant behavioral change. A nonjudgmental inquiring attitude on the part of the physician helps patients know that the physician will continue to work with them and help them find solutions to their problems. (*Chapter 3, Pages 17–18.*)

27.27 The traditional Western medical model

   (A) is an analytical tool to deal with illness
   (B) considers disease an intrusion imposed on humans from outside
   (C) assigns physicians responsibility for the care of persons with compromised function
   (D) places a high value on the social context of health and health care

Answer: (A-True, B-True, C-True, D-False). The Western medical model was developed in contemporary Western society as a powerful analytic tool to deal with illness. This model developed around the classical Greek myth of Pandora's box in which disease is an intrusion superimposed on humans from the outside. The concept defines the social system within which a defined professional group (i.e., physicians) takes responsibility for the care of persons with compromised function. The model determines the type of questions raised during the history-taking process. Emphasis on physical symptoms often predisposes the interviewer to neglect material of potentially great value (e.g., the social system of the patient). (*Chapter 4, Page 20.*)

27.28 True statements regarding clinical encounters involving the need for translation (e.g. language) include which of the following?

   (A) The physician should speak looking at the interpreter to be sure that subtleties of meaning are conveyed to the patient.
   (B) Body language is important and will be recognized by the patient.
   (C) Explaining to the interpreter in advance what you are trying to accomplish during the interview is demeaning to the patient and violates confidentiality.
   (D) From time to time during the interview, the physician should test the patient's understanding of what is being communicated.

Answer: (A-False, B-True, C-False, D-True). Special care is needed with interviews involving translators to ensure the accuracy and completeness of the information and the cooperation of the patient. Clinicians must view the translator as part of a team whose members collaborate to arrive at a competent plan for the patient.

   1. *Look at the patient when speaking.* Always address the patient, not the interpreter, and speak in the first person directly to the patient, asking the interpreter to interpret in a direct fashion.

   2. *Use comforting body language,* recognizing that it is instantaneously interpreted by the patient.
   3. Whenever possible, *explain to the interpreter in advance* what you are trying to say and accomplish during the interview.
   4. *Assume that there will be misunderstandings,* particularly when you are using nonprofessional interpreters.
   5. *Remain aware and test your patient's understanding.* Some patients may understand your language even if they choose to use an interpreter; or, conversely, patients who *speak* fairly well in the language of the clinician may not have the same level of comprehension. (*Chapter 4, Page 24.*)

27.29 Which of the following statements regarding an individual's symptoms and the family system is/are true?

   (A) An individual's symptoms may have a stabilizing function within the family.
   (B) An acute illness is more likely than a chronic problem to involve multiple family-level factors.
   (C) Questioning regarding the meaning of symptoms within the family system is a form of family therapy.
   (D) When chronic illness is present, FPs should listen respectfully to expressions of frustration by other family members.

Answer: (A-True, B-False, C-True, D-True). An individual's symptoms may have a stabilizing function within the family. This is not to say that such symptoms or illnesses are intentional or requested overtly by other family members. When an illness is chronic or persistently recurrent, it is more likely to involve such family-level factors. For example, parents may avoid discussing and resolving their marital discord if they remain focused on their asthmatic child's need for recurrent urgent and chronic medical treatment. Even when there is objective evidence that the child has improved and has less need for emergency treatment, the parents may continue to demand urgent treatment and complain about a lack of clinical progress. In this case, the FP may have to remain patient and respectfully probe into what the family and couple would be doing differently if the child were well. Such questioning is a form of family therapy and might be more than some FPs want to do. However, all FPs could listen respectfully to parental frustration and inquire about how the child's illness affects other members of the family. (*Chapter 5, Page 27.*)

27.30 Families generally have an "informal family health advisor." The FP

(A) should ignore the patient's informal family health advisor

(B) should identify the person in the family who has the strongest opinions on medical matters

(C) will generally find that the "informal family health advisor" has had some formal medical education or training

(D) will establish credibility by respectfully explaining the fallacies of cultural health belief systems

Answer: (A-False, B-True, C-False, D-False). Identify the "informal family health advisor" for your patients. To do so, just ask the identified patient, "Who in your family has the strongest opinions about medical matters?" or "Is there someone in your family or network of friends to whom your family turns for informal but trusted opinions about medical matters?" In most families, there is some long-trusted person (usually female) who either verifies the worthiness of medical clinicians and their recommended treatments or declares the practitioner and his or her treatments invalid. The family's trust in this "informal family health advisor" is usually not related to whether that person has any formal medical education or training. A clever clinician can identify this person and respectfully work to establish credibility as soon as possible. (*Chapter 5, Page 28.*)

27.31 For clinical guidelines constructed using explicit (evidence-based) methods, the terms *standard*, *guideline*, and *clinical option* are used. True statements regarding these descriptive terms include which of the following?

(A) There is virtual unanimity regarding the interventions preferred in *standard* practice policies.

(B) An appreciable majority agree which intervention is preferred in practice policies described as *guidelines*.

(C) Practice policies in which the health and economic consequences of a decision are not sufficiently well known to permit meaningful decisions are described as *options*.

(D) Most clinical guidelines are stated as *standards*.

Answer: (A-True, B-True, C-True, D-False). The following describes degrees of flexibility in clinical guidelines:

Standard—A practice policy is considered a standard if the health and economic outcomes of the alternative interventions are sufficiently well known to permit meaningful decisions and there is virtual unanimity about which intervention is preferred.

Guideline—A practice policy is considered a guideline if the health and economic outcomes of the interventions are sufficiently well known to permit meaningful decisions and an appreciable majority agree which intervention is preferred.

Option—A practice policy is considered a practice option if

1. the health and economic consequences of a decision are not sufficiently well known to permit meaningful decisions;

2. the preferences among the outcomes are not known;

3. the patients' preferences are divided among the alternative interventions; or

4. the patients are indifferent about the alternative interventions

Standards and guidelines are less common than clinical options because even if the science is fairly solid, there are few clinical conditions for which the outcomes are fully understood and even fewer for which patient preferences are known and uniform. (*Chapter 127, Page 1129.*)

27.32 True statements regarding hospital admitting privileges of FPs include which of the following?

(A) Approximately 87% of active members of the AAFP have hospital admission privileges.

(B) Most FPs report that their hospital privileges granted are less inclusive than they would wish.

(C) The percentage of FPs with hospital privileges tends to decrease each year.

(D) The types of hospital admission privileges held by FPs varies by census division and metropolitan area.

Answer: (A-True, B-False, C-False, D-True). Although FPs in the United States practice primarily in the office setting, approximately 87% of active members of the AAFP had hospital admission privileges in May 1995. Of these physicians, 86% indicated that the privileges they were granted were "generally about right." Both the percentage of FPs with hospital privileges and the satisfaction rates are similar to the results published in previous years. The types of privilege afforded FPs varied by census divisions, metropolitan area, and residency training. (*Chapter 130, Page 1150.*)

Index